Breaking the Silence on Cancer and Sexuality: A Handbook for Healthcare Providers

By
Anne Katz, RN, PhD

Oncology Nursing Society

ONS Publishing Division
Publisher: Leonard Mafrica, MBA, CAE
Director, Commercial Publishing/Technical Publications Editor: Barbara Sigler, RN, MNEd
Production Manager: Lisa M. George, BA
Staff Editor: Lori Wilson, BA
Copy Editor: Amy Nicoletti, BA
Graphic Designer: Dany Sjoen

Breaking the Silence on Cancer and Sexuality: A Handbook for Healthcare Providers

Library of Congress Control Number: 2007927023

ISBN-13: 978-1-890504-67-0

Publisher's Note
This book is published by the Oncology Nursing Society (ONS). ONS neither represents nor guarantees that the practices described herein will, if followed, ensure safe and effective patient care. The recommendations contained in this book reflect ONS's judgment regarding the state of general knowledge and practice in the field as of the date of publication. The recommendations may not be appropriate for use in all circumstances. Those who use this book should make their own determinations regarding specific safe and appropriate patient-care practices, taking into account the personnel, equipment, and practices available at the hospital or other facility at which they are located. The editors and publisher cannot be held responsible for any liability incurred as a consequence from the use or application of any of the contents of this book. Figures and tables are used as examples only. They are not meant to be all-inclusive, nor do they represent endorsement of any particular institution by ONS. Mention of specific products and opinions related to those products do not indicate or imply endorsement by ONS. Web sites mentioned are provided for information only; the hosts are responsible for their own content and availability.

ONS publications are originally published in English. Publishers wishing to translate ONS publications must contact the ONS Publishing Division about licensing arrangements. ONS publications cannot be translated without obtaining written permission from ONS. (Individual tables and figures that are reprinted or adapted require additional permission from the original source.) Because translations from English may not always be accurate or precise, ONS disclaims any responsibility for inaccuracies in words or meaning that may occur as a result of the translation. Readers relying on precise information should check the original English version.

Printed in the United States of America

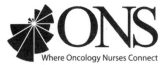

Oncology Nursing Society
Integrity • Innovation • Stewardship • Advocacy • Excellence • Inclusiveness

For Alan, Ayli and Zak
From A to Z: All that I will ever need.

Table of Contents

Acknowledgments

My heartfelt thanks to Jill Taylor-Brown, MSW, RSW, director of Patient and Family Support Services, who embraced the idea of sexuality counseling as one of the services offered at CancerCare Manitoba. Jill welcomed me into her department, and the psychosocial clinicians offered me support and, even more importantly, referred patients to me. I am immensely grateful to you all.

Thanks also to the librarians who photocopied countless articles for me over the years with good cheer, even when the subject matter caused raised eyebrows for some. I am indebted to the staff of the Carolyn Sifton Library and Donna Pacholok and Ruth Holmberg from the CancerCare Manitoba Library for their help. I apologize for the many trees that were felled in this endeavor.

I am also grateful to the patients and their partners who allowed me to hear their stories over the years and asked for my help as they tried to help themselves. The generosity of their spirit has been a source of inspiration and courage to me, and I am honored by their trust.

My family is central to everything that I have ever accomplished, and I do not have the words to express my gratitude. My husband, Alan, has read every word of every chapter of this book and anything else I have ever written. His ongoing enthusiasm for all my schemes and dreams truly meets the meaning of "unconditional," and while I probably could have done it without him, why would I want to? My children, Ayli and Zak, have grown into adulthood in spite of their mother and her rather embarrassing predilection for pushing the boundaries of what most would consider a "normal" career. I know that having a sexuality counselor for a mother has at times been very uncomfortable, but I hope that I have shown them what passion and drive mean in deeds as well as words.

Section I

Human Sexuality in the Context of Cancer

CHAPTER 1

Introduction: Why Is Sexuality Important in the Context of Cancer?

Sexuality has been defined in many different ways. It is described as "the ways in which we experience and express ourselves as sexual beings. Our awareness of ourselves as females and males is part of our sexuality as is the capacity we have for erotic experiences and responses. Our sexuality is an essential part of ourselves, whether or not we ever engage in sexual intercourse or sexual fantasy, or even if we lose sensation in our genitals because of injury" (Rathus, Nevid, & Fichner-Rathus, 2000, p. 5). It is seen as "a central aspect of being human throughout life and encompasses sex, gender, identities and roles, sexual orientation, eroticism, pleasure, intimacy, and reproduction" (Wagner et al., 2005, p. 167). People's views of themselves and others as sexual beings are influenced by cultural, ethnic, and religious beliefs and practices.

The definition of sexuality also encompasses peoples' relationships with others and how they are perceived by others as sexual beings (van der Riet, 1998). Perhaps more creatively, Weiss (1992) described sexuality as a connection between the heart and the gut and a means of joining pleasurable physical sensations with the spirit and a sense of serenity.

Sexuality is sometimes spoken of as *intimacy*, and the word *intimacy* may be used as a euphemism (Hughes, 2000). Intimacy often is equated with privacy and closeness, but in the context of human interactions, intimacy involves self-disclosure, partner disclosure, and partner responsiveness (Laurenceau, Barrett, & Pietromonaco, 1998).

This contrasts with individuals' understanding of sexual functioning, which is seen as what they *do* as sexual beings, and is further deconstructed to consist of the four phases of the sexual response cycle (excitement, plateau, orgasm, resolution) as conceived by Masters and Johnson (Barton, Wilwerding, Carpenter,

3

& Loprinzi, 2004). Sexual functioning thus equates to sexual behavior and is accompanied by the occurrence of sexual dysfunction when behavior does not follow some predetermined path and is seen as wrong, abnormal, or requiring intervention.

Sexual functioning also may be equated to sexual health. The World Health Organization (2004) provided a working definition of sexual health:

> A state of physical, emotional, mental and social well-being related to sexuality; it is not merely the absence of disease, dysfunction or infirmity. Sexual health requires a positive and respectful approach to sexuality and sexual relationships, as well as the possibility of having pleasurable and safe sexual experiences, free of coercion, discrimination and violence. For sexual health to be attained and maintained, the sexual rights of all persons must be respected, protected and fulfilled.

Cancer and Sexuality

In the context of cancer, sexuality is an important aspect of quality of life, and cancer affects quality of life in multiple dimensions, including psychological, functional, social, and physical (Hughes, 2000). The importance of sexuality in the lives of people with cancer is recognized by the Oncology Nursing Society, and sexuality is included as one of the standards of cancer nursing (Brant & Wickham, 2004). The cancer itself may affect both sexuality and sexual functioning, and the many different treatment modalities have an impact on individuals with physical, psychological, and social consequences (Bruner & Berk, 2004). For many people newly diagnosed with cancer, the diagnosis may feel like a death sentence, and the meaning that they ascribe to sexuality may be in stark contrast to this. For some, sexuality is something that is equated with health, life, and reproduction (Nishimoto, 1995). To even think about sex when the threat of death looms seems antithetical, so many give up on this aspect of their lives. Although the fight for survival is acute, sex itself, and even thinking of oneself as a sexual being, is relegated to the back burner. Sexual problems can occur as a result of psychological responses to the diagnosis and treatment. Cancer and the treatments offered can affect physical, endocrine, neurogenic, and vascular functioning. Iatrogenic consequences from any of the drugs used to treat the cancer or to treat side effects also may have an impact on sexual functioning.

Stages of Illness

Any illness, including cancer, has different stages associated with it (Rolland, 2005), and these stages affect sexuality and sexual functioning. In the crisis phase, individuals with cancer must reorganize their lives and adapt to the crisis. Patients have to learn to live with symptoms, adapt to treatments, and develop flexibility to the social demands of illness. In the chronic phase of the illness, patients must renegotiate relationships within the family, learn to live with uncertainty, and balance connectedness and separateness within social and familial relationships. The terminal phase requires individuals with cancer and their families to live with anticipatory grief.

However, many people now survive cancer and go on to lead normal lives. But survivorship is not always easy. Many myths are associated with surviving cancer, including the expectation that individuals should recover after treatment is over and also should return quickly to their prediagnosis sense of self (Stanton et al., 2005). It may take many months or years to recover from treatment and the physical and psychological changes that have occurred. Some of these survivors return to their previous level of sexual functioning; some do not. Many may not know that help is available because they have never been asked if they have experienced any changes. Whether this results in distress is extremely variable, and many patients/survivors never seek help for dealing with sexual changes. Almost half of cancer survivors report ongoing problems with sexual functioning (Baker, Denniston, Smith, & West, 2005). These issues are global and reflect changes in body image, sexual self-image, and reentering life as a cancer survivor (Holland & Reznik, 2005).

Conclusion

The intent of this text is to change the status quo of healthcare providers' knowledge related to sexual changes and cancer. Through discussion of a range of cancers and how they affect the sexual lives and feelings of patients and their sexual partners, readers of this book will learn how to initiate a discussion with patients and their partners. Readers also will learn about evidence-based interventions that can be used to help patients to minimize or recover from sexual difficulties. In particular, this book will help nurses and other healthcare professionals to break the silence on a topic that is real and important to patients but that has been shrouded in silence far too long.

References

Baker, F., Denniston, M., Smith, T., & West, M.M. (2005). Adult cancer survivors: How are they faring? *Cancer, 104,* 2565–2576.

Barton, D., Wilwerding, M., Carpenter, L., & Loprinzi, C. (2004). Libido as part of sexuality in female cancer survivors. *Oncology Nursing Forum, 31,* 599–609.

Brant, J.M., & Wickham, R.S. (Eds.). (2004). *Statement on the scope and standards of oncology nursing practice.* Pittsburgh, PA: Oncology Nursing Society.

Bruner, D.W., & Berk, L. (2004). Altered body image and sexual health. In C.H. Yarbro, M.H. Frogge, & M. Goodman (Eds.), *Cancer symptom management* (3rd ed., pp. 596–623). Sudbury, MA: Jones and Bartlett.

Holland, J., & Reznik, I. (2005). Pathways for psychological care of cancer survivors. *Cancer, 104,* 2624–2637.

Hughes, M.K. (2000). Sexuality and the cancer survivor: A silent coexistence. *Cancer Nursing, 23,* 477–482.

Laurenceau, J., Barrett, L., & Pietromonaco, P. (1998). Intimacy as an interpersonal process: The importance of self-disclosure, and perceived partner responsiveness in interpersonal exchanges. *Journal of Personality and Social Psychology, 74,* 1238–1251.

Nishimoto, P.W. (1995). Sex and sexuality in the cancer patient. *Nurse Practitioner Forum, 6,* 221–227.

Rathus, S., Nevid, J., & Fichner-Rathus, L. (2000). What is human sexuality? In S. Rathus, J. Nevid, & L. Fichner-Rathus (Eds.), *Human sexuality in a world of diversity* (4th ed., pp. 4–33). Boston: Allyn and Bacon.

Rolland, J. (2005). Cancer and the family: An integrative model. *Cancer, 104,* 2584–2595.

Stanton, A.L., Ganz, P.A., Rowland, J., Meyerwitz, B.E., Krupnick, J.L., & Sears, S. (2005). Promoting adjustment after treatment for cancer. *Cancer, 104,* 2608–2613.

van der Riet, P. (1998). The sexual embodiment of the cancer patient. *Nursing Inquiry, 5,* 248–257.

Wagner, G., Bondil, P., Dabees, K., Dean, J., Fourcroy, J., Gingell, C., et al. (2005). Ethical aspects of sexual medicine. *Journal of Sexual Medicine, 2,* 163–168.

Weiss, K. (1992). *Women's experiences of sex and sexuality.* City Centre, MN: Hazeldon.

World Health Organization. (2004). *Definition of sexual health.* Retrieved June 14, 2006, from http://www.who.int/reproductive-health/gender/sexual_health.html#3

CHAPTER 2

A Primer in Human Sexual Functioning

Human sexuality is a complex phenomenon. In part, it is based on the structure and function of sexual and reproductive organs acting in concert with and under the influence of hormones. It also is intimately connected to the brain through cognition, emotion, motivation, and memory. Over the past 50 years, the understanding of human sexuality has increased, but many unanswered questions still remain.

Sexual Anatomy

The structures that constitute the *female sexual organs* are the breasts, the mons pubis, the vulva (clitoris, labia majora and minora, and vaginal introitus), the vagina and cervix, and the uterus and uterine tubes. The ovaries are responsible for production of the hormones that affect target organs and influence sexual functioning.

The breasts are classified as secondary sex organs that grow and develop during puberty. The breasts are composed of mammary glands that produce milk and fatty tissue that gives breasts their size and shape. Each breast has a nipple that is surrounded by an areola. The nipples and areolae are well supplied with nerve endings and are generally regarded as important for sexual arousal.

The mons pubis is an area of fatty tissue over the pubic bone and from puberty is covered with hair. The cushioning of the fatty tissue protects the woman and her partner from experiencing pain during thrusting. The labia majora are two thick folds of skin that run from the mons in the front toward the perineum. They cover and protect the labia minora, the urethral opening, and the vaginal introitus. The labia minora are two thinner folds of tissue that lie underneath the labia majora.

All these structures are richly supplied with nerve endings and blood supply and respond to stimulation by swelling.

The clitoris is composed of a body that is about 0.5 inch wide and 1–2 inches long and two large wings (called *crura* in Latin) that extend sideways from the body and are 2–4 inches long. There are also two other structures made of the same erectile tissue, which are part of the internal structure of the clitoris. These are 1–3 inches in length and triangular in shape and are called the bulbs of the clitoris. They fill in the space between the clitoris, the crura, and the urethra. All these tissues are richly supplied with nerves and blood vessels and play an important role in sexual arousal; however, this has not been extensively studied. The part of the clitoris that is visible is partially covered by a hood, or prepuce.

The vaginal introitus, or opening, lies between the urethral meatus in the front and the perineum and the anus behind. The vagina extends upward and backward and is about 3–5 inches in length. At rest, it is a collapsed tube whose walls touch one another along their length. The vaginal walls are made up of three layers: the innermost mucosal layer, a middle muscular layer, and an outer fibrous layer. The mucosal layer is richly supplied with blood vessels but has relatively few nerve endings other than in the lower third, close to the introitus. The mucosal layer is characterized by numerous folds, or rugae, and secretes an acidic fluid that keeps the membranes moist.

The cervix is found at the top of the vagina and is the entry to the uterus. The cervix itself secretes fluid. Many of the nerves to the pelvic area run through a structure called the uterovaginal plexus, which is found on either side of the cervix. The uterus is a pear-shaped muscular organ that usually lies so that the uppermost part (the fundus) is tipped over or anteverted. The uterine tubes extend from the side of the uterus, and their ends lie close to the ovaries. The ovaries produce several hormones, including estrogen, progesterone, and testosterone.

The *external male sexual organs* are the penis and scrotum. The internal organs are the testicles, the vas deferens, the seminal vesicles, the Cowper glands, and the prostate. The penis consists of three cylinders of spongy tissue that run along its length. Two of these cylinders are called the corpora cavernosa, and they lie on either side of the urethra and fill with blood when the man is aroused. The corpus spongiosum is a single tube that lies along the length of the penis on the ventral surface. It contains the urethra and widens at the end of the penis to become the glans. The glans is separated from the body of the penis by a structure called the corona. The glans is covered loosely by the foreskin, which may be surgically removed in infancy (circumcision) or later in life. The base of the penis extends backward into the pelvis where it ends in the bulb of the penis that is anchored to the pelvic bones by two wings of tissue (crura).

The scrotum is a sac of tissue that houses the testicles and is covered with hair after puberty. The testicles lie in their own separate compartments in the scrotum and are held in place by the spermatic cords, which contain the vas deferens, nerves, blood vessels, and the cremaster muscles. The cremaster muscles raise and lower the testicles in response to sexual stimulation and temperature changes.

The testes are regarded as internal organs and are the site of sperm production and testosterone synthesis. Sperm are carried from the seminiferous tubules into the epididymis, which, in turn, empties into the vas deferens. The seminal vesicles produce a fluid rich in fructose that is needed to nourish the sperm. The prostate gland manufactures prostatic fluid, which combines with the sperm and fluid from the seminal vesicles to form the ejaculate. The Cowper glands (bulbourethral glands) lie below the prostate gland and empty their secretions directly into the urethra. During arousal, the fluids from these glands often appear at the tip of the penis prior to ejaculation.

Hormonal Influences

The hypothalamus and pituitary gland are found in the brain and regulate the secretion of hormones by the ovaries and testes through feedback loops involving luteinizing and follicle-stimulating hormones. The hormones produced by the ovaries and testes under this stimulation (estrogens, progesterone, and testosterone) are linked to various aspects of male and female sexuality and sexual functioning, as is prolactin (Regan, 1999). The bodies of both men and women contain estrogen and testosterone but in different levels, with men having more testosterone and less estrogen and women having the opposite.

Women produce three different estrogens in the ovaries under the influence of luteinizing hormone and follicle-stimulating hormone from the anterior pituitary gland. The three forms of estrogen are estradiol, estrone, and estriol. Estrogens are involved in maturation of the sexual organs, development of secondary sex characteristics, and regulation of the menstrual cycle. They are found in the body bound to sex hormone–binding globulin. Estrogen is regarded as the hormone of arousal and is involved in the secretion of vaginal lubrication. After menopause, the ovaries stop producing estradiol and estrone, and the majority of estrogen produced after this comes from extraovarian and extraglandular production of estrone (Robinson & Huether, 2002). Progesterone also is produced in the ovaries under the influence of luteinizing hormone, and small amounts are produced by the adrenal cortex. Progesterone is associated primarily with control of the menstrual cycle. Women produce small amounts of androgens in the ovaries and adrenal cortex. These hormones are involved in the growth of pubic and axillary hair, and a woman's libido is thought to be linked to testosterone levels; however, recent research has brought this into question (Davis, Davison, Donath, & Bell, 2005).

In women, testosterone together with estrogen is thought to be involved in what sensations are perceived by the brain to be sexual. Serum androgen levels have been found to decline steeply in the early reproductive years, and menopause does not appear to alter levels, as postmenopausal women continue to produce testosterone in the ovaries (Davison, Bell, Donath, Montalto, & Davis, 2005). No association has been found between specific androgen levels and low sexual function (Davis et al., 2005).

The primary male sex hormone is testosterone, and it is produced by the Leydig cells in the testes and, to a lesser extent, by the adrenal cortex. Testosterone is involved in the development of secondary sex characteristics and sperm. It also is involved in secretion of fluid from the prostate gland, seminal vesicles, and Cowper glands. As in the female, luteinizing hormone and follicle-stimulating hormone are involved in the production of testosterone. Almost all the circulating testosterone (98%) is bound to either albumin or sex hormone–binding globulin, and only 2% is free to enter cells. Men have a small amount of estrogen in their bodies, 25% of which is produced in the testes and the remainder by the peripheral conversion of testosterone and other androgens. Prolactin is secreted by the pituitary gland and maintains the production of testosterone; however, high levels suppress production in a negative feedback loop (Robinson & Huether, 2002).

Sex and the Brain

Parts of the brain are thought to play key roles in sexual functioning. The cerebral cortex and the limbic system are the structures that are deemed to be most important. The cerebral cortex is activated when people experience sexual thoughts or fantasies. Signals are sent to the sexual organs causing vasocongestion or arousal. The cerebral cortex also interprets stimuli as sexually stimulating or not and judges whether sexual behavior is pleasurable (Basson, 2001). The limbic system most likely plays a role in experiencing pleasure, but its exact role in human sexual functioning is not fully mapped out.

The Sexual Response Cycle

For many years, the sexual response cycle was not discussed or understood. However, this all changed in 1966 when Drs. William Masters and Virginia Johnson conducted a number of groundbreaking observations of humans and sexual functioning. They developed a four-stage model that suggested major similarities between males and females. The four stages of their model are excitement, plateau, orgasm, and resolution, and they represent episodes of vasocongestion and muscle contractions.

In the excitement stage, heart rate and blood pressure increase, and blood flows into the tissues of the sexual organs. For women, the breasts enlarge in size, and a reddish flush may appear on the chest and neck. The nipples become more erect and feel harder to the touch. Increased blood flow to the genitalia results in enlargement of the clitoris as it swells and grows wider and longer; engorgement of the labia majora, which flatten and spread outward; and simultaneous swelling of the labia minora. The upper two-thirds of the vagina grow bigger, and the walls of the entire vagina thicken. The walls of the vagina secrete a fluid that facilitates penetration. For men, the penis becomes erect as blood flows into the spongy tissues. The skin of the scrotum also thickens, the testicles grow bigger, and the entire scrotum elevates and moves in toward the body.

The plateau phase is essentially a state of advanced arousal. Blood pressure and heart rate continue to increase, and breathing becomes rapid. Some people have involuntary facial grimaces, and the hands and feet may contract as a result of myotonia. In women, the lower third of the vagina (at the vaginal introitus) swells, making the entry to the vagina tighter, presumably to grasp the penis. The upper two-thirds of the vagina continues to expand, and the uterus moves into an upright position. The labia minora become more engorged with blood, and the color changes to a darker hue. The clitoris shortens and withdraws below the clitoral hood. The breasts continue to increase in size, and the nipples may appear to flatten out as the areolae become engorged. In men, the testicles continue to enlarge and move closer to the inside of the abdomen. The head, or glans, of the penis shows evidence of vasocongestion by changing to a deeper color. The Cowper glands secrete some fluid that may be visible at the tip of the penis.

Orgasm is the phase of maximal muscular contractions. Respiration and heart rate peak during this phase, and subjective feelings of intense pleasure radiate throughout the body. Major muscles in the body contract and go into spasm. In women, the pelvic muscles contract between 3 and 15 times. The first contractions tend to be strong and close together. These are followed by three or more slower contractions. The muscles of the anal sphincter and the uterus itself contract.

Orgasm for men occurs in two stages and is accompanied by ejaculation, which has its own unique sensations. In the first phase, seminal fluid is forced into the bulb of the penis by contractions of the vas deferens, seminal vesicles, ejaculatory duct, and prostate gland. The bladder neck sphincter also closes off to prevent urine from mixing with the semen and semen from flowing into the bladder. Men experience a brief sensation called ejaculatory inevitability when the penile bulb swells to accommodate this buildup of fluid. The second stage of orgasm for men occurs with the opening of the second sphincter lower in the urethra. The muscles around the urethra contract, and the fluid is propelled along the urethra and out of the urethral meatus. Like in women, the first contractions are more intense and closer together than the later contractions. These contractions are accompanied be feelings of intense pleasure.

In the resolution phase, vasocongestion resolves, and the body returns to its normal nonaroused state. For both men and women, muscle tension dissipates within minutes, and heart rate, blood pressure, and respirations return to normal. During this phase in women, blood moves out of the pelvic organs, the labia return to their normal size and color, the uterus goes back to its usual size and position, and the vagina regains its usual size. The clitoris shrinks to its normal size. The breasts also return to their normal size, and any flushing of the skin disappears. In men, the penis loses its rigidity in two phases. In the first, about half the volume is lost as blood leaves the corpus cavernosum. A few minutes later, the remaining blood leaves the corpus spongiosum, and the testicles and scrotum also shrink in size. For men, the resolution phase is followed by a refractory period during which ejaculation and orgasm is physiologically not possible. This has a variable duration; in young men, the refractory period may last a few minutes. However, as men age, this period lasts longer, and older men may not be able to have another orgasm or ejaculation for hours or even days. Women do not experience a refractory period and may have multiple orgasms with continued stimulation. See Figures 2-1 and 2-2 for diagrams of the male and female sexual response cycles.

Helen Singer Kaplan (1979) introduced the idea of desire in her interpretation of the human sexual response cycle. Her model comprises three parts: desire, excitement, and orgasm, which are closely modeled on the work of Masters and Johnson. According to Kaplan, the psychological processes of emotion and cognition that lead to the subjective feeling of desire are an important part of the sexual response cycle. Excitement in this model follows much the same physiologic process as in the Masters and Johnson model, with vasocongestion causing erection for men and arousal and lubrication for women. Orgasm is a series of muscular contractions, and Kaplan does not address the topic of resolution in her model. Kaplan's model is not necessarily a linear process, such as the model suggested by Masters and Johnson. Kaplan poses her model as comprising three independent phases; according to this model, it is possible to experience excitement without first experiencing desire.

Zilbergeld and Ellison (1980) proposed a five-stage model that has both psychological and physiologic components, which they regard as relatively independent of one another. Their model contains the following phases: interest, arousal, physiologic readiness, orgasm, and satisfaction. Interest for them corresponds to the psychological processes introduced by Kaplan. Arousal is similar to that in the Masters and Johnson model, where vasocongestion is the primary physiologic process. For the readiness

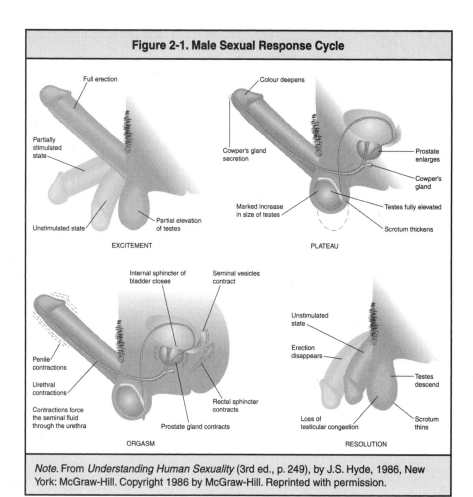

Figure 2-1. Male Sexual Response Cycle

Note. From *Understanding Human Sexuality* (3rd ed., p. 249), by J.S. Hyde, 1986, New York: McGraw-Hill. Copyright 1986 by McGraw-Hill. Reprinted with permission.

stage, Zilbergeld and Ellison propose that erection for men and lubrication or swelling for women are necessary for intercourse. Orgasm then is theorized to occur, and they suggest that orgasm has a physiologic component as well as subjective sensations. Finally, the last stage of this model is satisfaction, which is a psychological/cognitive reaction or appraisal to what has occurred.

Rosemary Basson (2005) has further refined the female sexual response cycle with a heavy emphasis on psychoemotional processes as opposed to the more physiologic basis of the other models described. In her model, libido (or innate desire) is theorized to occur at a number of places in the sexual response cycle, which is conceptualized as a circle rather than a linear process. She suggests that women have many reasons to be receptive to or instigators of sexual activity. These include rewards such as emotional intimacy, feelings of well-being, and lack of negative feelings resulting from avoiding

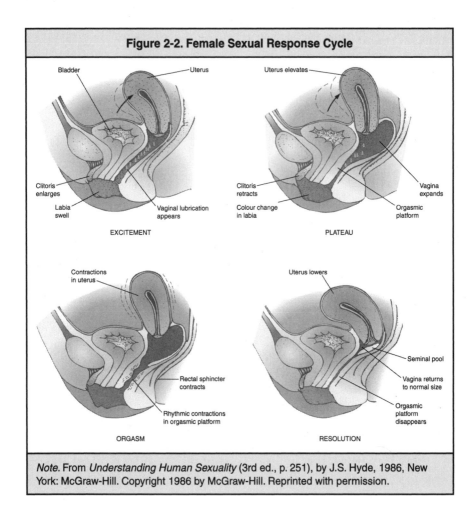

Figure 2-2. Female Sexual Response Cycle

Bladder | Uterus

Clitoris enlarges
Labia swell | Vaginal lubrication appears

EXCITEMENT

Uterus elevates

Clitoris retracts | Vagina expands
Colour change in labia | Orgasmic platform

PLATEAU

Contractions in uterus

Rectal sphincter contracts
Rhythmic contractions in orgasmic platform

ORGASM

Uterus lowers

Seminal pool
Vagina returns to normal size
Orgasmic platform disappears

RESOLUTION

Note. From *Understanding Human Sexuality* (3rd ed., p. 251), by J.S. Hyde, 1986, New York: McGraw-Hill. Copyright 1986 by McGraw-Hill. Reprinted with permission.

sex. This motivation leads to women being receptive to sexual stimuli from a partner if those stimuli are within an appropriate context. When the stimuli are perceived by women, they are processed psychologically and physically and lead to subjective feelings of arousal and a responsive feeling of desire. The occurrence of sexual satisfaction for women in this cycle is thought to further increase their motivation and willingness to be receptive in a future encounter. Arousal and desire also contribute to the rewards that women receive from being sexual with their partner. For Basson (2005), satisfaction does not necessarily mean that the woman has an orgasm; she contends that for many women, the feelings of closeness and intimacy and the knowledge that one's partner may have achieved orgasm and/or satisfaction may be enough to engender satisfaction.

Basson's (2005) model provides a useful way of explaining to women how mo-tivation (reasons and incentives to be sexually active) and psychological processing interplay when they are receptive to sexual stimuli even though innate desire or libido may be missing (see Figure 2-3). Educating women that although they may not feel spontaneous desire, if they are willing to be receptive to their partner's sexual stimulation, assuming that the context (time, place, and mood) is appropriate, feelings of arousal may occur. This, in turn, may cause them to feel responsive and, in fact, it may be at this point that desire occurs. The rewards for women may be sexual satisfaction or feelings of closeness to their partner and pleasure in his or her sexual satisfaction. These feelings then increase women's motivation and willingness to be receptive on future occasions. This model has not yet been tested for its application in males; however, it may apply to them and be a useful adjunct to treating low sexual desire in men as well as women.

Human Sexual Behavior

Sexual scripts are the learned behaviors, feelings, and meanings that people ascribe to sexual behavior. Each person has learned an individual set of thoughts and actions that dictate the *who, how, what, when,* and *where* related to sex. People start to learn these scripts by observing their parents and the way they display affection for one another. Societal norms and messages from peers further influence one's thinking and behavior. When people enter into an intimate relationship, they develop a set of behaviors that dictate what comes next. For example, one sexual script may involve sexual intercourse in the missionary position every Saturday night after dinner and a movie. The man and the woman have a set of actions that occur in the same pattern every week: she takes off her nightgown, and he stimulates her breasts for three minutes while she strokes his penis. He then inserts his penis into her vagina, thrusts for about five minutes, and ejaculates. She goes to the bathroom to clean up and returns to the bedroom to find him asleep. Anything outside of this regular activity would be noted by the couple to be highly unusual. Another sexual script may be more complicated. The woman may leave a note for her lesbian partner to suggest that she not make plans after work as she has something special planned. The partner comes home from work to find the house in darkness and a trail of lit candles leading toward the bedroom. In the bedroom, she finds her partner dressed in a black bustier and feather mask. She has never encountered this situation before, and the novelty arouses her. They spend two hours exploring each other's bodies in the dark, and the encounter ends in mutual orgasms. This couple has a far more inventive sexual script than the first couple. Neither is normal or abnormal; they are just different. For many adults, the normative (heterosexual) North American sexual script involves the male as the initiator of sexual activity and the female as the passive but eager recipient. Kissing, touching, and genital stimulation occur as a prelude to penetrative intercourse, after

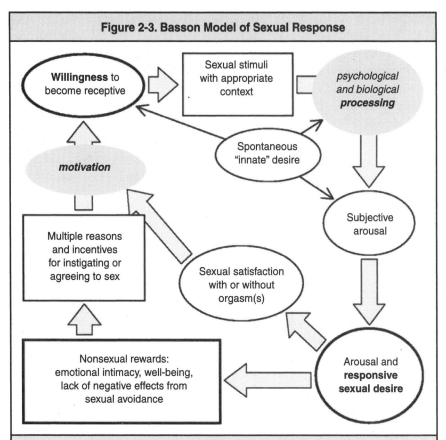

Figure 2-3. Basson Model of Sexual Response

Sex response cycle, showing responsive desire experienced during the sexual experience as well as variable initial (spontaneous) desire. At the "initial" stage (left) there is sexual neutrality, but with positive motivation. A woman's reasons for instigating or agreeing to sex include a desire to express love, to receive and share physical pleasure, to feel emotionally closer, to please the partner and to increase her own well-being. This leads to a willingness to find and consciously focus on sexual stimuli. These stimuli are processed in the mind, influenced by biological and psychological factors. The resulting state is one of subjective sexual arousal. Continued stimulation allows sexual excitement and pleasure to become more intense, triggering desire for sex itself: sexual desire, absent initially, is now present. Sexual satisfaction, with or without orgasm, results when the stimulation continues sufficiently long and the woman can stay focused, enjoys the sensation of sexual arousal and is free from any negative outcome such as pain.

Note. From "Women's Sexual Dysfunction: Revised and Expanded Definitions," by R. Basson, 2005, *Canadian Medical Association Journal, 172,* p. 1328. Copyright 2005 by CMA Media Inc. Reprinted with permission.

which some more cuddling occurs and the couple then go to sleep. Of course, many other scripts exist, each as unique as the individuals who have held them over the years. People tend to use the same script over and over, as that script tends to be reinforced by pleasurable encounters. When the individual or couple is challenged by an illness that has a consequence of temporary or permanent alteration of the anatomy or physiology of the sexual organs, some will not be able to alter their usual sexual script, and sexual activity may cease as a result.

Conclusion

Sexual functioning for human beings is a complex phenomenon comprising anatomic, hormonal, and behavioral aspects. A number of different models exist to explain this aspect of life, and these differ in their theoretical underpinnings. These models have shaped people's understanding of human sexuality for most of the latter part of the 20th century and continue to guide therapy and research in human sexuality.

References

Basson, R. (2001). Human sex-response cycles. *Journal of Sex and Marital Therapy, 27,* 33–43.

Basson, R. (2005). Women's sexual dysfunction: Revised and expanded definitions. *Canadian Medical Association Journal, 172,* 1327–1333.

Davis, S., Davison, S., Donath, S., & Bell, R. (2005). Circulating androgen levels and self-reported sexual function in women. *JAMA, 294,* 91–96.

Davison, S., Bell, R., Donath, S., Montalto, J., & Davis, S. (2005). Androgen levels in adult females: Changes with age, menopause, and oophorectomy. *Journal of Clinical Endocrinology and Metabolism, 90,* 3847–3853.

Kaplan, H.S. (1979). *Disorders of sexual desire.* New York: Simon and Schuster.

Masters, W.H., & Johnson, V.E. (1966). *Human sexual response.* Boston: Little, Brown.

Regan, P. (1999). Hormonal correlates and causes of sexual desire: A review. *Canadian Journal of Human Sexuality, 8,* 1–16.

Robinson, K., & Huether, S. (2002). Structure and function of the reproductive systems. In K. McCance & S. Huether (Eds.), *Pathophysiology: The biologic basis for disease in adults and children* (4th ed., pp. 670–704). Philadelphia: Mosby.

Zilbergeld, B., & Ellison, C. (1980). Desire discrepancies and arousal problems in sex therapy. In S. Leiblum & L. Pervin (Eds.), *Principles and practice of sex therapy* (pp. 65–101). New York: Guilford Press.

CHAPTER 3

Sexual Health Assessment

Nurses should include information about sexual health and the implications for sexuality when caring for patients and should question patients about any sexual concerns they have related to treatments (Albaugh & Kellog-Spadt, 2003). This is especially true in the oncology arena, where both the cancer itself and the treatments have anatomic and physiologic side effects (Andersen, 1990). However, this is frequently not done, and nurses are missing a valuable opportunity to be proactive and holistic in the care they provide (Haboubi & Lincoln, 2003).

Sexual Assessment by Nurses

Research indicates that nurses do not routinely inquire about sexual practices and are inconsistent in providing teaching or counseling in this area (Haboubi & Lincoln, 2003). Nurses may be reluctant to ask questions about patients' sexual functioning because they are embarrassed, they believe that sexuality is not part of the presenting problem, or they feel that they lack the necessary education and do not know appropriate nursing interventions for the problems that are identified. Fear of legal consequences also may play a role (Herson, Hart, Gordon, & Rintala, 1999; Maurice, 2000). Some healthcare professionals feel that asking about sexuality is an invasion of patients' privacy (Bartlik, Rosenfeld, & Beaton, 2005) or may think that gender is an issue (Burd, Nevadunsky, & Bachmann, 2006). Although patients have said that a discussion about sexual concerns is appropriate (Waterhouse, 1996), nurses are more likely to wait for patients to initiate the discussion rather than to assess sexual functioning routinely (Guthrie, 1999). Nurses may think that patients do not expect them to ask questions about sexuality (Magnan, Reynolds, & Galvin, 2005) and may believe that it is someone else's responsibility (Herson et al.). In some instances, this may result in sexual problems not being recognized or addressed at all. Some healthcare providers may presume that because of the seriousness of the disease or the patient's stage of life that sexuality is not an important issue (Huang, 1999). Even when the cancer site is one that is directly associated with sexual functioning—for example, ovarian cancer—healthcare providers may be derelict in their duty to ask about any problems or changes in sexual functioning (Stead, Brown, Fallowfield, & Selby, 2003).

Communicating About Sex

Why is it so difficult to talk to patients about this aspect of their lives? Personal history and family values and attitudes play an important role. Nurses bring to their professional lives the lessons, beliefs, and values that they were taught as children (Lewis & Bor, 1994). Nurses may not have the words or the comfort level to discuss this topic or the confidence to raise this issue with patients. People speak about sex in many different ways (Evans, 2000). Childhood language uses babyish terms that are designed to lessen embarrassment and are frequently euphemistic. For example, genitals may be referred to as a "pee pee." Common language is also euphemistic and vague, such as saying "down there" to refer to the genitals. Some may find that using medical terminology (e.g., "vulva" or "glans") provides some distance, but this might be a barrier for patients who do not know the meaning of the word. Some patients may use street language, generally regarded as coarse or crude, but this is the only way they know how to describe or name part of their anatomy.

Talking about sex can be embarrassing for many people. They may blush, reduce eye contact, alter their speech, or increase body movements (Meerabeau, 1999); all are typical behavior of someone who is embarrassed. If attention is drawn to this, such as if the patient comments on obvious embarrassment, secondary embarrassment merely adds to the discomfort. Most nurses learn very early to hide or manage embarrassment; however, novel experiences can occur at any time that can cause embarrassment. Fear of embarrassment often motivates people to avoid uncomfortable questions or situations, such as talking about sexuality.

One way of addressing any discomfort related to sexuality is to practice asking the necessary questions among colleagues. This can be done as part of a continuing education session where healthcare professionals can discuss personal barriers and attitudes in a supportive, nonjudgmental environment. Observing how expert nurses include questions about sexuality also may be helpful (O'Keefe & Tesar, 1999). In addition, attending sexuality workshops and self-study can be useful (Katz, 2003a). A number of college and online courses are available that address this topic (Weerakoon & Wong, 2003), and there are dedicated journals that address research and counseling across the life span (see Chapter 24 for resources). Including factual information about sexuality in nursing curricula is one part of the solution; however, incorporating this as part of routine practice is more of a challenge (Palmer, 1998).

Individuals should understand how they developed specific attitudes and values toward sexuality and sexual functioning. Think about the messages received about the body and sexuality as a child and teenager. How was affection shown in the family? What did religion teach about sex? How have those teachings contributed to personal feelings and practices as an adult? How does one communicate about sexuality in the family and culture? Sexual values clarification exercises also can help nurses to become attuned to their own personal sexual values and how these values may affect interactions with patients. Nurses should ask themselves what they think about oral sex; is it acceptable for them? For teens? For adults? For older adults? They also should ask themselves why they feel this way. What about anal sex or masturbation? What about homosexuality? Discussing these issues with a group of trusted colleagues can help nurses both in practicing saying the words and also in creating an opportunity to explore personal thoughts, feelings, and values (Longworth, 1997).

Although remaining true to oneself and not compromising personal integrity and beliefs are important, biases and judgments should not interfere with the provision of competent nursing care. If a healthcare professional feels that his or her personal values will be compromised by addressing the sexual issues concerning a patient, he or she should validate the patient's concerns and arrange for another staff member to address these concerns (Ekland & McBride, 1997).

How to Conduct a Sexual History

The goals of a sexual health history are to identify a sexual problem, to determine whether the problem is associated with the disease or treatment or if it is long-standing, to learn about the patient's sexual history, to make the patient feel comfortable with the conversation, and to take the necessary steps to manage the problem (Bartlik et al., 2005). Although many institutions include one or more questions about sexuality as part of a screening health history, these often are not completed by either the healthcare provider or the patient. Electronic health records can include a prompt to ask the questions, but these are frequently overridden or ignored (Katz, 2005). A number of assessment tools specifically related to sexuality exist, but they tend to be long and not well suited to the clinical setting (Katz, 2003a). Taking a sexual history is best done by nurses using well-honed communication and interpersonal skills (Warner, Rowe, & Whipple, 1999).

Privacy is essential when initiating the sexual history discussion, which is sometimes difficult in a busy outpatient clinic or in a shared room. However, nurses can use a general statement such as, "I would like to ask you some questions about sexual functioning when your infusion is over. We will move to a more private area to do this." Even if another patient overhears this statement, it indicates to the other patient that the nurse is open to discussing the topic, and this may encourage others to initiate the discussion with other nurses.

It often is easier to talk about sexuality once a rapport has been established. This topic usually is not discussed in an emergent or urgent situation. Using a phrase such as, "I always ask patients about any concerns they may have about sex" serves to normalize the discussion (Warner et al., 1999). The patient's age usually is not a reason to avoid this topic—the older adult population often is assumed to be nonsexual and therefore may have the greatest need for information because of ageist attitudes. Adolescents, even if not sexually active at the time, often have many questions about how a disease or treatment may affect their sexual life in the future. Nurses should be aware of cultural norms related to sexuality and should be mindful of these when beginning the discussion (Katz, 2003b). Being of the opposite sex than the patient is not necessarily a barrier; the important thing is that nurses demonstrate to patients that they are comfortable talking about this issue.

Nurses need to develop a systematic and consistent set of questions to screen for sexual issues. This will ensure that they are comfortable with the questions and that they ask the same questions of all patients. Using open-ended questions is suggested because they encourage discussion rather than a "yes" or "no" response. Silence is a valuable tool when discussing sensitive topics. Although people generally rush on to the next question, keeping quiet both encourages patients to fill the silence and also allows for some reflection on the part of patients. Healthcare professionals should use simple words and try to avoid medical jargon. If the patient appears to not understand what they are asking, they should rephrase the question or ask the patient what he or she is comfortable calling a body part or sexual activity. If the patient's partner is not present or the nurse does not know the patient's sexual orientation, it is best to use gender-neutral language until the patient indicates his or her orientation. Patients are not offended when nurses refer to their significant other as a "partner" and will quickly tell them that "my wife/husband" or "he/she" is named "Chris."

The presence of a partner can be helpful, or it may pose a barrier. Patients may be reluctant to disclose fully in front of their partner or may try to protect their partner from potentially hurtful statements. If a problem is identified, it is useful to ask patients to bring their partner to a subsequent visit to obtain the partner's perspective on the issue or to include him or her in education about the origins and/or solutions to the problem. Patients often regard a sexual problem as an individual problem; however, for the most part, sexual issues relate to the couple, and solutions will be found only if they are based on the couple.

So, how can nurses include questions about sexual functioning in their daily encounters with patients? A suggested set of four questions may be used to screen for sexual problems (Longworth, 1997).

1. Do you have any concerns about your sexual functioning?
2. Has there been any change in your sexual functioning?
3. How satisfied are you with your sex life?
4. Has your cancer or the treatments affected your sexual functioning?

An affirmative answer to any of the questions would lead to more in-depth questioning. One of the risks of this approach is that some of the questions are closed-ended and the patient can answer "yes" or "no" and effectively shut down a more detailed discussion. Questions that can elicit more detailed information include the following topics.

- The history of the present problem
  - Date of onset
  - Duration
  - Situational context
  - Attempted management
- Current sexual interaction
  - Frequency of intercourse or love play
  - Frequency preference of both partners
  - Influence of any fatigue or other symptoms
  - Verbal and nonverbal communication
  - Level of arousal
  - Frequency of orgasm and any changes
  - Pain or other symptoms during love play and/or intercourse
- Sexual history
  - Level of sexual knowledge
  - History of negative experiences
  - Body image
- Family history
  - Family attitudes toward sexuality
  - Parental modeling
  - Religious influences
- Relationship history
  - Development and stability of present relationship
  - Changes in feelings toward partner over time
  - Presence of unresolved conflict
  - Communication about feelings
- Current stressors
  - Strains associated with illness

- – Associated strains in the family
- – Extrafamilial strains (e.g., financial, occupational)
- Medical history
  - – History of current illness
  - – Past medical and surgical history
  - – Medications
  - – Recreational drug and alcohol use

Another way of asking the questions is to approach this from a more sociopolitical perspective, taking into consideration how men and women see themselves in the context of the family of origin, sexual orientation, partner relationship, etc. The Sexual History Questionnaire in Figure 3-1 addresses the four domains of sexual problems as identified in the "new view" of men's and women's sexual problems, which is described in detail in Chapter 22. The four domains are sociocultural, political, or economic; partner and relationship; psychological factors; and physiologic and medical factors.

Many nurses may not feel comfortable or have the time to conduct an in-depth assessment of sexual functioning. However, this list may be modified to elicit the basic information needed to decide whether patients need a referral to a sexuality counselor or sex therapist or whether they need clarification and education, which falls within the scope of practice of most nurses.

Sexual Assessment Models

One way nurses can include sexual health information and assess for problems or concerns is to use a model that allows for the incorporation of information related to sexuality in the general care that is given to patients with cancer. A number of models exist that can be helpful. The most frequently used model is the PLISSIT model (Annon, 1974). The first level of this model involves giving patients or clients *permission* to talk about sexual issues. The second level, *limited information,* refers to nurses giving patients factual information in response to a question or observation. The third level involves making a *specific suggestion* to clients or patients. Finally, the fourth level refers to the *intensive therapy* needed for severe or more long-standing sexual problems (see Figure 3-2).

Another model is the BETTER model (Mick, Hughes, & Cohen, 2003), which was developed to assist healthcare providers in including sexuality assessment in the care of patients with cancer. This model is comprehensive and the most highly recommended. It is similar to the PLISSIT model in that the first level of intervention involves *bringing up* the topic. The second step involves *explaining* that sexuality is part of quality of life, and patients should be aware that they can talk about this with

---

Figure 3-1. Sexual History Questionnaire

1. Some men and women worry about knowing the right words to use to talk about sex. Do you feel as if you have the right words and vocabulary to describe sexuality issues?
   - Are there any words, terms, or definitions you would like to learn?
2. What type of sex education have you ever had?
   - Would you like to have more knowledge of sexuality as it involves physiology, psychology, social norms and values, or any other topic?
3. Do you have information about how sexuality changes at different life stages (e.g., childhood, young adulthood, mid-life, old age)?
   - How do you feel about adapting to sexual changes that come with aging?
4. How have social ideas and requirements about "masculinity/femininity" and "manhood/womanhood" affected you and your sexual life?
5. Is there any conflict or disagreement between the messages you learned from the social/cultural group you grew up in and the social/cultural group you live in now?
6. What kinds of ideas about sexuality did you receive from religion in your past or present faith community?
7. Do you feel comfortable with how your body looks? Do you see yourself as sexually attractive?
8. Do you worry in any way about being punished for your sexual fantasies or activities?
9. Do you feel that there are conflicts between your family and work obligations and having a satisfactory sexual life?
10. Describe the sexual and intimate relationships you are currently involved with (long-term and casual).
11. How do you feel about your sexual partner(s)?
    - Do you like each other?
    - Do you feel intimate?
    - How do you communicate about sex?
12. In your primary sexual relationship, is there
    - A similar level of desire?
    - Similar preferences for various sexual activities?
    - An ability to communicate about initiating, pacing, or shaping sexual activities?
    - A history of violence or coercion?
    - Clear agreement about monogamy or non-monogamy?
13. Are you comfortable with nudity and physical touch?
14. Do you experience any anxiety or difficulty with sex because of any of the following?
    - Past physical or emotional abuse
    - Intimacy problems with your partner
    - Rejection or fear of rejection
    - Jealousy
15. Do you or your partner have disagreements over any of the following issues that affect your sexual life?
    - Money
    - Schedules
    - Children/childcare
    - Relatives
16. Do you have any problems with sex as a result of your partner's health status, attitudes, sexual preferences, or past sexual experiences?

(Continued on next page)

Figure 3-1. Sexual History Questionnaire *(Continued)*

17. How would you describe your sexual orientation/identity?
    - Heterosexual
    - Gay
    - Bisexual
    - Not sure
18. Do you have any problems with masturbation?
    - How often do you masturbate? Do you masturbate on a weekly basis?
    - Do you always have an orgasm when you want to?
    - Do you use masturbation to relieve tension? Does this occur at night before going to sleep, at work during the day, or at other times?
    - Do you masturbate to have an orgasm as quickly as possible, or do you take your time?
    - Do you use any fantasies or visual materials when you masturbate?
19. How do you feel about sexual activities?
    - Do you have a generally positive or negative attitude?
    - Are you afraid or disgusted in any way?
    - Do you try to avoid sex?
    - Does sex make you feel guilty or ashamed in any way?
    - Do you feel entitled to have a lot of physical pleasure?
    - Do you feel burdened by having to give another person physical pleasure?
    - What aspect of sex gives you the most pleasure?
20. Do you use alcohol or recreational drugs with sexual activities? Is this because they help you feel better or perform better?
21. Are you satisfied with your level of interest in sex? Your physical arousal including erection? Your orgasm and ejaculation? Give as much detail as you can about aspects of sex you are dissatisfied about.
22. Do you experience any kind of pain or lack of physical or emotional response with sexual activity?
    - Describe when and how this pain or lack of response occurs.
    - Are there any sexual experiences when you do not have this pain or lack of response?
23. Is your pain or lack of response associated with any of the following?
    - Anxiety or tension
    - A physical problem or health condition
    - Sexually transmitted infection
    - Side effects of drugs, medications, or medical treatments
    - What do you think are the causes of the pain or lack of response?

Note. Based on information from Kaschuk & Tiefer, 2001.

---

the nurse. Care providers then should *tell* patients that appropriate resources can be found to address their concerns and that, although the *timing* may not be appropriate now, they can ask for information at any time. Patients should be *educated* about the sexual side effects of their treatment, and, finally, a *recording* should be made in the patient chart to report that this topic has been discussed (see Figure 3-3).

Figure 3-2. The PLISSIT Model

- **Permission:** All nurses should be able to function at this level. An example of this level would be to include a general statement that normalizes the topic.
- **Limited information:** Most nurses should be able to give this kind of information. In the case of a couple in which one person has had surgery, nurses should be able to give general information about resuming intercourse following the surgery.
- **Specific suggestion:** This level of the model requires a deeper degree of nursing expertise. Information at this level includes anticipatory guidance related to possible sexual consequences of medications and other treatments.
- **Intensive therapy:** This level of the model usually requires a referral to a sex therapist or specially trained counselor. Nurses should know where to refer patients when problems or issues are disclosed that are beyond their scope of practice or expertise.

Figure 3-3. The BETTER Model

- **Bringing up the topic:** Nurses are encouraged to raise the issue of sexuality with patients.
- **Explaining that sex is a part of quality of life:** This helps to normalize the discussion and may help patients to feel less embarrassed or alone in having a problem.
- **Telling patients that resources will be found to address their concerns:** This step suggests to patients that even if the nurse does not have the immediate solution to the problem or question, there are others that can help.
- **Timing the intervention:** Patients may not be ready to deal with sexual issues at the time a problem is identified; however, patients can ask for information at any time in the future.
- **Educating patients about sexual side effects of treatment:** Educating patients about potential sexual side effects from treatments does not mean that they will occur. However, informing patients about sexual side effects is as important as informing them about any other side effects.
- **Recording:** It is not necessary to describe in detail what was discussed; however, a brief notation that a discussion about sexuality or sexual side effects occurred is important.

In Chapters 4–12, examples of disease-specific discussions using the PLISSIT and BETTER models will be discussed.

A third model is the ALARM model (Andersen, 1990), which was developed as a brief assessment of sexual activity and the sexual response cycle. It is based on Masters and Johnson's (1966) four-stage sexual response cycle and is more biomedical in its approach than the preceding two models (see Figure 3-4).

Conclusion

In this chapter, information about the importance of clarifying one's own attitudes and values toward sexuality, as well as information on how to take a sexual

---

Figure 3-4. The ALARM Model

- **Activity:** Frequency of current sexual activities (intercourse, kissing, masturbation)
- **Libido/desire:** Desire for sexual activity and interest in initiating or responding to partner
- **Arousal and orgasm:** Occurrence of erection/lubrication and orgasm accompanied with feelings of sexual excitement
- **Resolution:** Feelings of release of tension following sexual activity and satisfaction with current sexual life
- **Medical history:** Current age and medical, psychiatric, and substance abuse history, which may have caused acute or chronic disruption of sexual activity or response

---

health history, was presented. When and how to take a sexual health history, the importance of the choice of language when obtaining this information, and how to deal with personal discomfort as well as discomfort on the part of the patient also were addressed. A number of different models were presented, including one specifically developed for patients with cancer. No perfect model or method for taking a sexual history exists. Nurses must develop a level of comfort in discussing this topic, making it part of routine assessment of every patient, and then acting on the information gleaned from the patient and/or partner so that they can address this important quality-of-life issue.

References

Albaugh, J., & Kellog-Spadt, S. (2003). Sexuality and sexual health: The nurse's role and initial approach to patients. *Urologic Nursing, 23,* 227–228.

Andersen, B.L. (1990). How cancer affects sexual functioning. *Oncology, 4,* 81–94.

Annon, J. (1974). *The behavioral treatment of sexual problems.* Honolulu, HI: Enabling Systems.

Bartlik, B., Rosenfeld, S., & Beaton, C. (2005). Assessment of sexual functioning: Sexual history taking for health care practitioners. *Epilepsy and Behavior, 7*(Suppl. 2), S15–S21.

Burd, I., Nevadunsky, N., & Bachmann, G. (2006). Impact of physician gender on sexual history taking in a multispecialty practice. *Journal of Sexual Medicine, 3,* 194–200.

Ekland, M., & McBride, K. (1997). Sexual health care: The role of the nurse. *Canadian Nurse, 93*(7), 34–37.

Evans, D. (2000). Speaking of sex: The need to dispel myths and overcome fears. *British Journal of Nursing, 9,* 650–655.

Guthrie, C. (1999). Nurses' perceptions of sexuality relating to patient care. *Journal of Clinical Nursing, 8,* 313–321.

Haboubi, N.H., & Lincoln, N. (2003). Views of health professionals on discussing sexual issues with patients. *Disability and Rehabilitation, 25,* 291–296.

Herson, L., Hart, K.A., Gordon, M.J., & Rintala, D.H. (1999). Identifying and overcoming barriers to providing sexuality information in the clinical setting. *Rehabilitation Nursing, 24,* 148–151.

Huang, C. (1999). Discussing sex with disabled patients. *Western Journal of Medicine, 171,* 76–77.

Kaschuk, E., & Tiefer, L. (2001). *A new view of women's sexual problems.* New York: Haworth Press.

Katz, A. (2003a). Sexuality after hysterectomy: A review of the literature and discussion of nurses' role. *Journal of Advanced Nursing, 42,* 297–303.

Katz, A. (2003b). "Where I come from, we don't talk about that": Exploring sexuality and culture among Blacks, Asians and Hispanics. *AWHONN Lifelines, 6,* 533–536.

Katz, A. (2005). The sounds of silence: Sexuality information for cancer patients. *Journal of Clinical Oncology, 23,* 238–241.

Lewis, S., & Bor, R. (1994). Nurses' knowledge of and attitudes towards sexuality and the relationship of these with nursing practice. *Journal of Advanced Nursing, 20,* 251–259.

Longworth, J. (1997). Sexual assessment and counseling in primary care. *Nurse Practitioner Forum, 8,* 166–171.

Magnan, M.A., Reynolds, K.E., & Galvin, E.A. (2005). Barriers to addressing patient sexuality in nursing practice. *Medsurg Nursing, 14,* 282–289.

Masters, W.H., & Johnson, V.E. (1966). *Human sexual response.* Boston: Little, Brown.

Maurice, W.L. (2000). Talking about sexual matters with patients. Time to re-examine the CMPA's policy. *Canadian Family Physician, 46,* 1553–1560.

Meerabeau, L. (1999). The management of embarrassment and sexuality in health care. *Journal of Advanced Nursing, 29,* 1507–1513.

Mick, J., Hughes, M., & Cohen, M. (2003). Sexuality and cancer: How oncology nurses can address it BETTER. *Oncology Nursing Forum, 30*(Suppl. 2), 152–153.

O'Keefe, R., & Tesar, C.M. (1999). Sex talk: What makes it hard to learn sexual history taking? *Family Medicine, 31,* 315–316.

Palmer, H. (1998). Exploring sexuality and sexual health in nursing. *Professional Nurse, 14,* 15–17.

Stead, M.L., Brown, J.M., Fallowfield, L., & Selby, P. (2003). Lack of communication between healthcare professionals and women with ovarian cancer about sexual issues. *British Journal of Cancer, 88,* 666–671.

Warner, P.H., Rowe, T., & Whipple, B. (1999). Shedding light on the sexual history. *American Journal of Nursing, 99,* 34–40.

Waterhouse, J. (1996). Nursing practice related to sexuality: A review and recommendations. *Nursing Times Research, 1,* 412–418.

Weerakoon, P., & Wong, M. (2003, May 6). Sexuality education on-line for health professionals. *Electronic Journal of Human Sexuality, 6.* Retrieved December 20, 2006, from http://www.ejhs.org/volume6/SexEd.html

Section II

How Cancer Impacts Sexuality

CHAPTER 4

Breast Cancer

For many women, breasts are an important aspect of femininity and sexual persona. For others, breasts are more functional and are seen as a source of nourishment for babies. For women at increased risk for developing breast cancer because of genetic factors, breasts may be a medicalized body part, removed from sensuality (Langellier & Sullivan, 1998). A diagnosis of breast cancer and the subsequent treatment modalities may profoundly affect the way a woman sees herself and functions as a sexual being.

The Effect of Breast Cancer on Sexuality

Sexuality in the context of breast cancer must be viewed within the disease trajectory. A diagnosis of breast cancer can precipitate a physical, psychological, and emotional crisis. Around the time of diagnosis and during the treatment phase, fear of the cancer and of death overrides the potential loss of sexuality and intimacy (Anllo, 2000). Many women perceive that surviving the disease is enough, and this supersedes sex (Hordern, 2000). At this time, women need to focus their energy on coping with the diagnosis, decision making related to treatment options, and immediate health issues. Decisions made soon after diagnosis tend to focus on the best options for maximizing survival rather than on the potential for body image or sexual disturbances (Krauss, 1999). For women who are taking hormone therapy to treat menopausal symptoms, a breast cancer diagnosis means they have to stop this treatment, and the return of menopausal symptoms can be sudden and severe and may affect sexual functioning (Rogers & Kristjanson, 2002).

When treatment is over, many women are left to deal with sexual consequences, which are global, long-lasting, and related to the type of treatment (Mols, Vingerhoets,

Coebergh, & van de Poll-Franse, 2005; Stead, 2003). Women tend to return to sexual activity in spite of lack of libido, decreased arousal, dyspareunia, and fatigue. Some may fear abandonment if they do not resume sexual activity with their partners and thus endure physical pain and other problems associated with intercourse (Anllo, 2000). Others resume sexual activity as a way of expressing affection and maintaining intimacy in the relationship in spite of discomfort or lack of interest. After the treatment phase is over, many women realize the full impact of the cancer on other aspects of their lives, including sexuality. Sex, once a source of comfort for many women, may become a source of physical and emotional discomfort (Davis, Zinkand, & Fitch, 2000), and finding solutions that work can be difficult.

Treatment of Breast Cancer

Breast cancer is treated according to the stage of the cancer. The vast majority of women with early breast cancer can be treated with breast-conserving procedures (lumpectomy, partial mastectomy, segmental resection, or quadrectomy) and radiation therapy. However, some women may require more extensive surgery, with radical mastectomy involving removal of all breast tissue and the nipple areola complex and axillary node dissection. Breast reconstruction is common after mastectomy, and a variety of surgical techniques are used, including the transverse rectus abdominis musculocutaneous (also known as TRAM) flap procedure or the implantation of a saline prosthesis (Veiga et al., 2004).

Mastectomy and other surgical procedures do not have a direct effect on any aspect of the sexual response cycle. However, the resultant scarring, deformity, or absence of the breast can have far-reaching emotional consequences for both patients and their partners. Some may avoid sexual intimacy because of a fear of rejection of their new, cancer-scarred body. Body image changes are not only related to the scar on the breast from lumpectomy or mastectomy. Some women experience lymphedema in the arm or a shoulder disability of the affected side following lymph node dissection or sentinel lymph node biopsy (Morrell et al., 2005). Extensive removal of lymph nodes may result in persistent swelling, pain, limitation in movement, frustration at limitations leading to depression, and social isolation if women restrict social activity because of embarrassment (McWayne & Heiney, 2005).

Lumpectomy, although conserving much of the breast tissue, might leave one breast looking very different from the other. Women may experience alterations in sensation over the scar during the immediate postoperative period, and though these sensations can change over time, numbness and loss of sensation may persist. This can have significant sexual consequences for both patients and their partners. Some partners might be reluctant to touch the affected breast for fear of causing pain, and women may interpret this reluctance as rejection. Some women who have had breast reconstruction after mastectomy report that although the reconstructed breast is aesthetically pleasing, there is lack of sensation over the area, which affects sexual pleasure (Wilmoth & Ross, 1997).

Women who have undergone a mastectomy report negative body image more frequently than those who have had lumpectomy. Reconstruction after mastectomy affords some satisfaction in terms of how women view their body (Al-Ghazal, Fallowfield, & Blamey, 2000), and many women relate body image to sexual attractiveness. Immediate rather than delayed breast reconstruction results in less distress for women (Al-Ghazal, Sully, Fallowfield, & Blamey, 2000). However, fears of recurrence may be greater after breast-conserving treatment because women are not certain that all the cancer has been removed (Bredin, 1999).

Even with reconstruction, many women report that their breast looks and feels different (Nissen, Swenson, & Kind, 2002) and may be caressed less often by their sexual partner (Schover et al., 1995). Women report altered sensation in the reconstructed breast (such as pins and needles, numbness), and the surgical scar does not go away (Rowland et al., 2000).

Radiation therapy affects sexuality in a number of ways. Fatigue is a common side effect of radiation therapy, and this can profoundly affect sexual desire. Many women continue to work and maintain their normal family and household duties while undergoing radiation therapy. This can have a measurable effect on fatigue, which might affect their libido and ability to engage in sexual activity. Radiation damage to the skin can affect sexual response to caressing, and some women experience shooting pain in the breast, along with nipple discomfort (Wilmoth & Botchway, 1999). This therapy also can cause skin discoloration as a result of burning from the radiation, which might be both painful and disfiguring (Wilmoth & Botchway). The tattoo marks left on the patient's chest can be a constant reminder of the cancer and therefore can have long-lasting emotional and sexual side effects, as well.

The most profound impact on sexual activity for patients with breast cancer is related to hormonal changes caused by chemotherapy. Many women who receive chemotherapy, especially if an alkylating agent such as cyclophosphamide is used, will experience ovarian failure (Stead, 2003). The incidence of sexual dysfunction in women receiving adjuvant chemotherapy is significant. Sixty-four percent report having no sexual desire at all, and 48% report having low desire (Barni & Mondin, 1997). Dyspareunia is another common complaint caused by vaginal dryness associated with reduced estrogen levels (Knobf, 2001). Almost 80% of the women in one large study reported experiencing some change in sexual functioning up to five years after treatment (Meyerowitz, Desmond, Rowland, Wyatt, & Ganz, 1999). Not only does ovarian failure result in loss of circulating estrogen, but it also can cause the levels of testosterone to fall (Speer et al., 2005), thus creating problems with decreased libido.

Hair loss is a common side effect of chemotherapy. This can have a major impact on body image. Loss of pubic hair will occur as well, and this also might affect the woman's perception of herself as a sexual being. Many women are embarrassed by the loss of pubic hair and see it as a barrier to feeling and acting like an adult sexual partner.

For premenopausal women, chemotherapy-induced ovarian failure, which is experienced as the sudden onset of severe menopausal symptoms, is extremely distressing. Women report experiencing menstrual cycle changes, hot flashes, insomnia, vaginal dryness, dyspareunia, and weight gain (Knobf, 2001). Although many studies suggest that menopausal symptoms are worse for women who were premenopausal when diagnosed (Rogers & Kristjanson, 2002), a conflicting report stated that postmenopausal women are five to seven times more likely than younger women to suffer severe menopausal symptoms (Crandall, Petersen, Ganz, & Greendale, 2004). Breast cancer survivors who are treated with chemotherapy, particularly women younger than 50, have a greater risk of experiencing sexual dysfunction in arousal and orgasm. This did not appear to create problems in their intimate relationships, as women report satisfaction in these relationships in spite of ongoing sexual challenges (Ganz, Rowland, Desmond, Meyerowitz, & Wyatt, 1998). Long-term (i.e., more than five years) survivors have reported significant decreases in their libido, their ability to relax and enjoy sex, and their ability to become aroused and achieve orgasm. This was strongly associated with vaginal dryness (Broeckel, Thors, Jacobsen, Small, & Cox, 2002).

Furthermore, ovarian failure also causes decreased levels of circulating estrogen. Consequently, the vaginal mucosa thins and less lubrication is produced, thus causing vaginal dryness. As a result, women experience pain when penetration is attempted (dyspareunia), and this may become a chronic condition known as vaginismus (Barni & Mondin, 1997). Some women also experience urinary tract infections (UTIs) after attempts at sexual intercourse, most likely as a result of increased irritation of the urethra with the friction of penetration. The alteration in the vaginal pH level due to estrogen deficiency also predisposes women to UTIs (Ponzone et al., 2005). This can set up a negative feedback loop with decreased interest in sex if the result is a painful infection.

Fatigue, weight gain, and altered sexuality occur as a cluster of symptoms, which magnifies the impact of each more so than if they were viewed individually (Wilmoth, Coleman, Smith, & Davis, 2004). For many women, weight is an important body image issue and is closely connected to sexual self-schema and perception of sexual attractiveness. The weight gain experienced in the months and years after chemotherapy, usually in the range of 10 pounds or more (McInnes & Knobf, 2001), can have a significant impact on patients' sexual life and relationships.

Another factor associated with menopausal symptoms and sexual dysfunction in postmenopausal women is the incidence of urinary incontinence. In a study of postmenopausal women with breast cancer, investigators found that urinary incontinence was a significant predictor of problems in sexual functioning (Greendale, Petersen, Zibecchi, & Ganz, 2001). The role of urinary incontinence in avoidance of sexual intercourse has not been extensively studied, but its occurrence is associated with deep vaginal penetration, abdominal pressure, and clitoral stimulation and is a source of great embarrassment.

Endocrine manipulation of estrogen receptor–positive breast cancers as an adjuvant treatment is now the standard of care, which further affects menopausal symptoms and sexuality. Tamoxifen, a selective estrogen receptor modulator (SERM), lowers serum estrogen and progesterone levels and has proliferative effects on vaginal and uterine epithelial tissues (Angelopoulos, Barbounis, Livadas, Kaltsas, & Tolis, 2004). The side effects of tamoxifen appear to be most severe in premenopausal women with breast cancer, and postmenopausal women seem to experience a lesser degree of negative side effects from this drug (Ganz et al., 1998). Women taking tamoxifen commonly experience hot flashes (Young-McCaughan, 1996). Although a decrease in libido has been reported (Hunter et al., 2004), some healthcare professionals suggested that libido is a complex construct that is multifactorial and not related to the use of a SERM alone (Angelopoulos et al.). Tamoxifen has mildly estrogenic effects on the vaginal mucosa, and some women find that it provides relief from the vaginal dryness experienced as a result of chemotherapy-induced atrophy (Rogers & Kristjanson, 2002). Conversely, others think that dryness has resulted from tamoxifen use (Hunter et al.). A newer and more effective class of drug, aromatase inhibitors, now is being used subsequent to a period on tamoxifen. They appear to have similar estrogen-suppressive side effects as the SERMs, including hot flashes and vaginal dryness (Bentrem & Jordan, 2002).

Body Image

Breast cancer also has an effect on body image. Women with breast cancer have described their breasts as medicalized during the various stages of treatment. Breasts are gendered organs in that they denote femininity to some and are an essential aspect of female body image. Breasts also are considered sexual organs (Langellier & Sullivan, 1998). The daily exposure of the breasts during radiation therapy can cause women to become dissociated from their breasts as sexual organs. Many women comment that if a person in a white coat enters the room, their first action is to expose their breasts for examination. This contrasts with the usual notion of breasts as private parts of a woman's body that are for the nourishment of babies or are part of sexual play.

Studies of women who have had breast conservation surgery or reconstruction surgery after treatment for breast cancer report a more positive body image (Bukovic et al., 2005). These women report that they are more comfortable appearing nude in front of their sexual partner and are more satisfied with sex (Schover et al., 1995), but this is not universal. Some younger women describe feeling ashamed of their body (Bloom, Stewart, Chang, & Banks, 2004), which may reflect unrealistic expectations on the woman's part related to what the reconstructed breast would look and feel like. The ability to return to a healthy view of the sexual self is, in part, dependent on a woman's ability to engage in sexually pleasurable activities, her comfort with her body after treatment, and the reaction of her sexual partner to her body (Wilmoth & Ross, 1997). Body image problems are associated with mastectomy, hair loss from chemotherapy, alterations in weight, low self-esteem, and the partner having difficulty understanding the patient's feelings (Fobair et al., 2006).

Younger women, particularly women who do not have a partner at the time of diagnosis and treatment, have special needs. Unpartnered women with breast cancer suffer significant distress related to body image. Some of these women may have received negative messages about their bodies in previous relationships and might be anxious that this will happen in any future relationship, especially now that they have scars or asymmetrical breasts. Concerns about when and how to disclose their cancer history with prospective sexual partners are common, and these women often feel shame and loss of dignity, along with experiencing difficulty looking at their own bodies (Holmberg, Scott, Alexy, & Fife, 2001).

Consistent reports in the literature suggest that younger women experience more depression, greater distress and difficulty adjusting to the diagnosis, and lower quality of life (Sammarco, 2001; Wong-Kim & Bloom, 2005). Depression is well recognized in women with breast cancer, with alterations in desire, arousal, and ability to achieve orgasm (Clayton, 2001). Moreover, the treatment of depression, particularly with selective serotonin reuptake inhibitors (SSRIs), has been shown to affect sexuality, with approximately half of those who take this class of drugs experiencing a decrease in libido, difficulty becoming aroused, less vaginal lubrication, and difficulty reaching orgasm (Ferguson, 2001).

Women younger than 50 report experiencing more hot flashes, dyspareunia, and difficulty with bladder control (Avis, Crawford, & Manuel, 2005). Radiation side effects such as fatigue, insomnia, and emotional distress contribute to this (Hassey Dow & Lafferty, 2000), and fatigue has been shown to persist for 10 years after treatment (Bower et al., 2006). A decrease in perceived quality of life can persist for years after treatment, and again younger women fare worse than their older counterparts (Arndt, Merx, Stegmeier, Ziegler, & Brenner, 2005).

Younger women also may experience issues related to fertility. In one study, premenopausal women reported experiencing discord between what physicians regarded as important information for women and what the patients thought was important. Women felt bombarded by the amount of information given at the time of diagnosis but needed specific sexuality-related information later in the disease trajectory. For young women, fertility issues are more important at the time of diagnosis; however, a discussion about menopausal symptoms becomes important after surgery when adjuvant therapy is given and symptoms are pervasive (Thewes et al., 2005).

Women who carry the *BRCA1* and *BRCA2* genes may have a much higher risk of developing breast cancer. One of the preventive strategies suggested for these women is prophylactic mastectomy, which reduces their risk by at least 90%. In a study of women who had undergone this surgery, some expressed regret related to diminished sexual satisfaction and ghost pains where their breasts had been (Payne, Biggs, Tran, Borgen, & Massie, 2000).

Nursing Interventions in the Care of Women With Breast Cancer

Assessment of Expectations

For women who plan to have a mastectomy, a preoperative assessment is an important part of care and can identify the potential for maladaptive coping later in the disease trajectory (Nissen et al., 2002). Asking the woman (and her partner) what her expectations of the surgery are is vital to identifying and then correcting any misconceptions. This also will allow for an assessment of any discrepancy or discord between the couple. Women experience high levels of distress in the pretreatment phase and have to make complex treatment decisions under these conditions. The amount of information they have absorbed or assimilated in this process is unclear (Cimprich, 1999). The dominant drive is to survive the cancer at any cost, so quality-of-life issues such as sexuality may seem superfluous at this time but will increase in importance in the months and years of recovery.

Many women who have a lumpectomy assume that the affected breast will look the same as it did prior to surgery. However, significant distortion of the breast may occur depending on the amount of tissue removed and the location of the tumor. Women who have had a lot of tissue removed may find that the resulting shape of the breast makes it difficult to find a comfortable bra. Some women elect to have a mastectomy at a later date because it often is easier to deal with an external prosthesis than a partial breast.

Most women have no idea what physical changes to expect following surgery. Preparing patients by showing them photographs and diagrams will be helpful in explaining what is to come. Breast reconstruction may minimize the negative body image for women undergoing mastectomy (Rowland et al., 2000). However, women need a realistic picture of what the cosmetic results may be. Showing patients photographs of women before and after reconstruction as well as introducing them to other women who have had reconstruction may allow for a more detailed understanding of the procedure and results. Not all women will want to or be able to have reconstruction. Some women will prefer to wear an external prosthesis, whereas others will not replace the missing breast. Not replacing the weight of the breast may cause problems with back and neck pain, as the body will not be balanced properly without the natural breast weight on that side (Ehmann, 1997).

Information Sharing

A number of interventions may help women who are experiencing problems with sexual functioning associated with breast cancer and its treatments. Timely information is first and foremost and must be given at all stages of the disease trajectory (Rustoen & Begnum, 2000). Individual women will have unique needs for information at different points in time. Often a great deal of information is given at the time of diagnosis, when the woman cannot assimilate and integrate the new information (Koinberg, Holmberg, & Fridlund, 2001). The need for different types of information also changes throughout the cancer continuum. For example, younger women may be more interested in information about fertility in the early stages of diagnosis, but their needs will change as they begin treatment and need information about treatment-related side effects. Examples of questions to ask and information to discuss with patients are presented in Figure 4-1. This information is based on the PLISSIT model (Annon, 1974) described in Chapter 3 (see Figure 3-2).

The method of providing information also plays a role. Written information is not always effective for women with a low literacy level. Supportive phone calls and informational audiotapes have been shown to be more effective than written material in reducing anxiety and encouraging self-care behaviors in women with breast cancer (Williams & Schreier, 2004). Education, active support programs, and repeated phone calls by trained nurses also have been shown to reduce fatigue (Yates et al., 2005).

Healthcare providers often make assumptions about the type of information that patients and their partners need, and some healthcare providers are never comfortable discussing sexual issues with patients (Gray, Goel, Fitch, Franssen, & Labrecque, 2002; Rabinowitz, 2002). Barni and Mondin (1997) reported that only a small portion of women with breast cancer discussed sexual issues with their physician. Young-McCaughan (1996) found that most women had never been asked during treatment if sexual problems had occurred. Some women may be reluctant to talk

---

Figure 4-1. Example of the PLISSIT Model in Patients With Breast Cancer

- **Permission:** An example of this level would be to include a general statement that normalizes the topic.

  "Many couples are concerned about making love after the woman has had a mastectomy. Do you have any concerns that I can help you with?"

- **Limited information:** If the woman has had a mastectomy, the nurse should be able to give the couple some general information about resuming intercourse.

  "Once the sutures have been removed and you are no longer in pain, gentle love making is fine. You will need to tell your partner when you are uncomfortable, and in the beginning, you may want to protect that side of your body, as you are probably anxious that any pressure will cause you pain."

- **Specific suggestion:** Information at this level includes anticipatory guidance related to possible sexual consequences of medications and other treatments.

  "Taking tamoxifen for the prevention of breast cancer recurrence may have the side effect of reducing desire or libido. Often, women state that even when they do not feel the desire to have sex, gentle sexual stimulation can sometimes be exciting and cause you to become aroused and interested."

- **Intensive therapy:** Nurses should know where to refer patients when problems or issues are disclosed that are beyond the scope of practice or expertise of the nurse.

  "It seems to me that you are struggling with the side effects of chemotherapy, and perhaps a visit to a sexuality counselor would be helpful. We have one on staff. Would you like to have a name and number so that you can call to schedule an appointment?"

---

about intimate sexual matters with healthcare providers (Knobf, 2001). Furthermore, women have reported that their physicians were not understanding or helpful when sexual dysfunction was identified as a problem (Wilmoth & Ross, 1997). Older women may be more reluctant to state their need for information (Gray et al., 2002), particularly in the area of sexuality, where ageist attitudes are common and healthcare providers may assume that sexual relations are no longer possible or important after a certain age.

Specific programs designed to meet the information needs of women with breast cancer can be effective. In one program, a nurse practitioner's intervention with women led to significantly improved sexual functioning among those who participated. The program focused on symptom assessment, education, counseling, and specialist referral (Ganz et al., 2000). Even when supportive services are available from a range of allied healthcare professionals, many women with breast cancer do not use the services. Some possible reasons for this are that healthcare providers may not be aware of these other services, that they may forget to mention them or refer patients to them, or because information about these services was given early in the disease continuum and patients may not remember the information when they need the support (Gray et al., 2000). Nurses must know what services are available along with where and how to refer patients to them. This knowledge is part of both the PLISSIT and BETTER models discussed in Chapter 3.

Interventions for Treatment-Related Side Effects

Many of the menopausal symptoms may be amenable to pharmacotherapy, including progestogens, clonidine (an antihypertensive), and antidepressants for hot flashes, testosterone for decreased libido (Molina, Barton, & Loprinzi, 2005), and local estrogen therapy for vaginal atrophy (Loprinzi & Barton, 2000). However, no consensus exists on the safety of hormone therapy for women with breast cancer, especially if it is estrogen receptor positive (Hickey, Saunders, & Stuckey, 2005; Ponzone et al., 2005). As mentioned previously, SSRIs have shown effectiveness in reducing the frequency and severity of hot flashes, but women need to decide whether the risk of sexual side effects outweighs the benefits. Alternative/complementary therapies such as vitamin E, phytoestrogens, and black cohosh are frequently mentioned as treatments for menopausal symptoms, although their effectiveness and safety for women with breast cancer is not established (Graf & Geller, 2003; Hickey et al.).

Vaginal dryness can be significantly reduced with the use of a vaginal estrogen cream, pessary, or ring. Some systemic absorption occurs, but preliminary data suggest that the use of much lower doses can alleviate symptoms without increasing serum levels of estrogen (Ponzone et al., 2005). Vaginal moisturizers such as Replens® (Lil' Drug Store Products, Cedar Rapids, IA) also may help women who are experiencing vaginal dryness, as may a gradual resumption of sexual activity in the context of a loving relationship with a partner who is understanding and prepared to make changes in sexual activities based on the level of the woman's comfort (Davis et al., 2000).

Absence of libido can be a frustrating experience for many couples, particularly if in the past the woman was an eager and willing participant in sexual play and expression or was the initiator of sexual activity. The couple may mourn this change, and for some, this may mean the end of their usual sex life. Basson's model (2005) provides a useful way of explaining to women how motivation (reasons and incentives to be sexually active) and psychological processing interplay when the woman is receptive to sexual stimuli even though innate desire (libido) may be missing. Educating the woman that although she may not feel spontaneous desire, if she is willing to be receptive to her partner's sexual stimulation, assuming that the context (time, place, and mood) is appropriate, feelings of arousal may occur. In a practical sense, if she is receptive to her partner touching or kissing her, she may find that even though sex is the last thing on her mind, the feelings that this kissing or touching arouse in her allow her to continue with further sexual exploration, which may or may not end with intercourse or other sexual activity. The pleasure she experiences from this and the satisfaction of giving her partner pleasure make it more likely that the next time her partner approaches her and starts caressing her, she will be willing to encourage this activity.

Treatment of depression plays an important role in maximizing quality of life for women with breast cancer, especially because depression has such a global effect on how women function in their many different roles. Given the sexual side effects of many of the SSRIs, which may compound cancer treatment–associated side effects, alternative suggestions may be appropriate as first-line therapy for depression. Cognitive therapy, support groups, exercise, and alternative/complementary therapies may help some women, but patients always should be under professional care. If patients are taking SSRIs, a number of strategies may help to lessen the sexual side effects of treatment for depression, including careful choice of drug, drug holidays, and reductions in dose (Zajecka, 2001).

Numerous interventions have been suggested to improve body image and quality of life. Many women find that once treatment is complete, they need to reestablish a connection to their body and body image, which is now altered. As previously discussed, the body and specifically the breasts have been seen by many professionals and have been surgically altered or irradiated, and body and head hair may have disappeared. It can take many months for the woman to accept her changed body and its sensations.

The partner's acceptance of the woman's changed body is an important aspect of healing and adjustment; however, not all women enjoy having someone touching or caressing the area of the missing breast. Altered sensation and increased sensitivity of the skin following surgery or radiation therapy can make this very painful. Women do not always find this an easy subject to talk about, and the usual communication style of the couple may prevent an open and honest discussion about what feels pleasurable to her and what she does not enjoy.

Sometimes partners may be bothered by the incision, scar, or skin changes, and this can cause avoidance or secondary sexual dysfunction for them. Their response has a direct effect on how women see themselves, and inclusion of partners in preparatory information sessions can help them to anticipate what the physical changes to the breast, overlying tissue, and scarring may look like and the effect this may have on the partner immediately and in the future. For some women, sexual activity is less important than the interest that the partner shows in being sexual with them (Wimberly, Carver, Laurenceau, Harris, & Antoni, 2005). Women report that displays of affection and tenderness are vital for positive perception of their attractiveness and significantly reduce the fear of abandonment (Dorval et al., 2005).

A modified form of sensate focus exercises can help women and their partners to learn a new way of dealing with the changes from treatment (see Appendix A and Chapter 22). Instead of working toward penetrative intercourse as an end goal, the objectives are to work toward sensual touching of the breast(s) and to help women to accept the physical changes resulting from treatment. Women must be allowed to control the pace and extent of touching; the goal is to have them feel comfortable with touching to the extent that they define.

A dance program emphasizing sensual, rhythmic movements may improve perceived body image scores (Sandel et al., 2005). Women who participated in a half-day educational intervention targeting individuals with different types of cancer also showed a decrease in depressive symptoms (Golant, Altman, & Martin, 2003). In addition, women who were randomized to receive either education about nutrition or adjustment to the cancer experience showed improvement in self-concept scores (Scheier et al., 2005).

Many women also benefit from the opportunity to discuss fears or problems related to sexuality with healthcare providers. Normalizing the experience for patients can reduce anxieties and calm fears. Participation in support groups appropriate to the patient's age and/or cancer stage can be useful; however, not all women will want to do this or will be able to do this because of distance or conflicting family/work demands.

Case Study

J.R. is 55 years old and three weeks ago was diagnosed with breast cancer after a routine screening mammogram. She is scheduled for lumpectomy next week followed by radiation therapy. J.R. and her husband are seeking information on the side effects of radiation; they state that they are happy that J.R. will be having a lumpectomy but are concerned about radiation side effects.

Questions to consider:
- What information related to sexuality, if any, should the nurse give to this couple?
- What are some of the barriers to listening that women and their partners experience?
- What anticipatory guidance may be useful for women prior to lumpectomy for breast cancer?

Three weeks after her lumpectomy, J.R. returns to see the nurse. The patient is alone and very upset. Her major concern is that her husband seems reluctant to touch her at all. She states that he has barely made eye contact with her since the surgery and appears to be withdrawing. As a result, she is feeling very much alone and is anxious that there is something very wrong with his reaction. She is not sure how she will manage the weeks of radiation therapy without him.
- What advice can the nurse give J.R. at this time?
- What further questions should the nurse ask?
- Who is the best person to refer J.R. to, and when should this be done?
See Appendix B for answers to the case study questions.

Conclusion

Breasts for some women are an important aspect of femininity and sexual persona. A diagnosis of breast cancer and the subsequent treatment may profoundly affect the way women see themselves and function as sexual beings. Interventions to improve sexual adaptation include giving information in a timely manner and when patients and their partners need it most; specifically treating the side effects of surgery, radiation therapy, and chemotherapy; and providing supportive counseling.

References

Al-Ghazal, S.K., Fallowfield, L., & Blamey, R.W. (2000). Comparison of psychological aspects and patient satisfaction following breast conserving surgery, simple mastectomy and breast reconstruction. *European Journal of Cancer, 36,* 1938–1943.

Al-Ghazal, S.K., Sully, L., Fallowfield, L., & Blamey, R.W. (2000). The psychological impact of immediate rather than delayed breast reconstruction. *European Journal of Surgical Oncology, 26,* 17–19.

Angelopoulos, N., Barbounis, V., Livadas, S., Kaltsas, D., & Tolis, G. (2004). Effects of estrogen deprivation due to breast cancer treatment. *Endocrine-Related Cancer, 11,* 523–535.

Anllo, L.M. (2000). Sexual life after breast cancer. *Journal of Sex and Marital Therapy, 26,* 241–248.

Annon, J. (1974). *The behavioral treatment of sexual problems.* Honolulu, HI: Enabling Systems.

Arndt, V., Merx, H., Stegmeier, C., Ziegler, H., & Brenner, H. (2005). Persistence of restrictions in quality of life from the first to the third year after diagnosis in women with breast cancer. *Journal of Clinical Oncology, 22,* 4945–4953.

Avis, N.E., Crawford, S., & Manuel, J. (2005). Quality of life among younger women with breast cancer. *Journal of Clinical Oncology, 23,* 3322–3330.

Barni, S., & Mondin, R. (1997). Sexual dysfunction in treated breast cancer patients. *Annals of Oncology, 8,* 149–153.

Basson, R. (2005). Women's sexual dysfunction: Revised and expanded definitions. *Canadian Medical Association Journal, 172,* 1327–1333.

Bentrem, D., & Jordan, C. (2002). Role of antiestrogens and aromatase inhibitors in breast cancer treatment. *Current Opinion in Obstetrics and Gynecology, 14,* 5–12.

Bloom, J.R., Stewart, S.L., Chang, S., & Banks, P.J. (2004). Then and now: Quality of life of young breast cancer survivors. *Psycho-Oncology, 13,* 147–160.

Bower, J., Ganz, P.A., Desmond, K., Bernaards, C., Rowland, J., Meyerowitz, B.E., et al. (2006). Fatigue in long-term breast carcinoma survivors: A longitudinal investigation. *Cancer, 106,* 751–758.

Bredin, M. (1999). Mastectomy, body image and therapeutic massage: A qualitative study of women's experiences. *Journal of Advanced Nursing, 29,* 1113–1120.

Broeckel, J.A., Thors, C.L., Jacobsen, P.B., Small, M., & Cox, C.E. (2002). Sexual functioning in long-term breast cancer survivors treated with adjuvant chemotherapy. *Breast Cancer Research and Treatment, 75,* 241–248.

Bukovic, D., Fajdic, J., Hrgovic, Z., Kaufmann, M., Hojsak, I., & Stanceric, T. (2005). Sexual dysfunction in breast cancer survivors. *Onkologie, 28,* 29–34.

Cimprich, B. (1999). Pretreatment symptom distress in women newly diagnosed with breast cancer. *Cancer Nursing, 22,* 185–194.

Clayton, A.H. (2001). Recognition and assessment of sexual dysfunction associated with depression. *Journal of Clinical Psychiatry, 62*(Suppl. 3), 5–9.

Crandall, C., Petersen, L., Ganz, P.A., & Greendale, G.A. (2004). Association of breast cancer and its therapy with menopause-related symptoms. *Menopause, 11,* 519–530.

Davis, C., Zinkand, J., & Fitch, M. (2000). Cancer treatment-induced menopause: Meaning for breast and gynecological cancer survivors. *Canadian Oncology Nursing Journal, 10,* 14–21.

Dorval, M., Guay, S., Mondor, M., Masse, B., Falardeau, M., Robidoux, A., et al. (2005). Couples who get closer after breast cancer: Frequency and predictors in a prospective investigation. *Journal of Clinical Oncology, 23,* 3588–3596.

Ehmann, J. (1997). Rehabilitation. *Journal of Gynecologic Oncology Nursing, 7,* 27–37.

Ferguson, J.M. (2001). The effects of antidepressants on sexual functioning in depressed patients: A review. *Journal of Clinical Psychiatry, 62*(Suppl. 3), 22–34.

Fobair, P., Stewart, S.L., Chang, S., D'Onofrio, C., Banks, P.J., & Bloom, J.R. (2006). Body image and sexual problems in young women with breast cancer. *Psycho-Oncology, 15,* 579–594.

Ganz, P.A., Greendale, G.A., Petersen, L., Zibecchi, L., Kahn, B., & Belin, T.R. (2000). Managing menopausal symptoms in breast cancer survivors: Results of a randomized controlled trial. *Journal of the National Cancer Institute, 92,* 1054–1064.

Ganz, P.A., Rowland, J.H., Desmond, K., Meyerowitz, B.E., & Wyatt, G.E. (1998). Life after breast cancer: Understanding women's health-related quality of life and sexual functioning. *Journal of Clinical Oncology, 16,* 501–514.

Golant, M., Altman, T., & Martin, C. (2003). Managing cancer side effects to improve quality of life: A cancer psychoeducation program. *Cancer Nursing, 26,* 37–44.

Graf, M.C., & Geller, P.A. (2003). Treating hot flashes in breast cancer survivors: A review of alternative treatments to hormone replacement therapy. *Clinical Journal of Oncology Nursing, 7,* 637–640.

Gray, R., Goel, V., Fitch, M., Franssen, E., Chart, P., Greenberg, M., et al. (2000). Utilization of professional supportive care services by women with breast cancer. *Breast Cancer Research and Treatment, 64,* 253–258.

Gray, R., Goel, V., Fitch, M., Franssen, E., & Labrecque, M. (2002). Supportive care provided by physicians and nurses to women with breast cancer. *Supportive Care in Cancer, 10,* 647–652.

Greendale, G.A., Petersen, L., Zibecchi, L., & Ganz, P.A. (2001). Factors related to sexual function in postmenopausal women with a history of breast cancer. *Menopause, 8,* 111–119.

Hassey Dow, K., & Lafferty, P. (2000). Quality of life, survivorship, and psychosocial adjustment of young women with breast cancer after breast-conserving surgery and radiation therapy. *Oncology Nursing Forum, 27,* 1555–1564.

Hickey, M., Saunders, C.M., & Stuckey, B.G. (2005). Management of menopausal symptoms in patients with breast cancer: An evidence-based approach. *Lancet Oncology, 6,* 687–695.

Holmberg, S.K., Scott, L.L., Alexy, W., & Fife, B.L. (2001). Relationship issues of women with breast cancer. *Cancer Nursing, 24,* 53–60.

Hordern, A. (2000). Intimacy and sexuality for the woman with breast cancer. *Cancer Nursing, 23,* 230–236.

Hunter, M., Grunfeld, E., Mittal, S., Sikka, P., Ramirez, A., Fentiman, I., et al. (2004). Menopausal symptoms in women with breast cancer: Prevalence and treatment preferences. *Psycho-Oncology, 13,* 769–778.

Knobf, M.T. (2001). The menopausal symptom experience in young mid-life women with breast cancer. *Cancer Nursing, 24,* 201–210.

Koinberg, I., Holmberg, L., & Fridlund, B. (2001). Satisfaction with routine follow-up visits to the physician. *Acta Oncologica, 40,* 454–459.

Krauss, P. (1999). Body image, decision making, and breast cancer treatment. *Cancer Nursing, 22,* 421–427.

Langellier, K.M., & Sullivan, C.F. (1998). Breast talk in breast cancer narratives. *Qualitative Health Research, 8,* 76–94.

Loprinzi, C.L., & Barton, D. (2000). Estrogen deficiency: In search of symptom control and sexuality. *Journal of the National Cancer Institute, 92,* 1028–1029.

McInnes, J.A., & Knobf, M.T. (2001). Weight gain and quality of life in women treated with adjuvant chemotherapy for early-stage breast cancer. *Oncology Nursing Forum, 28,* 675–684.

McWayne, J., & Heiney, S.P. (2005). Psychologic and social sequelae of secondary lymphedema: A review. *Cancer, 104,* 457–466.

Meyerowitz, B.E., Desmond, K.A., Rowland, J.H., Wyatt, G.E., & Ganz, P.A. (1999). Sexuality following breast cancer. *Journal of Sex and Marital Therapy, 25,* 237–250.

Molina, J.R., Barton, D.L., & Loprinzi, C.L. (2005). Chemotherapy-induced ovarian failure: Manifestations and management. *Drug Safety, 28,* 401–416.

Mols, F., Vingerhoets, A.J., Coebergh, J.W., & van de Poll-Franse, L.V. (2005). Quality of life among long-term breast cancer survivors: A systematic review. *European Journal of Cancer, 41,* 2613–2619.

Morrell, R.M., Halyard, M.Y., Schild, S.E., Ali, M.S., Gunderson, L.L., & Pockaj, B.A. (2005). Breast cancer-related lymphedema. *Mayo Clinic Proceedings, 80,* 1480–1484.

Nissen, M.J., Swenson, K.K., & Kind, E.A. (2002). Quality of life after postmastectomy breast reconstruction. *Oncology Nursing Forum, 29,* 547–553.

Payne, D.K., Biggs, C., Tran, K.N., Borgen, P.I., & Massie, M.J. (2000). Women's regrets after bilateral prophylactic mastectomy. *Annals of Surgical Oncology, 7,* 150–154.

Ponzone, R., Biglia, N., Jacomuzzi, M.E., Maggiorotto, F., Mariani, L., & Sismondi, P. (2005). Vaginal estrogen therapy after breast cancer: Is it safe? *European Journal of Cancer, 41,* 2673–2681.

Rabinowitz, B. (2002). Psychosocial issues in breast cancer. *Obstetrics and Gynecology Clinics of North America, 29,* 233–247.

Rogers, M., & Kristjanson, L.J. (2002). The impact on sexual functioning of chemotherapy-induced menopause in women with breast cancer. *Cancer Nursing, 25,* 57–65.

Rowland, J.H., Desmond, K.A., Meyerowitz, B.E., Belin, T.R., Wyatt, G.E., & Ganz, P.A. (2000). Role of breast reconstructive surgery in physical and emotional outcomes among breast cancer survivors. *Journal of the National Cancer Institute, 92,* 1422–1429.

Rustoen, T., & Begnum, S. (2000). Quality of life in women with breast cancer. *Cancer Nursing, 23,* 416–421.

Sammarco, A. (2001). Psychosocial stages and quality of life of women with breast cancer. *Cancer Nursing, 24,* 272–277.

Sandel, S.L., Judge, J.O., Landry, N., Faria, L., Ouellette, R., & Majczak, M. (2005). Dance and movement program improves quality-of-life measures in breast cancer survivors. *Cancer Nursing, 28,* 301–309.

Scheier, M., Helgeson, V., Schulz, R., Colvin, S., Berga, S., Bridges, M., et al. (2005). Interventions to enhance physical and psychological functioning among younger women who are ending nonhormonal adjuvant treatment for early-stage breast cancer. *Journal of Clinical Oncology, 23,* 4298–4311.

Schover, L.R., Yetman, R., Tuason, L., Meisler, E., Esselstyn, C., Hermann, R., et al. (1995). Partial mastectomy and breast reconstruction: A comparison of their effects on psychosocial adjustment, body image, and sexuality. *Cancer, 75,* 54–64.

Speer, J.J., Hillenberg, B., Sugrue, D.P., Blacker, C., Kresge, C.L., Decker, V.B., et al. (2005). Study of sexual functioning determinants in breast cancer survivors. *Breast Journal, 11,* 440–447.

Stead, M.L. (2003). Sexual dysfunction after treatment for gynaecologic and breast malignancies. *Current Opinion in Obstetrics and Gynecology, 15,* 57–61.

Thewes, B., Meiser, B., Taylor, A., Phillips, K.A., Pendlebury, S., Capp, A., et al. (2005). Fertility- and menopause-related information needs of younger women with a diagnosis of early breast cancer. *Journal of Clinical Oncology, 23,* 5155–5165.

Veiga, D.F., Sabino, N.M., Ferreira, L.M., Garcia, E.B., Veiga, F.J., Novo, N.F., et al. (2004). Quality of life outcomes after pedicled TRAM flap delayed breast reconstruction. *British Journal of Plastic Surgery, 57,* 252–257.

Williams, S.A., & Schreier, A.M. (2004). The effect of education in managing side effects in women receiving chemotherapy for treatment of breast cancer [Online exclusive]. *Oncology Nursing Forum, 31,* E16–E23.

Wilmoth, M.C., & Botchway, P. (1999). Psychosexual implications of breast and gynecologic cancer. *Cancer Investigation, 17,* 631–636.

Wilmoth, M.C., Coleman, E.A., Smith, S.C., & Davis, C. (2004). Fatigue, weight gain, and altered sexuality in patients with breast cancer: Exploration of a symptom cluster. *Oncology Nursing Forum, 31,* 1069–1075.

Wilmoth, M.C., & Ross, J.A. (1997). Women's perception. Breast cancer treatment and sexuality. *Cancer Practice, 5,* 353–359.

Wimberly, S.R., Carver, C.S., Laurenceau, J.P., Harris, S.D., & Antoni, M.H. (2005). Perceived partner reactions to diagnosis and treatment of breast cancer: Impact on psychosocial and psychosexual adjustment. *Journal of Consulting and Clinical Psychology, 73,* 300–311.

Wong-Kim, E., & Bloom, J.R. (2005). Depression experienced by young women newly diagnosed with breast cancer. *Psycho-Oncology, 14,* 564–573.

Yates, P., Aranda, S., Hargraves, M., Mirolo, B., Clavarino, A., McLachlan, S., et al. (2005). Randomized controlled trial of an educational intervention for managing fatigue in women receiving adjuvant chemotherapy for early-stage breast cancer. *Journal of Clinical Oncology, 23,* 6027–6036.

Young-McCaughan, S. (1996). Sexual functioning in women with breast cancer after treatment with adjuvant therapy. *Cancer Nursing, 19,* 308–319.

Zajecka, J. (2001). Strategies for the treatment of antidepressant-related sexual dysfunction. *Journal of Clinical Psychiatry, 62*(Suppl. 3), 35–43.

CHAPTER 5

Prostate Cancer

Prostate cancer seldom occurs in people younger than 45, but the incidence and mortality of this form of cancer increase with each decade among aging men, with a peak at about 70 years of age. Suspicious signs and symptoms include alterations in urinary function (urinary frequency, nocturia, poor stream, and hesitancy) as well as an abnormal digital rectal exam and elevated serum prostate-specific antigen. However, most prostate cancers are detected through prostate-specific antigen screening as part of the annual health visit. The diagnosis is confirmed on transrectal ultrasound-guided biopsy (Billington, 1998).

The Effect of Prostate Cancer on Sexuality

As with any cancer diagnosis, the news of this illness is distressing. Patients see prostate cancer not only as a threat to survival but also as a threat to self-image and masculinity (Boehmer & Clark, 2001). The cancer itself threatens sexual functioning, and, additionally, the treatment has significant short- and long-term side effects, including urinary incontinence and erectile dysfunction (ED). Receiving the diagnosis itself may lead to erectile difficulties in the period before treatment begins (Incrocci et al., 2001), and many men in this age group will already have some degree of ED related to age, comorbidities, or medications (Karakiewicz, Aprikian, Bazinet, & Elhilali, 1997). Sexual concerns may not seem to be that important when a life-threatening condition has been diagnosed. However, the treatment for prostate cancer is generally effective, and most men will go on to live years after diagnosis and treatment. After recovery, sex becomes important again.

Treatment of Prostate Cancer

The treatment options for men with prostate cancer are dependent on the sever-ity of the disease. These include surgery to remove the prostate gland and seminal vesicles (radical prostatectomy), radiotherapy by means of external beam radiation or brachytherapy (the insertion of radioactive seeds into the prostate gland itself) for localized prostate cancer, cryotherapy, and hormone therapy or removal of the testicles (orchiectomy) to suppress testosterone production in more advanced cancer. In some instances, patients will receive a combination of treatments to maximize the chances of survival. Each of these treatments has the potential to cause significant sexual problems.

Prostatectomy involves the surgical removal of the prostate gland and seminal vesicles. The surgery may be accomplished via a surgical incision through the abdomen or perineum (less common) or by laparoscopic technique. Significant side effects occur following the surgery; the two most likely to affect sexual functioning are ED and urinary incontinence. Because the average age of men who are diagnosed with prostate cancer is 60–70 years, some men already may be experiencing changes in potency before the diagnosis, and subsequent treatment tends to worsen this.

In the 1980s, Dr. Patrick Walsh pioneered the nerve-sparing technique in which one or both neurovascular bundles that run on the outside of the prostate gland are preserved and not severed when the prostate gland is surgically removed (Walsh & Worthington, 2001). These nerves are responsible for erectile function, along with good blood flow and healthy penile tissue. Sexual outcomes for men who have either unilateral or bilateral nerve-sparing surgery are better than for those men whose nerves are cut during the surgery. Depending on the size of the tumor and its spread, it may not be possible to avoid excising one or both of the nerve bundles in order to remove all the malignant tissue (Vale, 2000).

The sexual outcomes following surgery reported in the literature vary based on how erectile function or dysfunction is defined, whether the patients were operated on in centers of excellence or in the community, and whether validated instruments were used in the studies. Between 30% and 85% of men who have bilateral nerve-sparing surgery will eventually regain the ability to have an erection sufficient for penetration (Burnett, 2005a; Gralnek, Wessells, Cui, & Dalkin, 2000; Stanford et al., 2000). However, most men will require some form of erectile aid to achieve this (Perez et al., 1997). Even with nerve-sparing surgical techniques, trauma to the nerve bundles may occur from instrumentation, cautery, ischemia, or inflammation, and erectile difficulties may result (Meuleman & Mulders, 2003). Trauma to the blood vessels of the penis may lead to vascular insufficiency, and penile rigidity may not occur even with satisfactory nerve function (Nehra & Goldstein, 1999). Shortening of the penis also has been reported following surgery, with 48% of men in one study experiencing shortening greater than 1 cm. Overall, 71% of men had some degree of shortening (Munding, Wessells, & Dalkin, 2001). Mulhall (2005) suggested that this is because of early changes from nerve damage resulting in a hypertonic penis in the first three to six months after surgery. Delayed structural changes to the corporal smooth muscle also occur, resulting in permanent damage to the nerves as well as hypoxia-induced collagen buildup.

Recovery of sexual function is dependent on age (younger men have greater success), erectile function before the surgery, size of prostate gland (smaller size has better outcomes), and surgical technique (Hollenbeck, Dunn, Wei, Montie, & Sanda, 2003). Sexual problems can persist for years following the surgery, and a trend toward improvement is seen up to five years later (Penson et al., 2005). Men report ongoing difficulty with ED (Stanford et al., 2000), which affects their general quality of life, self-confidence, and self-esteem (Clark et al., 2003). Changes in social and intimate relationships may result, and masculine self-concept also is changed (Bokhour, Clark, Inui, Silliman, & Talcott, 2001). However, men with prostate cancer may interpret ED differently, as they can rationalize this as being a result of cancer treatment and may have better psychological health than men with ED who do not have cancer (Penson et al., 2003).

After surgery, orgasm is still possible despite lack of erections (Hollenbeck et al., 2003), but men will no longer experience ejaculation because the source of fluid, the seminal vesicles, has been removed. Many men do not anticipate this, and the experience of orgasm can be a very welcome surprise to men who were anticipating total cessation of sexual pleasure. However, others will notice a qualitative change in the experience of orgasm, which will lack the propulsive sensation of ejaculation and may be accompanied by pelvic pain of variable duration.

The other major side effect of radical prostatectomy that can affect sexual functioning is urinary function. During the surgery to remove the prostate gland, the proximal urethral sphincter comprising the bladder neck, the prostate gland, and the upper part of the urethra are removed, leaving the man with only the distal urethral sphincter to help with control of urine flow (Carlson & Nitti, 2001). Modifications in surgical technique, with preservation of the bladder neck and retention of the anatomic structure of the sphincter mechanisms, have resulted in improved continence rates in recent years (Hassouna & Heaton, 1999). Leakage during sex is not uncommon, and men report that this can occur when aroused or when attempting to have penetrative intercourse. Embarrassment and fear of this happening may be enough to prevent the man from attempting intercourse or to stop dating (Palmer, Fogarty, Somerfield, & Powel, 2003). Continence is seen as an essential construct of adulthood and, in part, as control and masculinity; to lose that is infantilizing and a threat to manhood (Paterson, 2000).

Men will have an indwelling urinary catheter for a number of weeks after the surgery. This can cause swelling, excoriation, and pain at the urethral meatus.

Leakage of urine past the catheter is common because of the occurrence of bladder spasms. After removal of the catheter, urinary incontinence and urgency are common and may last from a few days to much longer. Men may feel unprepared for the amount of postoperative pain and discomfort they experience. The indwelling catheter can be a source of spasm and rectal pain and is described by some as the worst aspect of the prostatectomy experience (Burt, Caelli, Moore, & Anderson, 2005). After removal, the incontinence is a source of great distress for many (Moore & Estey, 1999). This can have long-term psychological consequences for men and their sexual self-image. Damage to the nerve supply of the distal urethral sphincter and the development of strictures at the site of the anastomosis of the urethra are the most common causes of postoperative incontinence (Carlson & Nitti, 2001).

Radiation therapy causes ED in up to 84% of patients, depending on the method of radiation used (external beam versus brachytherapy) (Incrocci, 2004). The same problems with the definition and measurement of ED apply to the studies of sexual functioning during and after radiation therapy. The cause of ED after radiation therapy is not clear, and there appears to be venous and arterial as well as neural etiologies (Incrocci, 2004, 2006; Mulhall, 2001). Tissue fibrosis is most likely an important contributor to ED, as it is usually caused by reduced blood flow to the corpora cavernosa with resultant oxygen deprivation (Fitzpatrick et al., 1998). It is postulated that radiation to the bulb of the penis is a contributing cause of tissue damage (Merrick et al., 2005). No definitive evidence exists to support the influence of radiation dose to the bulb of the penis in brachytherapy. However, trauma to the tissues during insertion of the needles used to place the radioactive seeds is thought to be associated with ED (Macdonald et al., 2005).

Erectile function tends to decline in the years following external beam radiation therapy, with a decline beginning at 12 months after treatment (Turner, Adams, Bull, & Berry, 1999) and a nadir being reached at 22–24 months (Zelefsky et al., 1999). Outcomes are not all that different from surgery, with 50% of men experiencing ED three years after treatment (Merrick et al., 2005) and further decline up to five years following treatment (Potosky et al., 2004). Those receiving brachytherapy tend to do better in their sexual functioning and are generally satisfied with their level of functioning three years after treatment (Mabjeesh, Chen, Beri, Stenger, & Matzkin, 2005; Stock, Stone, & Iannuzzi, 1996). Some men with more advanced prostate cancer receive a combination of brachytherapy and external beam radiation therapy, and this increases the risk for sexual dysfunction, as does the addition of hormone ablation therapy (Speight et al., 2004).

The ability to achieve an erection is one part of sexual functioning for men, and ejaculatory disturbances are common after both forms of radiation therapy with reduction in the volume of ejaculate, absence of ejaculation, and pain with orgasm being noted (Incrocci, Slob, & Levendag, 2002). Men often choose radiation therapy because of the lower side-effect profile (Hall, Boyd, Lippert, & Theodorescu, 2003), and it is important that they are informed not only about the risk for ED but also about the temporal nature of sexual decline.

Cryosurgery is increasingly being used to treat men with locally advanced prostate cancer or those who have experienced a recurrence after radiation therapy. Side effects include incontinence, urethral sloughing, perineal pain, and ED, but advancements in techniques have decreased these significantly (Ahmed & Davies, 2005; Rees, McDonagh, & Persad, 2004). Sexual side effects are significant, with less than 20% of those potent before the procedure regaining erectile functioning three years after the treatment (Robinson et al., 2002). Sexual dysfunction is the most significant and severe side effect of cryotherapy, but urinary symptoms also are important (Anastasiadis et al., 2003). Improved techniques with focal nerve sparing have shown some good preliminary outcomes with preservation of erectile function; however, the number of patients who have had this kind of procedure is limited (Onik, Narayan, Vaughan, Dineen, & Brunelle, 2002).

Men who are diagnosed with advanced prostate cancer generally are treated with medications to suppress testosterone in an attempt to slow down the growth of the cancer, which is androgen dependent. Although advanced disease once was treated with estrogen or surgical castration, since the advent of injectable luteinizing hormone-releasing hormone agonists and nonsteroidal antiandrogens, the former treatments are hardly used (Potosky et al., 2002). Androgen deprivation therapy has a global effect on all aspects of sexual functioning. Men report changes in body image, perception of masculinity, and alterations in their spousal relationship (Clark et al., 1997). The most profound of these is the impact of testosterone deprivation on sexual desire. Men taking these medications report cessation of sexual dreams and fantasies, lack of interest in anything sexual, and a complete cessation of any sexual pleasure (Navon & Morag, 2003). However, testosterone levels will rise to normal levels 18–24 weeks after treatment is stopped (Murthy et al., 2006). Men with low or no desire who cannot achieve an erection appear to experience less distress than men who still desire sex but cannot have an erection (Dahn et al., 2004). Side effects of the drugs used to suppress testosterone production also include feminization, hot flashes, and gynecomastia (increase in volume of breast tissue) (Anderson, 2001). These side effects are regarded as extremely bothersome (Lubeck, Grossfeld, & Carroll, 2001) and contribute to lower quality of life. Orchiectomy or surgical castration is an alternative to medical treatment, but the thought of being castrated is a source of extreme distress for many men (Cleary, Morrissey, & Oster, 1995). They may choose to refuse treatment rather than undergo this surgical procedure.

Treatment of Sexual Side Effects

Men may be reluctant to talk about sexual problems after treatment, believing that they are lucky to be alive and that the satisfaction of being cured of the cancer should take the place of the need for sex (Moore & Estey, 1999). Healthcare providers may assume that sexual function is one of the highest priorities for men after treatment for prostate cancer, but this may not be so, and it is important to ask if this is a problem rather than assuming so (Jacobs et al., 2002). Despite the widespread availability of medical treatments for ED, men with prostate cancer often do not seek help from healthcare providers for months or years (Galbraith, Arechiga, Ramirez, & Pedro, 2005; Litwin, Nied, & Dhanani, 1998). Although healthcare providers may explain the potential side effects, patients may not recall the conversations in any detail after the surgery (Clark, Wray, & Ashton, 2001).

A thorough assessment of prediagnostic and pretreatment sexual functioning is important to establish the man's current level of functioning. It is common for men 75 years and older who have prostate cancer to have diminished levels of sexual interest and functioning before treatment begins. Other men may have erectile difficulties before the diagnosis of cancer that are associated with cardiac disease, diabetes, and medications (Helgason et al., 1997; Iversen, Melezinek, & Schmidt, 2001). An accurate depiction of pretreatment erectile functioning and sexual activity is essential.

The presence of the partner is very important during assessment and discussion of sexual functioning. She or he brings a different perspective and may corroborate or contradict self-reports from the patient (Chun & Carson, 2001). Men may overestimate their sexual capacity or misinterpret questions about sexual functioning, and, therefore, the healthcare provider will not have an accurate baseline to predict changes to sexual functioning or suggest strategies for treatment-related dysfunction. Having the couple present also will allow for a discussion about the relative importance of sexual functioning for each individual, satisfaction with the relationship in the light of sexual changes, as well as relative motivation for the use of erectile aids in the future.

Several assessment tools are available for this purpose, including the Prostate Cancer Outcomes Survey (known as PCOS) and the Expanded Prostate Cancer Index Composite (known as EPIC) (see Chapter 23). Older men may have difficulty talking about sexual matters to healthcare providers and may underestimate their sexual problems or deny them altogether to avoid embarrassment. Figure 5-1 shows sample statements that nurses can use with patients as part of the BETTER model described in Chapter 3 (see Figure 3-3).

Treatment of Erectile Dysfunction

Treatment of ED from a biomedical perspective focuses on oral therapies (phosphodiesterase-5 [PDE5] inhibitors), vacuum devices, intraurethral pellets

---

Figure 5-1. Example of the BETTER Model in Patients With Prostate Cancer

- **Bringing up the topic:** Nurses are encouraged to raise the issue of sexuality with patients.

  "I am now going to ask you some questions about sexual functioning. I ask all my patients about this before they have treatment for prostate cancer. What changes have you noticed in your ability to have an erection?"

- **Explaining that sex is a part of quality of life:** This helps to normalize the discussion and may help patients to feel less embarrassed or alone in having a problem.

  "Many men find that as they age, they experience difficulty achieving or maintaining an erection. This may be partly due to aging, and because the surgery you have chosen may negatively impact this, I would like to talk to you about your expectations in this regard."

- **Telling the patient that resources will be found to address their concerns:** This step suggests to patients that even if the nurse does not have the immediate solution to the problem or question, others are available who can help.

  "If at some point in time you would like to explore some interventions for erectile functioning, you can talk to your urologist or ask for a referral to a sexual medicine expert."

- **Timing the intervention:** Patients may not be ready to deal with sexual issues at the time a problem is identified, but they can ask for information at any time in the future.

  "In the immediate postoperative period, return of erectile functioning may not be of prime importance to you. However, as you heal and as time passes, this may become something that you wish to talk about or learn more about. Please do not hesitate to ask for additional information."

- **Educating patients about the sexual side effects of treatment:** Educating patients about potential side effects from treatments does not mean that they will occur. However, informing patients about sexual side effects is as important as informing them about any other side effects.

  "Following radical prostatectomy, most men will be unable to achieve an erection. This is a result of nerve and blood vessel damage, which may or may not be permanent."

- **Recording:** A brief notation that a discussion about sexuality or sexual side effects occurred is important.

  "Patient was informed about the potential for erectile dysfunction following surgery. He was also given reading material and information about a referral to a sexual medicine specialist."

(medicated urethral system for erections [MUSE®, Vivus, Inc., Mountain View, CA]), intracorporeal injections (Caverject®, Pfizer Inc., New York, NY; Trimix combination [papaverine, phentolamine, alprostadil]), and penile implants. Each has benefits and disadvantages, and all require a prescription, extensive patient education, and a varied degree of motivation on the part of both patients and their partners. Men who used erectile aids after surgery (penile implants, PDE5 inhibitors such as sildenafil, tadalafil, or vardenafil, or vacuum devices) reported greater satisfaction with their sex lives than those who did not use any aids (Perez et al., 1997).

PDE5 inhibitors act by causing the relaxation of smooth muscle in the corpus cavernosa of the penis, thus allowing blood to enter this spongy tissue during sexual stimulation (Shabsigh, 2004). Three PDE5 inhibitors are available: sildenafil, tadalafil, and vardenafil. No specific comparisons have been done of the three PDE5 inhibitors in men after radical prostatectomy (Padma-Nathan, McCullough, & Forest, 2004). Contraindications for the PDE5 inhibitors include use in men who have had a stroke, myocardial infarction, or life-threatening arrhythmia in the preceding six months; patients with resting hypotension, hypertension, or cardiac failure; and those on nitrates or alpha-blockers such as doxazosin (Shabsigh).

Sildenafil (Viagra®, Pfizer Inc.) has been shown in a number of trials to be moderately effective in the treatment of ED following prostatectomy (Vale, 2000), although the rate of success is higher among younger men who have had nerve-bundle sparing surgery (Zagaja, Mhoon, Aikens, & Brendler, 2000). The side effects of this medication include headache, flushing, nasal congestion, and blue-tinted vision (Feng, Huang, Kaptein, Kaswick, & Abosief, 2000). However, men and their partners appear to be happy with this therapy when it is successful in treating their impotence (Raina et al., 2003). Reports in the literature have noted a serious but rare condition called nonarteritic anterior ischemic optic neuropathy, which has led to vision loss 24–36 hours after ingestion of sildenafil (Pomeranz & Bhavsar, 2005). The risk factors for this condition are mainly vascular, which are common in men of the age who use PDE5 inhibitors; therefore, a causal relationship cannot be established. However, men should be warned about the potential for this adverse event (Laties & Sharlip, 2006).

Most of the studies on the efficacy of this drug are industry sponsored and so must be viewed with caution. Response is mediated by the type of surgery, the patient's age, and preoperative erectile functioning (Raina et al., 2004). If both nerve bundles are spared and age is younger than 55 years, 80% of men will respond with an erection firm enough for penetration in more than 50% of attempts. Forty-five percent of men 56–65 years old will respond in similar fashion with bilateral nerve-sparing surgery, but this drops to 33% in men older than 66 (Zagaja et al., 2000). If one nerve bundle was spared, only 44% of men younger than 55 had a positive response, and when both nerve bundles were cut, no response occurred, regardless of age and previous erectile functioning.

Tadalafil (Cialis®, Lilly ICOS LLC, Indianapolis, IN) is another PDE5 inhibitor that works in a similar fashion as sildenafil but has a longer half-life (Carrier et al., 2005). The major benefit of this is that it allows for more spontaneity, with men theoretically being able to respond to sexual stimulation with an erection from 30 minutes after ingesting a tablet to 36 hours later (Brock, 2003). It also can be taken with food, in contrast to sildenafil, which must be taken on an empty stomach. The same caveats regarding industry-sponsored trials apply, as the clinical trials included only men who have had bilateral nerve-sparing surgery. Side effects include headache, dyspepsia, myalgia, stuffy nose, and back pain (Carson et al., 2004, 2005). For men who had bilateral nerve-sparing prostatectomy, 54% achieved an erection sufficient for penetration, and 41% were able to attempt intercourse successfully (Montorsi et al., 2004).

Vardenafil (Levitra®, Bayer Pharmaceuticals Corp., West Haven, CT) is the third PDE5 inhibitor approved for the treatment of ED. Vardenafil differs from the others in its rapid onset of action, noted in one study to be 16 minutes as opposed to the hour or more with the other drugs (Hellstrom, 2003). In men who had either unilateral or bilateral nerve-sparing prostatectomy, 34% were able to have intercourse (Brock, Taylor, & Seger, 2002). Men taking vardenafil report high levels of first-time success and similar side effects to the other PDE5 inhibitors (Casey, 2003). The rapid onset of action is suggested to allow more spontaneity.

The efficacy of PDE5 inhibitors after radiation therapy appears to be the same as for prostatectomy (Incrocci, Hop, & Slob, 2003; Kedia, Zippe, Agarwal, Nelson, & Lakin, 1999; Merrick et al., 1999; Valicenti et al., 2001; Weber, Bieri, Kurtz, & Miralbell, 1999), with a time dependence response showing a gradual decrease in response rate over three years (Ohebshalom, Parker, Guhring, & Mulhall, 2005).

Oral medications are preferred because they are easy to use, are not invasive, and theoretically allow for spontaneous intercourse once erection is achieved. Many men will use a PDE5 inhibitor once or twice, and if success is not achieved, they will discontinue use. Common reasons for discontinuation are the effect was less than expected, high cost, loss of interest in sex, and inconvenience in obtaining the medication (Jiann, Yu, Su, & Tsai, 2006). Success with these medications increases with continued use, and some men may have to take up to eight successive doses to achieve an erection sufficient for penetration (Schulman, Shen, Stothard, & Schmitt, 2004). Other treatments currently are under investigation, including a topical alprostadil cream (Yeager & Beihn, 2005), phentolamine tablets, and sublingual apomorphine tablets.

Alternatives to oral medication are the vacuum constriction device (pump), intraurethral prostaglandin, or intracavernosal injections of alprostadil or other medications. It is common for a graduated treatment plan to be suggested to patients, starting with an oral PDE5 inhibitor and moving through the alternatives of the vacuum pump and then intraurethral or intracavernosal injections. The treatment of last resort is usually surgical implants. Less than 20% of men will use any of these approaches one year after initiation of a treatment regimen (Gontero, Fontana, Zitella, Montorsi, & Frea, 2005).

The vacuum pump/constriction device consists of a plastic tube that has a hand pump attached to it. The lubricated penis is placed in the plastic tube, the air is pumped out, and blood is drawn into the penis. An erection usually results in about two minutes. The erection is maintained by placing special elastic bands at the base of the penis to prevent escape of the blood. These can remain in place for up to 30 minutes (Levine & Dimitriou, 2001). Although noninvasive, it can present some challenges to couples, as it requires some dexterity and may interfere with spontaneity. Side effects include bruising, pain caused by the elastic band, decreased sensation for the man, and sensation of a cold penis for the partner (Lewis, Rosen, & Goldstein, 2004). This treatment has shown effectiveness in men who can achieve an erection spontaneously but are not able to maintain it (Dutta & Eid, 1999). The addition of sildenafil concomitant with the use of the vacuum pump may improve rigidity and satisfaction (Raina, Agarwal, Allamaneni, Lakin, & Zippe, 2005). Figure 5-2 depicts the use of a vacuum pump device.

Intraurethral prostaglandin suppositories (MUSE) are somewhat effective in producing an erection, with 29%–55% of men achieving an erection sufficient for penetrative intercourse (Jaffe et al., 2004; Raina, Agarwal, Ausmundson, Mansour, & Zippe, 2005). A small pellet containing alprostadil is inserted into the urethra via a special applicator (see Figure 5-3). The man then rubs the penis between his two hands to disperse the medication and after about 30 minutes should experience a response. Alprostadil acts by relaxing the muscles of the penis and allowing blood to flow into the spongy tissues. Some men have reported pain and burning in the urethra where the pellet is situated (Lewis et al., 2004).

Intracavernosal injections of alprostadil or a combination of vasoactive substances (alprostadil plus papaverine and phentolamine [Trimix]) is an effective method of achieving an erection for men who do not respond to PDE5 inhibitors (Gutierrez, Hernandez, & Mas, 2005). Trimix is as effective as alprostadil and produces a longer-lasting erection with a greater chance of priapism (a prolonged and painful erection) (Seyam, Mohamed, Akhras, & Rashwan, 2005). A small amount of the medication is injected into the body of the penis using a small-gauge needle; this causes smooth muscle to relax and blood to flow into the tissues, thus producing an erection (see Figure 5-4). Men need to be taught how to do this, and although it produces a firm erection, many men find the thought of injecting themselves to be distasteful. Priapism can result, and men need to seek immediate medical attention for this medical emergency. Pain at the insertion site, bruising, and scarring are other side effects.

Penile implants generally are regarded as a third-line treatment for ED. Although very effective, they are not commonly used (Stephenson et al., 2005). There are a number of different models of these devices. Some are semirigid and require the man to bend the device to a certain angle for intercourse and then return it to its usual position. These are not easy to conceal but have the least moving parts and thus are less likely to

Figure 5-2. Use of a Vacuum Constriction Device

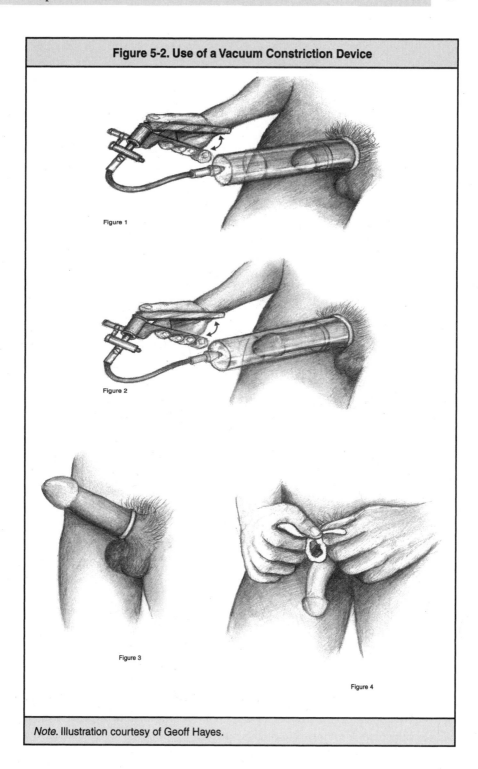

Figure 1

Figure 2

Figure 3

Figure 4

Note. Illustration courtesy of Geoff Hayes.

Figure 5-3. Intraurethral Prostaglandin Suppository Use

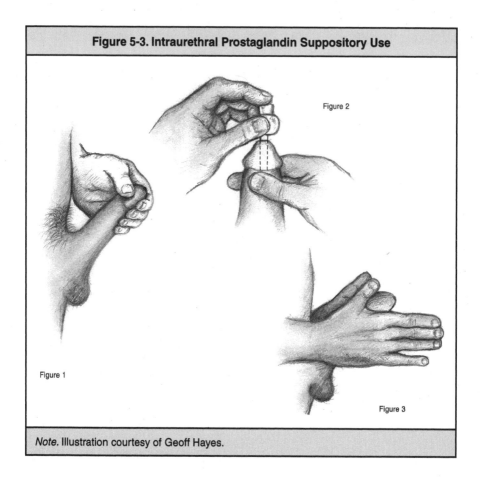

Figure 2

Figure 1

Figure 3

Note. Illustration courtesy of Geoff Hayes.

malfunction. A number of inflatable devices are available, which involve the implantation of a cylinder along the length of the penis on each side. These are connected to a pump, which is placed in the scrotum. The pump is connected to a reservoir containing saline, which is implanted in the abdomen. When the man wants to have an erection, he pumps saline from the reservoir into the cylinders using the scrotal pump. The flow of saline is reversed after intercourse (Hafez & Hafez, 2005). Placement of this device at the time of radical prostatectomy has been suggested for men in whom nerve-sparing surgery is not possible (Ramsawh, Morgentaler, Covino, Barlow, & DeWolf, 2005).

A relatively new intervention to optimize erectile functioning after surgery is called erectile rehabilitation. The theory supporting this is the apparently unique properties of sildenafil in improving endothelial function and nerve regeneration and protection. The regimen requires a nightly dose of sildenafil for months after surgery. Improvement in spontaneous return of erections occurs in up to 27% of those receiving this treatment, a seven-fold increase compared to those on placebo (Padma-Nathan et al., 2004). An

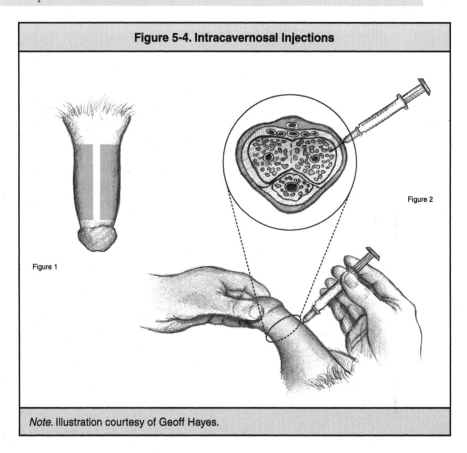

Figure 5-4. Intracavernosal Injections

Figure 1

Figure 2

Note. Illustration courtesy of Geoff Hayes.

alternative way of doing this is to have the man take 100 mg of sildenafil three times a week with the aim of achieving an erection with at least 60% of full rigidity. Intercourse and/or orgasm are not necessary; the aim is to have an erection three times a week. If the man is able to do this, he should continue with this regimen until spontaneous erections occur with regularity. If he is unable to achieve an erection with sildenafil alone, he can add intracavernosal injections of Trimix to the regimen. The dose of Trimix is titrated to achieve an erection with 60% rigidity. The man is instructed to challenge himself with 100 mg of sildenafil every four months to see if he has become responsive to the medication. If he has, he can stop using the injections and continue to use only the sildenafil three times a week. Men who use the combined regimen appear to become more responsive to sildenafil after treatment with injections and also are more likely to have intercourse without the use of medication in the future (Mulhall, Land, Parker, Waters, & Flanigan, 2005). A similar regimen has been shown to be effective when either sildenafil or vardenafil are used in combination with an alprostadil injection (Mydlo, Viterbo, & Crispen, 2005). Both of these protocols require high motivation, involve financial costs to the patient, and are required to continue for many months, sometimes with no visible success to increase compliance or motivation to continue. They also require specialized teaching, ongoing monitoring, and appointments with the sexual medicine specialist. Some concern exists that repeated exposure to a prescribed treatment will lower its effectiveness so that men who use a nightly dose of sildenafil, for instance, may become less responsive to a therapeutic dose when attempting intercourse (Burnett, 2005b).

Nursing Interventions in the Care of Men With Prostate Cancer

Sexuality is a complex issue and comprises relationship issues, self-esteem, gender issues, and moral values (Tiefer & Schuetz-Mueller, 1995). ED in the context of prostate cancer often is seen as a mechanical problem for the man alone and, since the advent of the PDE5 inhibitors, relatively easy to treat. Advertising in the media and attention in the lay press suggest that treatment of ED is as simple as taking a single pill and is highly effective. This is not necessarily the case for men with prostate cancer who have been treated with modalities known to cause anatomic and physiologic damage to nerves and blood vessels essential to erectile functioning. The success of these medications varies, and only a minority of men may be helped, depending on the type of treatment, their age, pretreatment erectile functioning, and adjuvant therapy.

A number of psychological factors can play a part in post-treatment ED, including fear of pain, a belief and fear that sexual activity will stimulate the cancer or spread it to a partner, and depression (Fitzpatrick et al., 1998). Men with prostate cancer are more likely to seek help for sexual dysfunction, especially if they had treatment that was purported to preserve sexual functioning, such as nerve-sparing prostatectomy or brachytherapy (Schover et al., 2004). Younger men tend to have higher needs for support in the area of sexual functioning. However, this is an unmet need in more than half of all men with prostate cancer regardless of age or marital status (Lintz et al., 2003).

Information Sharing

Lack of knowledge about male sexual functioning is fairly common. Men and their partners need explicit information before any treatment is initiated as to what can realistically be expected from the cancer treatment and any strategies for improving erectile functioning (Fitzpatrick et al., 1998). Healthcare providers often assume that men and their partners know about the use of PDE5 inhibitors because of the extensive amount of advertising of these products; however, many couples do not know about the other available treatments, and many want more information than they were given by their urologists (Davison, Keyes, Elliott, Berkowitz, & Goldenberg, 2004; Mishel et al., 2002). Some couples have unrealistic expectations of the treatments available for ED and may expect the man to attain a level of functioning that he had as a young man. The changes brought on by age, comorbidities, concurrent medications for these comorbidities, and other factors will continue to affect men's ability to both achieve and maintain an erection, and medication or an erectile aid is not the magical answer to a preexisting problem. Men may not be given sufficient information about how to take PDE5 inhibitors (e.g., the need to take sildenafil on an empty stomach, the need for sexual stimulation at the appropriate interval after taking the pill). The most common reason for failure of PDE5 inhibitor treatment is incorrect drug administration (Atiemo, Szostak, & Sklar, 2003). Men also may not discuss the use of the medication with their partner and may take a pill without discussing the potential for sexual activity later. If the partner has other plans or does not want to engage in such activity, the pill is wasted and the man may become demoralized or disinterested.

Education and support in a group setting has been shown to improve optimism about future functioning, normalize the experience, and reduce distress (Lepore, Helgeson, Eton, & Schulz, 2003), and it decreases depression in the short term (Weber et al., 2004). Wives of men with prostate cancer also can benefit from group education sessions where they can learn alternative coping mechanisms (Manne, Babb, Pinover, Horwitz, & Ebbert, 2004).

Couples Counseling

Incorporating couples counseling in the treatment for sexual problems is suggested as one way of improving both sexual and relationship outcomes (Schover et al., 2002). Men with prostate cancer frequently receive written information about sexual functioning, but this information tends to be generic and overly optimistic and may not answer the specific questions or concerns for that man and his partner. Men may, in fact, be interested in more in-depth sexuality counseling but will not necessarily request it (Kirby & Newling, 1998). Very often, patient education material is produced with the financial support of the pharmaceutical industry and may be biased in favor of one particular drug or device.

Communication issues between men and their partners related to sexual changes have the potential to cause long-term consequences that can negatively affect the relationship. Women may not be helpful in encouraging their male partners to find help for sexual problems. This may be a reflection of the woman's level of sexual interest (Neese, Schover, Klein, Zippe, & Kupelian, 2003) and her belief that this aspect of life is over for them. Couples often will not talk about their feelings for fear of increasing the distress of the partner or not wanting to bring up painful topics (Boehmer & Clark, 2001). Hiding feelings from each other is not an effective strategy; the resulting isolation and estrangement further increases the couple's distress. Couples should be encouraged to voice their concerns about any and all aspects of care from diagnosis through treatment and to seek information wherever possible, as this may be an effective coping mechanism (Heyman & Rosner, 1996).

Couples counseling can help people who are struggling with altered patterns of communication or sexual behavior. Although American society uses sex to sell products, it still is a difficult topic for many couples to talk about because it is not merely a mechanical act but one that is embedded in values, emotions, hopes, and memories. The presence of a professional, objective outsider is often the catalyst that the couple needs to begin talking about this topic in a nonthreatening atmosphere where there can be gentle prompting from the therapist or counselor. This will prevent the couple from falling back into ineffective or nonproductive communication patterns.

It is appropriate to refer a couple for counseling at any point in the disease or treatment trajectory. However, people often are more receptive at about nine months after treatment, which is the point when they realize that things may not get better spontaneously and that they need some help. Although erectile rehabilitation appears to offer some benefit to highly motivated men, a penis that can become engorged is but one aspect of a much more complex set of expectations, beliefs, and practices.

Asking both patients and their partners about the importance of sexuality, penetrative intercourse, and interest in alternatives to intercourse can be helpful both in assessing the concordance of the couple's sexual interest and in allowing for each member of the couple to hear the wishes and desires of the other. ED is a couple's issue, and problems need to be solved from a couple's perspective. Many couples are restricted in their sexual repertoire after years of doing the same things, at the same time, in the same place, and in the same order. Challenges to this usual pattern of behavior can seem overwhelming, and people's natural instinct may be to simply give up and not attempt anything else because of fear or lack of information or imagination, or because if the old or usual way is not possible, then nothing is possible.

Talking about feelings can be helpful for some couples, whereas others miss their usual sexual activities and want to find a way of regaining the physical and emotional intimacy that resulted from a regular and satisfying sex life. Some couples are able to adapt to the changes that ED and, to a lesser extent, the lack of ejaculation present. Many women say that they are content as long as their partner continues to display physical affection through hugging, kissing, and other displays of affection, including verbal messages of love and need. Men, on the other hand, may feel that anything other than penetrative intercourse is not satisfactory and may find it frustrating to touch their partner with no hope of intercourse. The couple must understand and believe that they can feel those feelings of intimacy again, but they have to change their sexual scripts.

One way of doing this is through the use of sensate focus exercises. Through these activities, the couple can relearn the pleasure of sensual touching without the pressure of intercourse. Because intercourse is prohibited in the first three stages of this therapy, the couple is forced to rely on the experiences of nongenital stroking, massage, and other kinds of touch. Although genital exploration eventually is allowed, many couples find that the other activities are as pleasurable, and intercourse may become less important. Communicating about what feels good for both partners is an essential part of the exercises, and this verbal exchange can further reinforce the pleasure that the partner is experiencing as a result of the efforts of their mate. Furthermore, many women experience sexual pleasure through noncoital activities, and this exercise can be very real proof to the man that he can provide her with a great deal of pleasure without an erection and penetration.

Interventions for Treatment-Related Side Effects

A number of educational interventions to enhance sexual outcomes for men with prostate cancer have been tested. These programs are not widely available and often are seen as too resource-intensive for institutions to support. However, there are lessons to be learned from those that are successful and have benefited couples. One program involved four sessions of counseling for the man with or without his partner. Information presented in the sessions included education about prostate cancer and sexual functioning and options for treatment. Communication about sexual issues was emphasized, and participants were expected to complete homework assignments. Those who participated appeared to benefit, and the presence of a partner was not significant in this study (Canada, Neese, Sui, & Schover, 2005). In another program, nurses provided a range of activities designed to provide information to couples after prostatectomy in a step-wise fashion based on the PLISSIT model. Suggestions from this program include that healthcare providers should be comfortable discussing sexual issues with patients, should know how to perform a sexual history, and should be able to differentiate between verbal and nonverbal cues (Monturo, Rogers, Coleman, Robinson, & Pickett, 2001). Davison, Elliott, Ekland, Griffin, and Wiens (2005) evaluated a sexual rehabilitation clinic in which trained nurses and a sexual medicine specialist provided information about treatment for sexual dysfunction after prostate cancer treatment. Most of the men did not bring their partners to appointments, attended only once, and did not present for follow-up.

Some success has been reported from using pelvic floor exercises in the treatment of post-prostatectomy urinary incontinence (Moore & Gray, 2004). These exercises involve contracting the pelvic floor muscles that control bladder emptying and are essentially the same as the Kegel exercises taught to women during pregnancy. They should be done five times every hour during waking hours and usually are effective after four to six weeks, with peak effectiveness reached after three months. Anticholinergic and antispasmodic medications also can be useful in treating urge incontinence; however, the evidence for effectiveness in men is moderate at best, as most of the studies have been done in women.

Case Study

> B.W. is 65 years old and was recently diagnosed with prostate cancer. He reports experiencing problems with urination for about six months prior to the diagnosis. B.W. is waiting to have nerve-sparing surgery and has come to the preoperative clinic to see the nurse and the anesthetist. His wife is with him at the preoperative appointment. The nurse informs the couple that sexual problems may occur as a result of the surgery or other treatments. B.W. attempts to change the topic of conversation. His wife persists in asking questions about potential sexual problems, and B.W. gets up and leaves the room.
>
> Questions to consider:
> - Why is B.W. apparently reluctant to discuss the topic?
> - How should the nurse address this?
> - What information can the nurse give his wife that may be helpful?
>
> After the surgery, B.W. is discharged home with an indwelling catheter. His wife calls the unit two days after his discharge with questions about his level of pain and some bloody discharge from the urethral meatus. She asks about when they may be able to resume sexual relations and seems surprised when the nurse states that it may be a number of months before the patient is able to have an erection sufficient for penetration.
> - Based on these details, would the nurse think that the patient's wife has forgotten what was discussed in the preoperative visit?
>
> *See Appendix B for answers to the case study questions.*

Conclusion

As with any cancer diagnosis, the news of this illness is disturbing. Men view prostate cancer as a threat to survival, self-image, and masculinity. Not only does the cancer itself threaten sexual functioning, but the treatment also has potential short- and long-term consequences, including urinary incontinence and ED. Both men and their partners will be affected in the short and long term; interventions to address sexual difficulties should include both patients and their partners. Although a number of pharmaceutical and mechanical treatments are available for the treatment of ED in this population, their success is limited, and nurses should provide realistic guidance.

References

Ahmed, S., & Davies, J. (2005). Managing the complications of prostate cryosurgery. *BJU International, 95,* 480–481.

Anastasiadis, A.G., Sachdev, R., Salomon, L., Ghafar, M.A., Stisser, B.C., Shabsigh, R., et al. (2003). Comparison of health-related quality of life and prostate-associated symptoms after primary and salvage cryotherapy for prostate cancer. *Journal of Cancer Research and Clinical Oncology, 129,* 676–682.

Anderson, J. (2001). Quality of life aspects of treatment options for localized and locally advanced prostate cancer. *European Urology, 40*(Suppl. 2), 24–30.

Atiemo, H., Szostak, M., & Sklar, G. (2003). Salvage of sildenafil failures referred from primary care physicians. *Journal of Urology, 170,* 2356–2358.

Billington, A. (1998). Prostate cancer and its effect on sexuality. *Community Nurse, 4,* 33–34.

Boehmer, U., & Clark, J.A. (2001). Communication about prostate cancer between men and their wives. *Journal of Family Practice, 50,* 226–231.

Bokhour, B.G., Clark, J.A., Inui, T.S., Silliman, R.A., & Talcott, J.A. (2001). Sexuality after treatment for early prostate cancer: Exploring the meanings of "erectile dysfunction." *Journal of General Internal Medicine, 16,* 649–655.

Brock, G. (2003). Tadalafil: A new oral therapy for erectile dysfunction. *Journal of Sexual and Reproductive Medicine, 3,* 123–127.

Brock, G., Taylor, T., & Seger, M. (2002). Efficacy and tolerability of vardenafil in men with erectile dysfunction following radical prostatectomy. *European Urology Supplements, 1*(1), 152.

Burnett, A.L. (2005a). Erectile dysfunction following radical prostatectomy. *JAMA, 293,* 2648–2653.

Burnett, A.L. (2005b). Vasoactive pharmacotherapy to cure erectile dysfunction: Fact or fiction? *Urology, 65,* 224–230.

Burt, J., Caelli, K., Moore, K., & Anderson, M. (2005). Radical prostatectomy: Men's experiences and postoperative needs. *Journal of Clinical Nursing, 14,* 883–890.

Canada, A.L., Neese, L.E., Sui, D., & Schover, L.R. (2005). Pilot intervention to enhance sexual rehabilitation for couples after treatment for localized prostate carcinoma. *Cancer, 104,* 2689–2700.

Carlson, K., & Nitti, V. (2001). Prevention and management of incontinence following radical prostatectomy. *Urologic Clinics of North America, 28,* 595–612.

Carrier, S., Brock, G., Pommerville, P., Shin, J., Anglin, G., Whitaker, S., et al. (2005). Efficacy and safety of oral tadalafil in the treatment of men in Canada with erectile dysfunction: A randomized, double-blind, parallel, placebo-controlled clinical trial. *Journal of Sexual Medicine, 2,* 685–698.

Carson, C.C., Rajfer, J., Eardley, I., Carrier, S., Dennes, J., Walkers, D., et al. (2004). The efficacy and safety of tadalafil: An update. *BJU International, 93,* 1276–1281.

Carson, C., Shabsigh, R., Segal, S., Murphy, A., Fredlund, P., & Kuepfer, C. (2005). Efficacy, safety, and treatment satisfaction of tadalafil versus placebo in patients with erectile dysfunction evaluated at tertiary-care academic centers. *Urology, 65,* 353–359.

Casey, R. (2003). Vardenafil—a new and effective treatment for erectile dysfunction. *Journal of Sexual and Reproductive Medicine, 3,* 128–132.

Chun, J., & Carson, C.C. (2001). Physician-patient dialogue and clinical evaluation of erectile dysfunction. *Urologic Clinics of North America, 28,* 249–258.

Clark, J.A., Inui, T.S., Silliman, R.A., Bokhour, B.G., Krasnow, S.H., Robinson, R.A., et al. (2003). Patients' perceptions of quality of life after treatment for early prostate cancer. *Journal of Clinical Oncology, 21,* 3777–3784.

Clark, J.A., Wray, N.P., & Ashton, C.M. (2001). Living with treatment decisions: Regrets and quality of life among men treated for metastatic prostate cancer. *Journal of Clinical Oncology, 19,* 72–80.

Clark, J.A., Wray, N., Brody, B., Ashton, C., Giesler, B., & Watkins, H. (1997). Dimensions of quality of life expressed by men treated for metastatic prostate cancer. *Social Science and Medicine, 45,* 1299–1309.

Cleary, P., Morrissey, G., & Oster, G. (1995). Health-related quality of life in patients with advanced prostate cancer: A multinational perspective. *Quality of Life Research, 4,* 207–220.

Dahn, J.R., Penedo, F.J., Gonzalez, J.S., Esquiabro, M., Antoni, M.H., Roos, B.A., et al. (2004). Sexual functioning and quality of life after prostate cancer treatment: Considering sexual desire. *Urology, 63,* 273–277.

Davison, B.J., Elliott, S., Ekland, M., Griffin, S., & Wiens, K. (2005). Development and evaluation of a prostate sexual rehabilitation clinic: A pilot project. *BJU International, 96,* 1360–1364.

Davison, B.J., Keyes, M., Elliott, S., Berkowitz, J., & Goldenberg, S.L. (2004). Preferences for sexual information resources in patients treated for early-stage prostate cancer with either radical prostatectomy or brachytherapy. *BJU International, 93,* 965–969.

Dutta, T.C., & Eid, J.F. (1999). Vacuum constriction devices for erectile dysfunction: A long-term, prospective study of patients with mild, moderate, and severe dysfunction. *Urology, 54,* 891–893.

Feng, M., Huang, S., Kaptein, J., Kaswick, J., & Abosief, S. (2000). Effect of sildenafil citrate on post-radical prostatectomy erectile dysfunction. *Journal of Urology, 164,* 1935–1938.

Fitzpatrick, J.M., Kirby, R.S., Krane, R.J., Adolfsson, J., Newling, D.W., & Goldstein, I. (1998). Sexual dysfunction associated with the management of prostate cancer. *European Urology, 33,* 513–522.

Galbraith, M., Arechiga, A., Ramirez, J., & Pedro, L. (2005). Prostate cancer survivors' and partners' self-reports of health-related quality of life, treatment symptoms, and marital satisfaction 2.5–5.5 years after treatment [Online exclusive]. *Oncology Nursing Forum, 32,* E30–E41.

Gontero, P., Fontana, F., Zitella, A., Montorsi, F., & Frea, B. (2005). A prospective evaluation of efficacy and compliance with a multistep treatment approach for erectile dysfunction in patients after non-nerve sparing radical prostatectomy. *BJU International, 95,* 359–365.

Gralnek, D., Wessells, H., Cui, H., & Dalkin, B.L. (2000). Differences in sexual function and quality of life after nerve sparing and nonnerve sparing radical retropubic prostatectomy. *Journal of Urology, 163,* 1166–1169.

Gutierrez, P., Hernandez, P., & Mas, M. (2005). Combining programmed intracavernous PGE1 injections and sildenafil on demand to salvage sildenafil nonresponders. *International Journal of Impotence Research, 17,* 354–358.

Hafez, E.S., & Hafez, S.D. (2005). Erectile dysfunction: Anatomical parameters, etiology, diagnosis, and therapy. *Archives of Andrology, 51,* 15–31.

Hall, J.D., Boyd, J.C., Lippert, M.C., & Theodorescu, D. (2003). Why patients choose prostatectomy or brachytherapy for localized prostate cancer: Results of a descriptive survey. *Urology, 61,* 402–407.

Hassouna, M.M., & Heaton, J.P. (1999). Prostate cancer: 8. Urinary incontinence and erectile dysfunction. *Canadian Medical Association Journal, 160,* 78–86.

Helgason, A.R., Adolfsson, J., Dickman, P., Arver, S., Fredrikson, M., & Steineck, G. (1997). Factors associated with waning sexual function among elderly men and prostate cancer patients. *Journal of Urology, 158,* 155–159.

Hellstrom, P. (2003). Vardenafil: A new approach to the treatment of erectile dysfunction. *Current Urology Reports, 4,* 479–487.

Heyman, E.N., & Rosner, T.T. (1996). Prostate cancer: An intimate view from patients and wives. *Urologic Nursing, 16,* 37–44.

Hollenbeck, B.K., Dunn, R.L., Wei, J.T., Montie, J.E., & Sanda, M.G. (2003). Determinants of long-term sexual health outcome after radical prostatectomy measured by a validated instrument. *Journal of Urology, 169,* 1453–1457.

Incrocci, L. (2004). Radiotherapy for prostate cancer and sexual functioning. *Hospital Medicine, 65,* 605–608.

Incrocci, L. (2006). Sexual function after external-beam radiotherapy for prostate cancer: What do we know? *Critical Reviews in Oncology/Hematology, 57,* 165–173.

Incrocci, L., Hop, W.C., & Slob, A.K. (2003). Efficacy of sildenafil in an open-label study as a continuation of a double-blind study in the treatment of erectile dysfunction after radiotherapy for prostate cancer. *Urology, 62,* 116–120.

Incrocci, L., Madalinska, J.B., Essink-Bot, M.L., Van Putten, W.L., Koper, P.C., & Schroder, F.H. (2001). Sexual functioning in patients with localized prostate cancer awaiting treatment. *Journal of Sex and Marital Therapy, 27,* 353–363.

Incrocci, L., Slob, A.K., & Levendag, P.C. (2002). Sexual (dys)function after radiotherapy for prostate cancer: A review. *International Journal of Radiation Oncology, Biology, Physics, 52,* 681–693.

Iversen, P., Melezinek, I., & Schmidt, A. (2001). Nonsteroidal antiandrogens: A therapeutic option for patients with advanced prostate cancer who wish to retain sexual interest and function. *BJU International, 87,* 47–56.

Jacobs, J.R., Banthia, R., Sadler, G.R., Varni, J.W., Malcarne, V.L., Greenbergs, H.L., et al. (2002). Problems associated with prostate cancer: Differences of opinion among health care providers, patients, and spouses. *Journal of Cancer Education, 17,* 33–36.

Jaffe, J.S., Antell, M.R., Greenstein, M., Ginsberg, P.C., Mydlo, J.H., & Harkaway, R.C. (2004). Use of intraurethral alprostadil in patients not responding to sildenafil citrate. *Urology, 63,* 951–954.

Jiann, B., Yu, C., Su, C., & Tsai, J. (2006). Compliance of sildenafil treatment for erectile dysfunction and factors affecting it. *International Journal of Impotence Research, 18,* 146–149.

Karakiewicz, P.I., Aprikian, A.G., Bazinet, M., & Elhilali, M.M. (1997). Patient attitudes regarding treatment-related erectile dysfunction at time of early detection of prostate cancer. *Urology, 50,* 704–709.

Kedia, S., Zippe, C.D., Agarwal, A., Nelson, D.R., & Lakin, M.M. (1999). Treatment of erectile dysfunction with sildenafil citrate (Viagra) after radiation therapy for prostate cancer. *Urology, 54,* 308–312.

Kirby, R., & Newling, D. (1998). Prostate cancer and sexual function. *Prostate Cancer and Prostatic Diseases, 1,* 179–184.

Laties, A., & Sharlip, I. (2006). Ocular safety in patients using sildenafil citrate therapy for erectile dysfunction. *Journal of Sexual Medicine, 3,* 12–27.

Lepore, S.J., Helgeson, V., Eton, D.T., & Schulz, R. (2003). Improving quality of life in men with prostate cancer: A randomized controlled trial of group education interventions. *Health Psychology, 22,* 443–452.

Levine, L.A., & Dimitriou, R.J. (2001). Vacuum constriction and external erection devices in erectile dysfunction. *Urologic Clinics of North America, 28,* 335–341.

Lewis, J.H., Rosen, R., & Goldstein, I. (2004). Erectile dysfunction in primary care. *Nurse Practitioner, 29*(12), 42–50, 55.

Lintz, K., Moynihan, C., Steginga, S., Norman, A., Eeles, R., Huddart, R., et al. (2003). Prostate cancer patients' support and psychological care needs: Survey from a non-surgical oncology clinic. *Psycho-Oncology, 12,* 769–783.

Litwin, M.S., Nied, R.J., & Dhanani, N. (1998). Health-related quality of life in men with erectile dysfunction. *Journal of General Internal Medicine, 13,* 159–166.

Lubeck, D., Grossfeld, G., & Carroll, P. (2001). The effect of androgen deprivation therapy on health-related quality of life in men with prostate cancer. *Urology, 58,* 94–100.

Mabjeesh, N., Chen, J., Beri, A., Stenger, A., & Matzkin, H. (2005). Sexual function after permanent 125I-brachytherapy for prostate cancer. *International Journal of Impotence Research, 17,* 96–101.

Macdonald, A.G., Keyes, M., Kruk, A., Duncan, G., Moravan, V., & Morris, W.J. (2005). Predictive factors for erectile dysfunction in men with prostate cancer after brachytherapy: Is dose to the penile bulb important? *International Journal of Radiation Oncology, Biology, Physics, 63,* 155–163.

Manne, S., Babb, J., Pinover, W., Horwitz, E., & Ebbert, J. (2004). Psychoeducation group intervention for wives of men with prostate cancer. *Psycho-Oncology, 13,* 37–46.

Merrick, G.S., Butler, W.M., Lief, J.H., Stipetich, R.L., Abel, L.J., & Dorsey, A.T. (1999). Efficacy of sildenafil citrate in prostate brachytherapy patients with erectile dysfunction. *Urology, 53,* 1112–1116.

Merrick, G.S., Butler, W.M., Wallner, K.E., Galbreath, R.W., Anderson, R.L., Kurko, B.S., et al. (2005). Erectile function after prostate brachytherapy. *International Journal of Radiation Oncology, Biology, Physics, 62,* 437–447.

Meuleman, E.J., & Mulders, P.F. (2003). Erectile function after radical prostatectomy: A review. *European Urology, 43,* 95–101.

Mishel, M.H., Belyea, M., Germino, B.B., Stewart, J.L., Bailey, D.E., Jr., Robertson, C., et al. (2002). Helping patients with localized prostate carcinoma manage uncertainty and treatment side effects: Nurse-delivered psychoeducational intervention over the telephone. *Cancer, 94,* 1854–1866.

Montorsi, F., Nathan, H.P., McCullough, A., Brock, G.B., Broderick, G., Ahuja, S., et al. (2004). Tadalafil in the treatment of erectile dysfunction following bilateral nerve sparing radical retropubic prostatectomy: A randomized, double-blind, placebo controlled trial. *Journal of Urology, 172,* 1036–1041.

Monturo, C.A., Rogers, P.D., Coleman, M., Robinson, J.P., & Pickett, M. (2001). Beyond sexual assessment: Lessons learned from couples post radical prostatectomy. *Journal of the American Academy of Nurse Practitioners, 13,* 511–516.

Moore, K.N., & Estey, A. (1999). The early post-operative concerns of men after radical prostatectomy. *Journal of Advanced Nursing, 29,* 1121–1129.

Moore, K.N., & Gray, M. (2004). Urinary incontinence in men: Current status and future directions. *Nursing Research, 53,* S36–S41.

Mulhall, J.P. (2001). Minimizing radiation-induced erectile dysfunction. *Journal of Brachytherapy International, 17,* 221–227.

Mulhall, J.P. (2005). Penile length changes after radical prostatectomy. *BJU International, 96,* 472–474.

Mulhall, J.P., Land, S., Parker, M., Waters, W., & Flanigan, R. (2005). The use of an erectogenic pharmacotherapy regimen following radical prostatectomy improves recovery of spontaneous erectile function. *Journal of Sexual Medicine, 2,* 532–542.

Munding, M., Wessells, H., & Dalkin, B. (2001). Pilot study of changes in stretched penile lengths 3 months after radical retropubic prostatectomy. *Urology, 58,* 567–569.

Murthy, V., Norman, A., Shahidi, M., Parker, C., Horwich, A., Huddart, R., et al. (2006). Recovery of serum testosterone after neoadjuvant androgen deprivation therapy and radical radiotherapy in localized prostate cancer. *BJU International, 97,* 476–479.

Mydlo, J.H., Viterbo, R., & Crispen, P. (2005). Use of combined intracorporal injection and a phosphodiesterase-5 inhibitor therapy for men with a suboptimal response to sildenafil and/or vardenafil monotherapy after radical retropubic prostatectomy. *BJU International, 95,* 843–846.

Navon, L., & Morag, A. (2003). Advanced prostate cancer patients' relationships with their spouses following hormonal therapy. *European Journal of Oncology Nursing, 7,* 73–80.

Neese, L.E., Schover, L.R., Klein, E.A., Zippe, C., & Kupelian, P.A. (2003). Finding help for sexual problems after prostate cancer treatment: A phone survey of men's and women's perspectives. *Psycho-Oncology, 12,* 463–473.

Nehra, A., & Goldstein, I. (1999). Sildenafil citrate (Viagra) after radical retropubic prostatectomy: Con. *Urology, 54,* 587–589.

Ohebshalom, M., Parker, M., Guhring, P., & Mulhall, J.P. (2005). The efficacy of sildenafil citrate following radiation therapy for prostate cancer: Temporal considerations. *Journal of Urology, 174,* 258–262.

Onik, G., Narayan, P., Vaughan, D., Dineen, M., & Brunelle, R. (2002). Focal "nerve-sparing" cryosurgery for treatment of primary prostate cancer: A new approach to preserving potency. *Urology, 60,* 109–114.

Padma-Nathan, H., McCullough, A., & Forest, C. (2004). Erectile dysfunction secondary to nerve-sparing radical retropubic prostatectomy: Comparative phosphodiesterase-5 inhibitor efficacy for therapy and novel prevention strategies. *Current Urology Reports, 5,* 467–471.

Palmer, M., Fogarty, L., Somerfield, M., & Powel, L. (2003). Incontinence after prostatectomy: Coping with incontinence after prostate cancer surgery. *Oncology Nursing Forum, 30,* 229–238.

Paterson, J. (2000). Stigma associated with postprostatectomy urinary incontinence. *Journal of Wound, Ostomy, and Continence Nursing, 27,* 168–173.

Penson, D.F., Latini, D.M., Lubeck, D.P., Wallace, K., Henning, J.M., & Lue, T. (2003). Is quality of life different for men with erectile dysfunction and prostate cancer compared to men with erectile dysfunction due to other causes? Results from the ExCEED data base. *Journal of Urology, 169,* 1458–1461.

Penson, D.F., McLerran, D., Feng, Z., Li, L., Albertsen, P.C., Gilliland, F.D., et al. (2005). 5-year urinary and sexual outcomes after radical prostatectomy: Results from the prostate cancer outcomes study. *Journal of Urology, 173,* 1701–1705.

Perez, M.A., Meyerowitz, B.E., Lieskovsky, G., Skinner, D.G., Reynolds, B., & Skinner, E.C. (1997). Quality of life and sexuality following radical prostatectomy in patients with prostate cancer who use or do not use erectile aids. *Urology, 50,* 740–746.

Pomeranz, H., & Bhavsar, A. (2005). Nonarteritic ischemic optic neuropathy developing soon after use of sildenafil (Viagra): A report of seven new cases. *Journal of Neuro-Ophthalmology, 25,* 9–13.

Potosky, A.L., Davis, W.W., Hoffman, R.M., Stanford, J.L., Stephenson, R.A., Penson, D.F., et al. (2004). Five-year outcomes after prostatectomy or radiotherapy for prostate cancer: The prostate cancer outcomes study. *Journal of the National Cancer Institute, 96,* 1358–1367.

Potosky, A.L., Reeve, B.B., Clegg, L.X., Hoffman, R.M., Stephenson, R.A., Albertsen, P.C., et al. (2002). Quality of life following localized prostate cancer treated initially with androgen deprivation therapy or no therapy. *Journal of the National Cancer Institute, 94,* 430–437.

Raina, R., Agarwal, A., Allamaneni, S.S., Lakin, M.M., & Zippe, C.D. (2005). Sildenafil citrate and vacuum constriction device combination enhances sexual satisfaction in erectile dysfunction after radical prostatectomy. *Urology, 65,* 360–364.

Raina, R., Agarwal, A., Ausmundson, S., Mansour, D., & Zippe, C.D. (2005). Long-term efficacy and compliance of MUSE for erectile dysfunction following radical prostatectomy: SHIM (IIEF-5) analysis. *International Journal of Impotence Research, 17,* 86–90.

Raina, R., Lakin, M.M., Agarwal, A., Mascha, E., Montague, D., Klein, E., et al. (2004). Efficacy and factors associated with successful outcome of sildenafil citrate use for erectile dysfunction after radical prostatectomy. *Urology, 63,* 960–966.

Raina, R., Lakin, M.M., Agarwal, A., Sharma, R., Goyal, K.K., Montague, D.K., et al. (2003). Long-term effect of sildenafil citrate on erectile dysfunction after radical prostatectomy: 3-year follow-up. *Urology, 62,* 110–115.

Ramsawh, H.J., Morgentaler, A., Covino, N., Barlow, D.H., & DeWolf, W.C. (2005). Quality of life following simultaneous placement of penile prosthesis with radical prostatectomy. *Journal of Urology, 174,* 1395–1398.

Rees, J., McDonagh, R., & Persad, R. (2004). Cryosurgery for prostate cancer. *BJU International, 93,* 710–714.

Robinson, J.W., Donnelly, B.J., Saliken, J.C., Weber, B.A., Ernst, S., & Rewcastle, J.C. (2002). Quality of life and sexuality of men with prostate cancer 3 years after cryosurgery. *Urology, 60,* 12–18.

Schover, L.R., Fouladi, R.T., Warneke, C.L., Neese, L., Klein, E.A., Zippe, C., et al. (2002). The use of treatments for erectile dysfunction among survivors of prostate carcinoma. *Cancer, 95,* 2397–2407.

Schover, L.R., Fouladi, R.T., Warneke, C.L., Neese, L., Klein, E.A., Zippe, C., et al. (2004). Seeking help for erectile dysfunction after treatment for prostate cancer. *Archives of Sexual Behavior, 33,* 443–454.

Schulman, C., Shen, W., Stothard, D., & Schmitt, H. (2004). Integrated analysis examining first-dose success, success by dose, and maintenance of success among men taking tadalafil for erectile dysfunction. *Urology, 64,* 783–788.

Seyam, R., Mohamed, K., Akhras, A.A., & Rashwan, H. (2005). A prospective randomized study to optimize the dosage of trimix ingredients and compare its efficacy and safety with prostaglandin E1. *International Journal of Impotence Research, 17,* 346–353.

Shabsigh, R. (2004). Therapy of ED: PDE-5 inhibitors. *Endocrine, 23,* 135–141.

Speight, J.L., Elkin, E.P., Pasta, D.J., Silva, S., Lubeck, D.P., Carroll, P.R., et al. (2004). Longitudinal assessment of changes in sexual function and bother in patients treated with external beam radiotherapy or brachytherapy, with and without neoadjuvant androgen ablation: Data from CaPSURE. *International Journal of Radiation Oncology, Biology, Physics, 60,* 1066–1075.

Stanford, J.L., Feng, Z., Hamilton, A.S., Gilliland, F.D., Stephenson, R.A., Eley, J.W., et al. (2000). Urinary and sexual function after radical prostatectomy for clinically localized prostate cancer: The Prostate Cancer Outcomes Study. *JAMA, 283,* 354–360.

Stephenson, R.A., Mori, M., Hsieh, Y.C., Beer, T.M., Stanford, J.L., Gilliland, F.D., et al. (2005). Treatment of erectile dysfunction following therapy for clinically localized prostate cancer: Patient reported use and outcomes from the Surveillance, Epidemiology, and End Results Prostate Cancer Outcomes Study. *Journal of Urology, 174,* 646–650.

Stock, R.G., Stone, N.N., & Iannuzzi, C. (1996). Sexual potency following interactive ultrasound-guided brachytherapy for prostate cancer. *International Journal of Radiation Oncology, Biology, Physics, 35,* 267–272.

Tiefer, L., & Schuetz-Mueller, D. (1995). Psychological issues in diagnosis and treatment of erectile disorders. *Urologic Clinics of North America, 22,* 767–773.

Turner, S.L., Adams, K., Bull, C.A., & Berry, M.P. (1999). Sexual dysfunction after radical radiation therapy for prostate cancer: A prospective evaluation. *Urology, 54,* 124–129.

Vale, J. (2000). Erectile dysfunction following radical therapy for prostate cancer. *Radiotherapy and Oncology, 57,* 301–305.

Valicenti, R.K., Choi, E., Chen, C., Lu, J.D., Hirsch, I.H., Mulholland, G.S., et al. (2001). Sildenafil citrate effectively reverses sexual dysfunction induced by three-dimensional conformal radiation therapy. *Urology, 57,* 769–773.

Walsh, P.C., & Worthington, J. (2001). *Dr. Patrick Walsh's guide to surviving prostate cancer.* New York: Warner Books.

Weber, B.A., Roberts, B.L., Resnick, M., Deimling, G., Zauszniewski, J.A., Musil, C., et al. (2004). The effect of dyadic intervention on self-efficacy, social support, and depression for men with prostate cancer. *Psycho-Oncology, 13,* 47–60.

Weber, D.C., Bieri, S., Kurtz, J.M., & Miralbell, R. (1999). Prospective pilot study of sildenafil for treatment of postradiotherapy erectile dysfunction in patients with prostate cancer. *Journal of Clinical Oncology, 17,* 3444–3449.

Yeager, J., & Beihn, R.M. (2005). Retention and migration of alprostadil cream applied topically to the glans meatus for erectile dysfunction. *International Journal of Impotence Research, 17,* 91–95.

Zagaja, G., Mhoon, D., Aikens, J., & Brendler, C. (2000). Sildenafil in the treatment of erectile dysfunction after radical prostatectomy. *Urology, 56,* 631–634.

Zelefsky, M.J., Wallner, K.E., Ling, C.C., Raben, A., Hollister, T., Wolfe, T., et al. (1999). Comparison of the 5-year outcome and morbidity of three-dimensional conformal radiotherapy versus transperineal permanent iodine-125 implantation for early-stage prostatic cancer. *Journal of Clinical Oncology, 17,* 517–522.

CHAPTER 6

Gynecologic Cancer

Most healthcare providers can contemplate the sexual consequences of gynecologic cancer. Given that the organs involved are responsible for both reproductive and sexual functioning, it may seem obvious that cancer of this organ system will have profound effects on global sexual functioning. Although some controversy exists about whether the symptoms of the disease itself have sexual consequences, there is no doubt that the treatments for gynecologic cancer have significant sexual side effects (Lagana, McGarvey, Classen, & Koopman, 2001).

The Effect of Gynecologic Cancer on Sexuality

Physical side effects from the treatment of gynecologic cancers include pain; loss of sensation, sensitivity, and sexual desire; shortening and stenosis of the vagina; and atrophic vaginitis (Weijmar Schultz & van de Wiel, 2003). These may be related to anatomic changes resulting from treatment or from hormonal changes resulting from loss of ovarian function because of surgery, radiation, or chemotherapy. Fatigue is a frequent side effect of both radiation and chemotherapy (de Groot et al., 2005).

Sexual self-concept or identity, body image, and relationship changes also are common (Lagana et al., 2001). Body image plays an important role for many women in how they view themselves as female, and the presence of scarring, edema, or weight gain can affect this self-image and have long-lasting effects on women and their roles in their intimate relationships. The loss of reproductive potential also may have an impact on how women see themselves (Wilmoth & Spinelli, 2000).

Treatment of Gynecologic Cancer

Cervical Cancer

Women with cervical cancer often are diagnosed early in the disease process, have an excellent prognosis, and can live for many years after treatment. However, these women will have some degree of sexual dysfunction following treatment, which may last for the rest of their lives. Sexual problems may arise even before the diagnosis. Complaints of fatigue, postcoital bleeding, vaginal discharge, pain, and resultant sexual dysfunction related to these symptoms may prompt women to seek medical attention, where the diagnosis of cervical cancer is made (Andersen, 1987; Selo-Ojeme, Dayoub, Patel, & Metha, 2004). Treatment with either hysterectomy or radiation therapy for cervical cancer leads to wide-ranging problems with sexual functioning after treatment. These problems include decreased vaginal lubrication and vaginal swelling during sexual stimulation, perception of a shortened and/or inelastic vagina, and pain during intercourse because of these and other factors, as well as distress with these sexual changes. This can result in a general dissatisfaction with sexual functioning and occur irrespective of the type of treatment (Bergmark, Avall-Lundqvist, Dickman, Henningsohn, & Steineck, 1999).

Hysterectomy is known to cause disruption of sensory nerves in the pelvic area, with associated alteration in feelings of sexual arousal. Damage to autonomic nerves affects vasocongestion, lubrication, and enlargement of the vagina; these are all signs of physiologic arousal (Gruhmann, Robertson, Hacker, & Sommer, 2001). Many women experience sexual dysfunction in the months following surgery, but consequences also can be experienced many years later. This is particularly relevant as women often are diagnosed with cervical cancer at a young age. Cervical cancer survivors report sexual problems 5–10 years after treatment, which include vaginal dryness leading to pain with sexual activity and hot flashes irrespective of whether the ovaries were removed (Wenzel et al., 2005). Women may anticipate pain with intercourse, and many are bothered by altered body image following radiation or surgery (Bukovic et al., 2003). Some report an awareness of the physical sensation of a shortened vagina, and many experience vaginal dryness leading to dyspareunia (Juraskova et al., 2003). Women are less sensitive to heat and vibration in the vagina following hysterectomy; however, the enervation of the vagina is through the hypogastric nerve, which is commonly injured during surgery. The clitoris is supplied by the pudendal nerve, which usually is untouched during hysterectomy, so orgasmic capacity is preserved (Lowenstein et al., 2005). Radical surgery also precludes future pregnancies, and some women may wish to discuss the option of removing only the cervix to preserve childbearing potential (Carter, Auchincloss, Sonoda, & Krychman, 2003).

Radiation therapy has been used for many years to treat cervical cancer. Radiation can be given externally and/or internally (brachytherapy). When brachytherapy is performed, applicators are inserted into the vagina, and the radiation source (either high or low dose) is loaded into the applicator. This remains in place for a predetermined period of time and then is removed. The treatment may be repeated a number of times depending on the radiation source (Lancaster, 2004). The tissues of the vagina react to this treatment with changes in the blood vessels in the walls, leading to fibrosis of tissues (Katz et al., 2001). Moreover, the vaginal epithelium may be destroyed during the active phase of radiation treatment (Pras et al., 2003). This reduces the length of the vagina, which can lead to pain during intercourse. In addition, the vagina will not become lubricated during stimulation, which also leads to pain. Radiation may affect the ovaries, thus resulting in estrogen deficiency and further thinning of the vaginal walls (Lamb, 1998). Anecdotal reports of the consequences of radiation therapy include extreme sensitivity to touch, especially at the vaginal introitus, friable mucous membranes, and local burning with exposure to semen when intercourse was attempted (Jenkins, 1986).

Radiation of adjacent tissues has the potential to affect both the bladder and bowel, which also may have an impact on sexual functioning (Burke, 1996). Andersen, Anderson, and deProsse (1989) found that women with cervical cancer experienced significant dysfunction in all phases of the sexual response cycle after treatment. Over time, these negative changes may decline, but they do not return to pretreatment levels. Women with cervical cancer treated with both hysterectomy and radiotherapy describe feeling sexually unattractive and also report pain on intercourse and concern that sexual activity might provoke a recurrence or spread of their disease (Cull et al., 1993; Kritcharoen, Suwan, & Jirojwong, 2005).

Psychological consequences from both the diagnosis and treatment also are common. Some women may associate past sexual activity with being a source of their cancer and may equate the diagnosis with punishment for perceived promiscuity. Some women do not resume sexual activity after treatment, and marital problems are common as a result (Corney, Crowther, Everett, Howells, & Shepherd, 1993). The treatment for cervical cancer is invasive and can provoke feelings of violation in some women. In women who have experienced past sexual abuse, the repeated examinations necessary for diagnosis, treatment, and follow-up may increase their sense of violation and can reactivate the psychological trauma (Bergmark, Avall-Lundqvist, Dickman, Steineck, & Henningsohn, 2005).

Cancer of the Vulva or Vagina

Primary cancer of the vagina is relatively uncommon, and most of the lesions found in the vagina are thought to be metastatic from either the cervix or the endometrium. Cancer of the vulva also is relatively rare and predominately affects women older than 60 (Goodman, 1998). Radical surgery has been the treatment of choice, which has far-reaching implications for sexual functioning but also for sexual self-image, body image, self-esteem, and feminine identity (Carter et al., 2003). More recently, tissue-sparing surgery has become more commonly performed, especially for early-stage cancer of the vulva, and sentinel node biopsy is performed instead of conventional lymphadenectomy (Gotlieb, 2003).

Vulvectomy involves a wide excision of the vulva with removal of the distal urethra. Fatty tissue and pelvic lymph nodes also are removed, and the clitoris often is excised (Wallace, 1987; Willibrord et al., 1990). After surgery for cancer of the vulva, women report significant alteration in body image, a decrease in the frequency of sexual activity, a lack of interest in sex, and avoidance behaviors (Green et al., 2000). They may experience scarring at the vaginal introitus that causes pain with attempted penetration, and removal of the clitoris essentially destroys orgasmic capacity. Loss of fatty tissue on the mons pubis and absence of the labia also contribute to altered, absent, or painful sensations. Lymphadenectomy may lead to edema of the legs, and removal of the urethra can cause incontinence and dysuria. Despite the extensive damage done to tissue and self-image, women who have had this surgery do not report dissatisfaction with the quality of their primary intimate relationships (Green et al.; Willibrord et al.).

Ovarian Cancer

Ovarian cancer usually is diagnosed late in the disease process and requires aggressive multimodal treatment. Very little exists in the research literature about the sexual effects of the cancer and its treatment, as most of the studies have not separated women with ovarian cancer from women with other kinds of gynecologic cancer. However, surgical removal of the ovaries (usually the first stage of treatment) profoundly affects the hormonal milieu of premenopausal women, in whom immediate menopause is triggered with resulting symptoms of hot flashes, irritability, vaginal dryness and atrophy, fatigue, and increased incidence of urinary tract infections (Carmack Taylor, Basen-Engquist, Shinn, & Bodurka, 2004). Removal of the ovaries and uterus also ends the patient's reproductive potential. This can bring about significant emotional effects and role changes, particularly for women who have not started or completed their family. Some women may be diagnosed at an early stage, which may allow for the sparing of an ovary (Fitch & Turner, 2006). The premature loss of ovarian androgens causes lack of desire and can contribute to fatigue.

Surgery usually involves not only removal of the ovaries, uterus, and uterine tubes but also debulking of visible tumor in the pelvis and sampling of pelvic lymph nodes and omentum (Mannix, Jackson, & Raftos, 1999). The effects of this extensive surgery on energy levels and body image compound the effects of surgically induced menopause. Psychological well-being is significantly affected by the real threat of death for women with this type of cancer, which has high morbidity and mortality. Younger women report being more concerned about sexual issues after diagnosis and are fearful that they will be sexually unattractive after treatment (Stewart, Wong, Duff, Melancon, & Cheung, 2001). Scars from surgery serve as a visible reminder of the cancer. Weight loss or edema following surgery also can affect how women see themselves as sexual beings. Women commonly will avoid being naked in front of their partner when they experience an alteration in body image, and this can cause distancing between the couple.

Most women with ovarian cancer begin chemotherapy shortly after surgery, and the global effects of this treatment on mood, fatigue, and nausea can further affect well-being and sexual functioning, particularly sexual desire (Carmack Taylor et al., 2004). Fatigue is a well-described symptom in women with ovarian cancer that can persist months after completion of treatment. Fatigue is associated with decreased quality of life and increased anxiety and depression, which all have an impact on sexuality (Holzner et al., 2003). Hair loss during chemotherapy has a major impact on body image (Fitch, 2003), and women may not expect that they will lose all their body hair, including pubic hair. This can be devastating to how the woman and her partner view her sexuality. Women report that without pubic hair, they feel like "little girls" who are not sexual, and so sexual touching in this circumstance is difficult. Ovarian cancer can leave a woman feeling inadequate in her role as a wife, mother, sexual partner, or even as a "whole" woman (Lammers, Schaefer, Ladd, & Echenberg, 2000). This causes distress for women, especially those who are in committed relationships who may be fearful that lack of sexual activity will cause problems in the relationship (Sun et al., 2005).

Pelvic Exenteration

Women with centrally recurring cervical or vaginal cancer can be offered pelvic exenteration with the hope of increasing survival. This radical surgery involves removal of all of the pelvic organs, including the uterus, ovaries, vagina, bladder, colon, and adjacent tissue. It is used to treat advanced and/or recurrent cervical, vaginal, or vulvar cancer. Traditionally, women who had this surgery were left with an ostomy for elimination; however, newer surgical techniques allow for a urinary diversion and anal-sparing surgery, which avoids the need for ostomies and continence devices (Carter et al., 2004). The construction of a neovagina using the myocutaneous flap procedure has greatly reduced the incidence of sexual dysfunction and has improved quality of life (Hawighorst-Knapstein, Schonefub, Hoffmann, & Knapstein, 1997; Mirhashemi et al., 2002; Ratliff et al., 1996). This radical surgery has enormous effects on body image, and many women are reluctant to talk to anyone about this or let family members see the changes to their bodies (Carter et al., 2004). Some women report that stimulation of the neovagina causes the sensation to be felt on the thigh, a result of the innervation of the flap used to create the neovagina. This tissue does not produce lubrication.

Nursing Interventions in the Care of Women With Gynecologic Cancer

The first step in providing care in the context of sexuality for women with gynecologic cancer is a sensitive assessment of their attitudes, knowledge, beliefs, and need for information. This can be done using any of the models suggested in Chapter 3. Figure 6-1 is an example of how to do this using the BETTER model (see Figure 3-3) in the case of a woman with vulvar cancer (see the case study later in this chapter).

Nurses and other healthcare providers can perform a number of interventions to assist women in coping with the sexual consequences of gynecologic cancer and its treatments. These interventions focus on information and some specific suggestions for coping with fatigue, vaginal dryness, the need for vaginal dilatation after radiation therapy, and alterations in body image.

Information Sharing

Women diagnosed with any of the cancers discussed previously commonly remember very little of the information they received at the time of diagnosis. They also may not have much knowledge of the anatomy and physiology of the reproductive system (Juraskova et al., 2003) and may not recall the details of what treatment they are to have or the associated sexual side effects. Nurses must review normal anatomy and physiology with patients, preferably with their partners present because they may have similar knowledge needs. Furthermore, nurses should ask patients and their partners what they understand about the diagnosis, staging, and treatment plan. The timing of this is critical, as women will need support in the immediate period following diagnosis but may not be emotionally or cognitively able to absorb factual information related to treatment side effects. Also, patients may have only a short period of time between the diagnosis and surgical intervention, so both the amount and content of any education should be carefully tailored to meet the individual needs of the patients, their partners, and families.

While still in shock about the diagnosis of gynecologic cancer, many women will state that sexual functioning is not important at all, as the focus is on the immediate threat

---

Figure 6-1. Example of the BETTER Model in Patients With Gynecologic Cancer

- **Bringing up the topic:** Nurses are encouraged to raise the issue of sexuality with patients.

  "Women who have this type of surgery often have questions about what this will mean for their sex life in the future. What are your thoughts about this?"

- **Explaining that sex is a part of quality of life:** This helps to normalize the discussion and may help patients to feel less embarrassed or alone in having a problem.

  "It may feel like sex is the last thing on your mind right now; however, as you recover over the next few months, you will probably find yourself once again becoming interested in that aspect of your life."

- **Telling patients that resources will be found to address their concerns:** This step suggests to patients that even if the nurse does not have the immediate solution to the problem or question, others are available who can help.

  "As your body heals, you may want to meet with a counselor who can talk to you more about how to deal with the changes in your body. I have some reading material that you may find helpful, and I will leave this with you to read when you feel like it."

- **Timing the intervention:** Patients may not be ready to deal with sexual issues at the time a problem is identified, but they can ask for information at any time in the future.

  "I wanted you to be aware that we have a number of books and videos that deal with sexual problems after treatment. Here is the phone number and address of the Resource Center where you can borrow these if you want."

- **Educating patients about the sexual side effects of treatment:** Educating patients about potential side effects from treatments does not mean that they will occur. However, informing patients about sexual side effects is as important as informing them about any other side effects.

  "Some women find that after the surgery, they experience altered sensations in the vulvar area. These may feel like electric shocks and are a result of the nerves being cut and then very slowly growing back. You may also feel numb in that area. You may not experience this, but I wanted to inform you that this is possible."

- **Recording:** A brief notation that a discussion about sexuality or sexual side effects occurred is important.

  "Potential side effects related to the planned surgery were discussed. Patient was given reading material as well as contact information for the Resource Center."

---

to survival. Nurses should acknowledge this but also should tell patients that although this is a common response, sexual consequences may become more important at a later stage in their treatment. The partner's needs may be different than those of the woman, and sometimes the partner wants information on sexuality even if the woman is not ready to discuss it. By raising the topic, the healthcare provider indicates to patients and their partners that sexuality is recognized as an important subject, and ideally they will be able to talk about this with the care team at a time that is appropriate for them.

Asking patients and their partners to describe what they understand from their discussions with members of the healthcare team also will allow for correction of misunderstandings or confusion. Many people subscribe to myths and beliefs that are not factual, particularly in the area of sexuality. People commonly think that sexual activity caused the cancer or that sexual activity after treatment may cause the cancer to spread.

Women should be counseled on what to expect in terms of sexual changes following hysterectomy. Informing patients about what to expect can help them to anticipate and then react in an appropriate and timely manner rather than becoming anxious if they experience something unexpected. Changes in all aspects of the sexual response cycle are to be expected in the face of radical surgery, so it is not unusual for women who have had a total hysterectomy to have no interest in sex (lack of libido), to have difficulty becoming aroused, and to experience changes in the frequency and quality of orgasm. These changes may improve over time. However, if radiation and/or chemotherapy is part of the treatment plan, women can expect further changes or, at the very least, no improvement.

Interventions for Treatment-Related Side Effects

Specific interventions are related to the type of cancer and treatment. Depression and anxiety can be treated with oral medication. However, many of the most popular antidepressants have sexual side effects specifically related to desire, arousal, and orgasm that can further compound symptoms that patients are already experiencing (Lagana et al., 2001). Fatigue often responds well to exercise, but it can be difficult to persuade patients—who are exhausted and having difficulty coping with the usual role demands—that exercising actually will help to alleviate this.

The changes associated with the loss of ovarian function resulting from any of the treatment modalities can be dealt with by prescribing hormone therapy. However, this may not be possible if the cancer is estrogen dependent. Local estrogen in the form of creams or pessaries is highly effective in treating vaginal atrophy. Vaginal dryness responds well to a vaginal lubricant such as Replens® (Lil' Drug Store Products, Cedar Rapids, IA), which may help to alleviate burning and itching of vaginal and vulval tissues not associated with sexual activity. A number of lubricants are available to help women to feel more comfortable with sexual activity. Water- and silicone-based lubricants are the safest to use, and several are free of dyes and perfumes. Women should avoid using oil-based products and anything that is colored, scented, or not designed specifically for sexual activity, such as hand lotion.

Pain with intercourse can result from vaginal dryness, muscle tension, scar tissue, or anxiety. The experience of pain can start a cycle of vaginismus, which can last a lifetime and has implications not only for the woman's sexual life but also for pelvic examinations. This is a reflex response to the anticipation of pain with penetration in which the woman contracts the pubococcygeal muscle, thus narrowing the vaginal opening. Women can learn to relax the vaginal muscles in much the same way that they learn to do Kegel exercises, which deliberately contract the same pubococcygeal muscle. A multimodality approach combining pharmacotherapy, sex therapy, and suggestions for specific problems is usually effective in enabling patients to return to a satisfying level of sexual functioning (Amsterdam & Krychman, 2006).

Vaginal Dilatation

Women who have had radiation therapy are required to perform regular vaginal dilatation to maintain patency for both sexual activity and pelvic examinations in follow-up care. Although there is little consensus on when to begin dilatation, how often it should be performed, and for how long (Lancaster, 2004), it is generally agreed that women should start as soon as it is comfortable to do so but certainly within four weeks of completion of therapy. Initially, patients should use a dilator with a narrow diameter (0.5–1 inch) and gradually increase the diameter up to a maximum of 1.5 inches. Women should be encouraged to use the dilator daily, but three times a week is the minimum. They should continue with this regimen for at least three years, and possibly longer (Lancaster). A lubricant should be used to ease insertion. An estrogen cream provides both lubrication and relief of vaginal dryness and may be used unless contradicted. An alternative to a mechanical dilator is regular penetrative intercourse; however, for women without a partner, this may not be a viable option. Women may not be ready for intercourse soon after cessation of treatment and may be afraid of pain or tissue damage. Therefore, a dilator may be preferable, especially in the short term. Healthcare providers must reinforce the instructions and rationale for using a dilator. A specific intervention focusing on education, motivation, and behavioral skills related to dilator use has been shown to be more effective than merely providing patients with written information (Robinson, Faris, & Scott, 1999). Written information often is given early in the treatment process, and patients may not recall the discussion or may not pay attention because at that time they are more concerned about survival.

Body Image and Integrity

After treatment for gynecologic cancer, many women report a fundamental change in the way they see their body. The presence of a hysterectomy scar can be a glaring reminder of the cancer and treatment. Women need reassurance that the scar will fade with time. However, the reassurance from their sexual partner that they are still attractive and desirable most likely will be of more comfort. Some women find it difficult to even hear and believe those words from the partner. It may be helpful to ask the women if their partner still looks the same as he or she did 10 or more years ago. Most women will laugh and comment that their partner has gained a few pounds, has lost some hair, and developed some wrinkles. But when asked, they will say that they love their partner just as much if not more than they did all those years ago. They can then see that their partner still loves them in spite of the physical changes that they find so bothersome.

After treatment, women may report a sense of violation because of the many invasive procedures and examinations they have endured. Women frequently distance themselves from their bodies in an attempt to cope with the procedures and maintain bodily integrity. Unfortunately, this does not encourage the woman to experience her body as a source of pleasure when she is with her partner or alone. Women can be encouraged to talk about their feelings of exposure and vulnerability during procedures. This often allows them to express grief and pain over what they have experienced and may be the beginning of healing. They also can be encouraged to relearn that the body can be a source of pleasure through touching that is enjoyable. A manicure or pedicure is a good place to start because it is nonthreatening to most women and does not involve exposure of the body. Some women enjoy spending time in a warm bath with soft music playing. She can use hypoallergenic bath products and lotions and learn from her own touch what feels pleasurable. This obviously is to be done only when wound healing is complete. A massage also may be a good idea, but only when the woman feels comfortable with another person touching her.

Another intervention that sex therapists teach is the use of sensate focus exercises (see Chapter 22), which help women to reconnect with their body as a source of pleasure and also allow for their partner to participate in giving them pleasure and to receive pleasure in return. This allows the couple to resume an intimate connection. It may take some time for women to be ready for penetrative intercourse, and some women find that this is not comfortable or pleasurable. The couple then will need to find alternative ways of expressing their sexual feelings. Level three of the sensate focus exercise may be as far as the couple goes, and this may be satisfactory to both of them.

Case Study

G.L. is a 19-year-old student who presented to her primary care provider with a small lesion on her labia that had been there for six months. She thought it was an ingrown hair and was not concerned. The primary care provider biopsied the lesion, and the result showed that it was malignant. G.L. comes from a very close Hispanic family, and her mother is struggling to cope with the diagnosis and has approached the nurse. It is apparent that the surgeon, who will perform a radical vulvectomy next week, has not given the family much information.

Questions to consider:

- When is the most appropriate time to give information to this family?
- How much should the nurse involve the family in teaching about the surgery and the consequences the patient may be faced with?
- What should the nurse tell them?

G.L. has the surgery and recovers well in the hospital. She is very quiet and does not ask many questions. On the day she is discharged, the nurse must make sure that she understands the plan for follow-up.

- How should the nurse help G.L. to look at her altered genitalia?
- What questions should the nurse expect the patient to ask?
- She asks about the need for birth control. How should the nurse reply?

See Appendix B for answers to the case study questions.

Conclusion

Gynecologic cancer and its treatments can have profound effects on sexual functioning in all phases of the sexual response cycle as well as on body image and sexual self-concept. A cancer diagnosis and the associated distress may have a profound effect on the emotional status of both patients and their partners. This psychological impact combined with the physical sensations of the disease and treatment side effects may lower women's interest in sex as well as the frequency of sexual activity.

References

Amsterdam, A., & Krychman, M. (2006). Sexual dysfunction in patients with gynecologic neoplasms: A retrospective pilot study. *Journal of Sexual Medicine, 3,* 646–649.

Andersen, B. (1987). Sexual functioning complications in women with gynecological cancer: Outcomes and directions for prevention. *Cancer, 15*(Suppl. 8), 2123–2128.

Andersen, B.L., Anderson, B., & deProsse, C. (1989). Controlled prospective longitudinal study of women with cancer: I. Sexual functioning outcomes. *Journal of Consulting and Clinical Psychology, 6,* 683–691.

Bergmark, K., Avall-Lundqvist, E., Dickman, P.W., Henningsohn, L., & Steineck, G. (1999). Vaginal changes and sexuality in women with a history of cervical cancer. *New England Journal of Medicine, 340,* 1383–1389.

Bergmark, K., Avall-Lundqvist, E., Dickman, P.W., Steineck, G., & Henningsohn, L. (2005). Synergy between sexual abuse and cervical cancer in causing sexual dysfunction. *Journal of Sex and Marital Therapy, 31,* 361–383.

Bukovic, D., Strinic, T., Habek, M., Hojsak, I., Silovski, H., Krhen, I., et al. (2003). Sexual life after cervical carcinoma. *Collegium Antropologicum, 27,* 173–180.

Burke, L. (1996). Sexual dysfunction following radiotherapy for cervical cancer. *British Journal of Nursing, 5,* 239–244.

Carmack Taylor, C.L., Basen-Engquist, K., Shinn, E.H., & Bodurka, D.C. (2004). Predictors of sexual functioning in ovarian cancer patients. *Journal of Clinical Oncology, 22,* 881–889.

Carter, J., Auchincloss, S., Sonoda, Y., & Krychman, M. (2003). Cervical cancer: Issues of sexuality and fertility. *Oncology (Williston Park), 17,* 1229–1234.

Carter, J., Chi, D.S., Abu-Rustum, N., Brown, C.L., McCreath, W., & Barakat, R.R. (2004). Brief report: Total pelvic exenteration—a retrospective clinical needs assessment. *Psycho-Oncology, 13,* 125–131.

Corney, R., Crowther, M., Everett, H., Howells, A., & Shepherd, J. (1993). Psychosexual dysfunction in women with gynaecological cancer following radical pelvic surgery. *British Journal of Obstetrics and Gynaecology, 100,* 73–78.

Cull, A., Cowie, V., Farquharson, D., Livingstone, J., Smart, G., & Elton, R. (1993). Early stage cervical cancer: Psychosocial and sexual outcomes of treatment. *British Journal of Cancer, 68,* 1216–1220.

de Groot, J.M., Mah, K., Fyles, A., Winton, S., Greenwood, S., Depetrillo, A.D., et al. (2005). The psychosocial impact of cervical cancer among affected women and their partners. *International Journal of Gynecological Cancer, 15,* 918–925.

Fitch, M.I. (2003). Psychosocial management of patients with recurrent ovarian cancer: Treating the whole patient to improve quality of life. *Seminars in Oncology Nursing, 19,* 40–53.

Fitch, M.I., & Turner, F. (2006). Ovarian cancer. *Canadian Nurse, 102,* 16–20.

Goodman, A. (1998). Primary vaginal cancer. *Surgical Oncology Clinics of North America, 7,* 347–361.

Gotlieb, W. (2003). The assessment and surgical management of early-stage vulvar cancer. *Best Practice and Research: Clinical Obstetrics and Gynaecology, 17,* 557–569.

Green, M., Naumann, W., Elliot, M., Hall, J., Higgins, R., & Grigsby, J. (2000). Sexual dysfunction following vulvectomy. *Gynecologic Oncology, 77,* 73–77.

Gruhmann, M., Robertson, R., Hacker, N., & Sommer, G. (2001). Sexual functioning in patients following radical hysterectomy for stage IB cancer of the cervix. *International Journal of Gynecological Cancer, 11,* 372–380.

Hawighorst-Knapstein, S., Schonefub, G., Hoffmann, S., & Knapstein, P. (1997). Pelvic exenteration: Effects of surgery on quality of life and body image—a prospective longitudinal study. *Gynecologic Oncology, 94,* 495–500.

Holzner, B., Kemmler, G., Meraner, V., Maislinger, A., Kopp, M., Bodner, T., et al. (2003). Fatigue in ovarian carcinoma patients: A neglected issue? *Cancer, 97,* 1564–1572.

Jenkins, B.Y. (1986). Sexual healing after pelvic irradiation. *American Journal of Nursing, 86,* 920–922.

Juraskova, I., Butow, P., Robertson, R., Sharpe, L., McLeod, C., & Hacker, N. (2003). Post-treatment sexual adjustment following cervical and endometrial cancer: A qualitative insight. *Psycho-Oncology, 12,* 267–279.

Katz, A., Njuguna, E., Rakowsky, E., Sulkes, A., Sulkes, J., & Fenig, E. (2001). Early development of vaginal shortening during radiation therapy for endometrial or cervical cancer. *International Journal of Gynaecological Cancer, 11,* 234–235.

Kritcharoen, S., Suwan, K., & Jirojwong, S. (2005). Perceptions of gender roles, gender power relation-ships, and sexuality in Thai women following diagnosis and treatment for cervical cancer. *Oncology Nursing Forum, 32,* 682–688.

Lagana, L., McGarvey, E., Classen, C., & Koopman, C. (2001). Psychosexual dysfunction among gynecological cancer survivors. *Journal of Clinical Psychology in Medical Settings, 8,* 73–84.

Lamb, M. (1998). Questions women ask about gynecologic cancer and sexual functioning. *Developments in Supportive Cancer Care, 1,* 11–13.

Lammers, S.E., Schaefer, K.M., Ladd, E.C., & Echenberg, R. (2000). Caring for women living with ovarian cancer: Recommendations for advanced practice nurses. *Journal of Obstetric, Gynecologic, and Neonatal Nursing, 29,* 567–573.

Lancaster, L. (2004). Preventing vaginal stenosis after brachytherapy for gynaecological cancer: An overview of Australian practices. *European Journal of Oncology Nursing, 8,* 30–39.

Lowenstein, L., Yarnitsky, D., Gruenwald, I., Deutsch, M., Sprecher, E., Gedalia, U., et al. (2005). Does hysterectomy affect genital sensation? *European Journal of Obstetrics, Gynecology, and Reproductive Biology, 119,* 242–245.

Mannix, J., Jackson, D., & Raftos, M. (1999). Ovarian cancer: An update for nursing practice. *International Journal of Nursing Practice, 5,* 47–50.

Mirhashemi, R., Averette, H., Lambrou, N., Penalver, M., Mendez, L., Ghurani, G., et al. (2002). Vaginal reconstruction at the time of pelvic exenteration: A surgical and psychosexual analysis of techniques. *Gynecologic Oncology, 87,* 39–45.

Pras, E., Wouda, J., Willemse, P., Midden, M., Zwart, M., de Vries, E., et al. (2003). Pilot study of vaginal plethysmography in women treated with radiotherapy for gynecological cancer. *Gynecologic Oncology, 91,* 540–546.

Ratliff, C., Gershenson, D., Morris, M., Burke, T., Levenback, C., Schover, L., et al. (1996). Sexual adjustment of patients undergoing gracilis myocutaneous flap vaginal reconstruction in conjunction with pelvic exenteration. *Cancer, 78,* 2229–2235.

Robinson, J.W., Faris, P.D., & Scott, C.B. (1999). Psychoeducational group increases vaginal dilation for younger women and reduces sexual fears for women of all ages with gynecological carcinoma treated with radiotherapy. *International Journal of Radiation Oncology, Biology, Physics, 44,* 497–506.

Selo-Ojeme, D., Dayoub, N., Patel, A., & Metha, M. (2004). A clinico-pathological study of postcoital bleeding. *Archives of Gynecology and Obstetrics, 270,* 34–36.

Stewart, D., Wong, F.W., Duff, S., Melancon, C., & Cheung, A. (2001). "What doesn't kill you makes you stronger": An ovarian cancer survivor survey. *Gynecologic Oncology, 83,* 537–542.

Sun, C.C., Bodurka, D.C., Weaver, C.B., Rasu, R., Wolf, J.K., Bevers, M.W., et al. (2005). Rankings and symptom assessments of side effects from chemotherapy: Insights from experienced patients with ovarian cancer. *Supportive Care in Cancer, 13,* 219–227.

Wallace, L. (1987). Psychological aspects of physical illness: Sexual adjustment after radical genital surgery. *Nursing Times, 83*(51), 41–43.

Weijmar Schultz, W., & van de Wiel, H. (2003). Sexuality, intimacy, and gynecological cancer. *Journal of Sex and Marital Therapy, 29,* 121–128.

Wenzel, L., DeAlba, I., Habbal, R., Kluhsman, B., Fairclough, D., Krebs, L., et al. (2005). Quality of life in long-term cervical cancer survivors. *Gynecologic Oncology, 97,* 310–317.

Willibrord, C., Weijmar Schultz, W., van de Wiel, H., Bouma, J., Hanssens, J., & Littlewood, J. (1990). Psychosexual functioning after the treatment of cancer of the vulva. *Cancer, 66,* 402–407.

Wilmoth, M.C., & Spinelli, A. (2000). Sexual implications of gynecologic cancer treatments. *Journal of Obstetric, Gynecologic, and Neonatal Nursing, 29,* 413–421.

CHAPTER 7

Testicular Cancer

Testicular cancer primarily affects young men at the peak of their sexual lives. Because of the importance of the role of male genitalia in a sexuality, a diagnosis of this cancer is both shocking and fear provoking, particularly for young men.

The Effect of Testicular Cancer on Sexuality

Men treated for testicular cancer experience both physiologic and psychological effects. The discovery of a lump or swelling in a testicle usually precipitates a diagnosis. However, fear may dissuade some men from seeking help, so diagnosis and treatment may be delayed (Gascoigne, Mason, & Roberts, 1999). The first stage of treatment involves surgical removal of the affected testicle (hemiorchiectomy) for staging and pathology. This has the potential for both immediate and long-range problems associated with shame, feeling less of a man, and feeling sexually unattractive. The diagnosis itself may cause sexual difficulties, with men reporting the onset of lack of libido at this time. Loss of one testicle should not result in sexual dysfunction, but the psychological impact of both the diagnosis and resultant treatment can precipitate significant consequences, which might resolve over time. After staging of the cancer is complete, the need for further treatment will be established.

Treatment of Testicular Cancer

Generally, stage I seminomas will require radiation therapy after orchiectomy. Stage I nonseminomas will have lymph node dissection in addition to orchiectomy and will be actively followed for progression. Higher-grade tumors usually are treated with cisplatin-based chemotherapy in combination with bleomycin and etoposide (Brown, 2003). The type of treatment has a direct effect on sexuality and fertility.

Treatment-Related Side Effects

Generally, orchiectomy does not interfere with physiologic functioning. However, although testosterone levels remain within the normal range (Lackner et al., 2005), up to 25% of men will experience loss of libido following orchiectomy (Jonker-Pool et al., 2001). This may be psychological in nature and related to the stress of the cancer diagnosis, anxiety, and fear of the unknown. Men also report orgasmic dysfunction following the surgery. The cause of this dysfunction is not known, as the surgical removal of one testicle should not interfere with either the physical sensation of orgasm or the reflex arc involved. Once again, this may be psychological in nature (Fegg et al., 2003).

Lymph node dissection at the time of diagnosis and secondary resection of a retroperitoneal tumor mass are associated with significantly greater ejaculatory problems (Jonker-Pool et al., 2001). Many men experience "dry ejaculation," especially if bilateral lymph node dissection was performed (Aass, Grunfeld, Kaalhus, & Fossa, 1993), which interrupts retroperitoneal sympathetic nerves (Hartmann et al., 1999). More modern, nerve-sparing surgical techniques may reduce the incidence and severity of this side effect (Jonker-Pool et al., 2001).

The addition of radiation therapy has significant effects on erectile capacity and ejaculation (Jonker-Pool et al., 2001). Men who have undergone radiation therapy tend to have fewer morning erections, and erections achieved with sexual stimulation are often insufficient for penetration or do not last long enough for penetration (Tinkler, Howard, & Kerr, 1992). These men also may experience a reduced volume of ejaculate (Arai, Kawakita, Okada, & Yoshida, 1997).

Chemotherapy has the most global impact on sexual functioning, with one-quarter to one-third of men experiencing loss of libido, orgasmic and ejaculatory problems, and a decrease in amount of sexual activity (Jonker-Pool et al., 2001). These side effects are expected to occur in the period during and immediately after chemotherapy, when nausea and fatigue are at their worst (Brown, 2003). Furthermore, these problems appear to persist for at least the first six months after completion of treatment (Heidenreich & Hofmann, 1999).

The combination of any of these treatments tends to exacerbate sexual side effects. In addition, older men report more problems, most likely a result of age and preexisting sexual problems and/or comorbidities that also can affect sexual functioning (Incrocci, Hop, Wijnmaalen, & Slob, 2002).

In general, men treated by any modality for testicular cancer report a decline in their sexual satisfaction (Joly et al., 2002). However, this is not related to satisfaction with their relationships (Jonker-Pool et al., 2001). Most men find that their marital or partner relationships are strengthened by their cancer diagnosis and treatment and that the level of support from partners increased during the treatment and then returned to pretreatment levels (Fleer, Hoekstra, Sleijfer, & Hoekstra-Weebers, 2004; Heidenreich & Hofmann, 1999).

Fertility issues are important considerations for men with testicular cancer. This type of cancer is most prevalent in men who are young and who are either at the peak of their reproductive years or have not yet thought about starting a family. Subfertility is an important issue for men with testicular cancer; 75% of men with this cancer will have decreased sperm production at the time of diagnosis. This is thought to be associated with cryptorchidism (condition in which one or both testicles fail to descend normally), among other factors. Radiation and chemotherapy further degrade spermatogenesis in a dose-related manner, and for those who have lymph node dissection or tumor resection, ejaculatory disturbances further affect fertility (Spermon et al., 2003). Some men may be able to impregnate their partners naturally; however, most will require some form of fertility assistance. All men diagnosed with testicular cancer may be offered the option of cryopreservation of sperm before treatment (Spermon et al.).

One of the most important issues related to fertility is the timing of diagnosis and treatment. Because testicular cancer primarily is diagnosed in young men, many patients are not in a relationship at the time of diagnosis, and thoughts of parenthood may be remote and not a priority. Men who are young, unmarried, and childless experience more infertility-related distress than those who have fathered children and are in a supportive relationship. Very little information has been reported on single men with testicular cancer, so information about their experiences with coping with the potential and actual loss of fertility remains speculative. Often the diagnosis is complicated by the emergent nature of testicular cancer, which without treatment can progress at a fairly rapid rate (Richie, 1993). Younger men may not have the opportunity to consider and discuss the potential for loss of fertility or may find it difficult to discuss with their parents or care providers. Treatment may be initiated without consideration of cryopreservation and sperm banking, and years later, the man and his partner will have to deal with the consequences of this lack of forethought and planning.

At the time of diagnosis, most men will experience the full range of emotions that any newly diagnosed patient with cancer must deal with. However, a testicular cancer diagnosis carries with it some unique social and cultural characteristics. Body image and masculinity are profoundly affected by a diagnosis of testicular cancer. For many, the testicles are both an anatomic structure as well as a symbol of masculinity and normalcy. Being a "normal" man is associated with being able to perform sexually with erections as visible proof of functioning masculinity (Gurevich, Bishop, Bower, Malka, & Nyhof-Young, 2004). Loss of a testicle threatens all this, in addition to the cancer being a threat to life itself. Some men who have had an orchiectomy reported body image alterations and were distressed by the sight of the surgical scar and felt unattractive (Arai et al., 1997). Men may be reluctant to undress in front of other men in the locker room or may feel embarrassed using a public urinal.

Treating Sexual Problems

Management of sexual difficulties related to treatment begins with providing patients with information appropriate for their age and developmental stage. Multiple studies report that men are not given adequate information about sexual consequences of treatment or that they do not recall the information they were given (Caffo & Amichetti, 1999; Heidenreich & Hofmann, 1999). As with other cancers, information often is given around the time of the diagnosis and not again unless the patient specifically requests it. Providing information at follow-up visits is especially important in the case of younger men who may not have regarded fertility as a priority at the time of diagnosis but years later will place more importance on it as their developmental stage changes (Jonker-Pool et al., 2004). This also applies to information about sexuality and sexual functioning, which may not be a priority for either patients or healthcare providers during the diagnostic period but becomes important to men as they return to their usual lives and find that sexual functioning is altered. Somewhat surprisingly, many men are not aware that a prosthesis can be implanted in the scrotum after treatment is complete, which reduces much of the psychosocial distress related to body image (Incrocci, Bosch, & Slob, 1999; Incrocci et al., 2002).

Erectile difficulties have both a physiologic and psychogenic etiology, and although medications such as phosphodiesterase-5 inhibitors (sildenafil, tadalafil, and vardenafil) may be useful in the treatment of age-related erectile dysfunction, it is not known whether they are effective in men with testicular cancer, where nerve and blood vessel damage may be contributing to the difficulty. Also, the psychological component may be significant and cause resistance to pharmaceutical solutions.

Ejaculation changes cannot be corrected. However, accurate information about the cause and consequences is an important aspect of coping with the treatment side effects. Many men find it difficult to express themselves and then suffer in silence. Although patients cannot be forced to verbalize their deep-seated fears and emotions, nurses can acknowledge that they may be suffering, and this recognition may allow the patients to express their thoughts and feelings.

Nursing Interventions in the Care of Men With Testicular Cancer

Information Sharing

Ideally, counseling for patients should begin early in the diagnostic process. Men may have significant anxiety stemming from erroneous beliefs about the cause of testicular cancer and the consequences of treatment. They may believe that too much (or too little) sex or masturbation caused the cancer. Others may fear that treatment, especially radiation, may harm their sexual partner or cause harm to a fetus in a future pregnancy (Schover & von Eschenbach, 1984). Counseling should take into consideration the context of the man's life; his life stage, coping skills, strengths and weaknesses, and support systems all will be factors as he moves from being a patient with cancer to a cancer survivor.

Nurses must inform patients that sexual problems and associated distress tend to decline in the six months following the end of treatment (Tamburini et al., 1989), but some issues persist for a longer period, and patients must seek help for these. Generally, testicular cancer survivors can expect normal sexual desire or libido and erections. Alterations in orgasmic sensation can occur, and men treated with radiation and/or lymph node and tumor dissection may experience alterations in ejaculation.

Cancer generally is regarded as an assault on one's sense of self (Rieker, 1996), and testicular cancer has the additional significance of being associated with a sense of masculinity and potency. This may be very difficult for men to deal with, and they may do so by either denying the type of cancer (calling it a germ cell cancer rather than testicular cancer) or using humor to challenge the assumptions of others in work or social settings. Humor also can be used with healthcare providers to lessen embarrassment and manage feelings (Chapple & Ziebland, 2004). Healthcare providers must be attuned to displays of humor and be sensitive to the fact that patients may be using humor as a cover for deeper feelings of distress. Asking a man directly if he finds something humorous or if, in fact, he is using humor to deflect painful feelings, rather than merely accepting the humor at face value, can open the door to a therapeutic conversation.

The cancer experience tends to strengthen intimate relationships, which also is the case with testicular cancer. Partners tend to be supportive and take on some of the emotional burden of the cancer and its treatment (Rieker, 1996). Marital distress is more likely to occur in newly married couples who are still negotiating their roles. Some women find that during the treatment phase they take on a more maternal role in contrast to the expected role of sexual partner, and men find that their role of provider and sexual partner is taken away by the illness (Schover & von Eschenbach, 1984). This may be extremely challenging to the couple. Anticipatory guidance in the early stages of the disease trajectory and follow-up may help the couple to negotiate new, and hopefully temporary, roles during treatment and then allow them to return to more normal roles in recovery. Men often become quite isolated during treatment and do not communicate their thoughts and feelings to their significant others. This can cause distancing and emotional distress for the female partner (Rieker). Assisting the couple in expressing themselves—their fears, hopes, and feelings—is an important component of any counseling strategy. If the nurse does not feel competent to deal with these sorts of issues, referral to a marital therapist or social worker is appropriate and can be very helpful to the couple.

Management of fertility-related issues must begin at the time of diagnosis. All men, regardless of age, need to receive accurate information about the risk of infertility following treatment. Ideally, cryopreservation and sperm banking should be part of the immediate treatment plan, but this does not always occur. In the haste to begin treatment, it may be assumed that there is not time for collection of sperm samples for freezing. Modern techniques allow adequate sperm samples to be collected with only 24–48 hours between collections (Brown, 2003), and new in vitro fertilization techniques allow for increased success even with suboptimal fertility (Hartmann et al., 1999). However, men should be counseled realistically, and cryopreservation does not guarantee success despite advances in technique (Schmidt et al., 2004). This topic is very important but difficult for younger men who are not in a relationship, who consider a cancer diagnosis to be life-threatening and may not be able to anticipate future feelings related to infertility. In the case of minors, the patient's parents may have to make the decision, and they may be too distraught to give this topic the consideration it deserves. Advising and encouraging a teenager to collect semen samples may be too embarrassing for the parents and very challenging for healthcare providers, but it is a vital conversation, given the long-term consequences for the young man. Figure 7-1 provides an example of possible questions and dialogue using the PLISSIT model (see Figure 3-2) (Annon, 1974).

Case Study

B.R. is 32 years old and engaged to be married. He presented to his family physician two weeks ago with a painful swelling in his scrotum that he thought was related to a sports injury. His physician ordered an ultrasound that demonstrated a suspicious mass in the left testicle. The patient was referred to an oncologist, who scheduled a hemiorchiectomy three days later. The clinical nurse specialist offered to meet with B.R. and his fiancée to discuss the treatment plan and, more specifically, his options for cryopreservation of sperm.

The patient reacted strongly to this suggestion and stated that there was no point, as his life was essentially over and his fiancée would most likely leave him for a "real" man.

Questions to consider:

- What can the nurse offer to this man who is obviously greatly distressed at this early stage?
- How much or how little information is appropriate at this time?
- What strategies may be helpful for this young couple?

See Appendix B for answers to the case study questions.

Figure 7-1. Example of the PLISSIT Model in Patients With Testicular Cancer

- **Permission:** An example of this level would be to include a general statement that normalizes the topic.

  "I realize that you are overwhelmed by the diagnosis and you are probably finding it hard to think right now. One of the most common questions men have when they are diagnosed with testicular cancer is what it is going to do to their sex life. When you feel able to talk about this, please raise the topic with any of the nurses or the medical team."

- **Limited information:** In the case of a couple where the man has had an orchiectomy, the nurse should be able to give general information about resuming intercourse.

  "The loss of one testicle should not cause you difficulties with your sex life. However, in the months following the surgery, you may find that your desire is lessened, and this may have more to do with what you have been through than anything physical related to the surgery."

- **Specific suggestion:** Information at this level includes anticipatory guidance related to possible sexual consequences of medications and other treatments.

  "I know how difficult it must be for you to have to make long-term decisions for a 15-year-old son. At this time, you are probably not thinking about 10 years from now, when the question of becoming a father will be important to your son. Something that we ask men with testicular cancer to consider is banking sperm for future use. Can I give you some written information about this and schedule a time to meet with you and your son in the next few days to discuss this further before he starts his radiation therapy?"

- **Intensive therapy:** Nurses should know where to refer patients when problems or issues are disclosed that are beyond their scope of practice or expertise.

  "Your wife has told me that you have been trying to conceive for 18 months now. Many men who have been treated for testicular cancer experience problems with fertility, and before more time passes, perhaps you would like to consult with our staff in the Assisted Reproduction Clinic who can explain some options to both of you."

Conclusion

Testicular cancer primarily affects young men at the peak of their sexual lives. Because of the importance of the role of male genitalia in sexuality, diagnosis of this cancer is shocking and fear provoking. Treatment includes removal of the affected testicle and possible lymph node dissection with the addition of radiation therapy and/or chemotherapy, depending on the type and stage of the cancer. Loss of one testicle should not result in sexual dysfunction per se; however, the psychological impact of both the diagnosis and resultant treatment may precipitate significant consequences, which ideally will resolve over time. Fertility issues may be a priority for the patient, but many patients are diagnosed at a young age when they are not thinking about becoming a father. The parents of the young man may have to make the decision about preserving sperm, and this can be very difficult. These families require a great deal of support to cope with all the issues facing them and the decisions they need to make in a short period of time.

References

Aass, N., Grunfeld, B., Kaalhus, O., & Fossa, S.D. (1993). Pre- and post-treatment sexual life in testicular cancer patients: A descriptive investigation. *British Journal of Cancer, 67,* 1113–1117.

Annon, J. (1974). *The behavioral treatment of sexual problems.* Honolulu, HI: Enabling Systems.

Arai, Y., Kawakita, M., Okada, Y., & Yoshida, O. (1997). Sexuality and fertility in long-term survivors of testicular cancer. *Journal of Clinical Oncology, 15,* 1444–1448.

Brown, C.G. (2003). Testicular cancer: An overview. *Medsurg Nursing, 12,* 37–43.

Caffo, O., & Amichetti, M. (1999). Evaluation of sexual life after orchidectomy followed by radiotherapy for early-stage seminoma of the testis. *BJU International, 83,* 462–468.

Chapple, A., & Ziebland, S. (2004). The role of humor for men with testicular cancer. *Qualitative Health Research, 14,* 1123–1139.

Fegg, M.J., Gerl, A., Vollmer, T.C., Gruber, U., Jost, C., Meiler, S., et al. (2003). Subjective quality of life and sexual functioning after germ-cell tumour therapy. *British Journal of Cancer, 89,* 2202–2206.

Fleer, J., Hoekstra, H.J., Sleijfer, D.T., & Hoekstra-Weebers, J.E. (2004). Quality of life of survivors of testicular germ cell cancer: A review of the literature. *Supportive Care in Cancer, 12,* 476–486.

Gascoigne, P., Mason, M., & Roberts, E. (1999). Factors affecting presentation and delay in patients with testicular cancer. *Psycho-Oncology, 8,* 144–154.

Gurevich, M., Bishop, S., Bower, J., Malka, M., & Nyhof-Young, J. (2004). (Dis)embodying gender and sexuality in testicular cancer. *Social Science and Medicine, 58,* 1597–1607.

Hartmann, J.T., Albrecht, C., Schmoll, H.J., Kuczyk, M.A., Kollmannsberger, C., & Bokemeyer, C. (1999). Long-term effects on sexual function and fertility after treatment of testicular cancer. *British Journal of Cancer, 80,* 801–807.

Heidenreich, A., & Hofmann, R. (1999). Quality-of-life issues in the treatment of testicular cancer. *World Journal of Urology, 17,* 230–238.

Incrocci, L., Bosch, J., & Slob, A. (1999). Testicular prostheses: Body image and sexual functioning. *BJU International, 84,* 1043–1045.

Incrocci, L., Hop, W.C., Wijnmaalen, A., & Slob, A.K. (2002). Treatment outcome, body image, and sexual functioning after orchiectomy and radiotherapy for stage I–II testicular seminoma. *International Journal of Radiation Oncology, Biology, Physics, 53,* 1165–1173.

Joly, F., Heron, J.F., Kalusinski, L., Bottet, P., Brune, D., Allouache, N., et al. (2002). Quality of life in long-term survivors of testicular cancer: A population-based case-control study. *Journal of Clinical Oncology, 20,* 73–80.

Jonker-Pool, G., Hoekstra, H.J., van Imhoff, G.W., Sonneveld, D.J., Sleijfer, D.T., Van Driel, M.F., et al. (2004). Male sexuality after cancer treatment—needs for information and support: Testicular cancer compared to malignant lymphoma. *Patient Education and Counseling, 52,* 143–150.

Jonker-Pool, G., van de Wiel, H.B., Hoekstra, H.J., Sleijfer, D.T., Van Driel, M.F., Van Basten, J.P., et al. (2001). Sexual functioning after treatment for testicular cancer—review and meta-analysis of 36 empirical studies between 1975–2000. *Archives of Sexual Behavior, 30,* 55–74.

Lackner, J., Schatzl, G., Koller, A., Mazal, P., Waldhoer, T., Marberger, M., et al. (2005). Treatment of testicular cancer: Influence on pituitary-gonadal axis and sexual function. *Urology, 66,* 402–406.

Richie, J. (1993). Advances in the diagnosis and treatment of testicular cancer. *Cancer Investigation, 11,* 670–675.

Rieker, P.P. (1996). How should a man with testicular cancer be counseled and what information is available to him? *Seminars in Urologic Oncology, 14,* 17–23.

Schmidt, K., Larsen, E., Bangsboll, S., Meinertz, H., Carlsen, E., & Andersen, A. (2004). Assisted reproduction in male cancer survivors: Fertility treatment and outcome in 67 couples. *Human Reproduction, 19,* 2806–2810.

Schover, L., & von Eschenbach, A. (1984). Sexual and marital counseling with men treated for testicular cancer. *Journal of Sex and Marital Therapy, 10,* 29–40.

Spermon, J.R., Kiemeney, L.A., Meuleman, E.J., Ramos, L., Wetzels, A.M., & Witjes, J.A. (2003). Fertility in men with testicular germ cell tumors. *Fertility and Sterility, 79*(Suppl. 3), 1543–1549.

Tamburini, M., Filiberti, A., Barbieri, A., Zanoni, F., Pizzocaro, G., Barletta, L., et al. (1989). Psychological aspects of testis cancer therapy: A prospective study. *Journal of Urology, 142,* 1487–1489.

Tinkler, S.D., Howard, G.C., & Kerr, G.R. (1992). Sexual morbidity following radiotherapy for germ cell tumours of the testis. *Radiotherapy and Oncology, 25,* 207–212.

CHAPTER 8

Colorectal Cancer

Colorectal cancer treatment has significant potential for causing sexual consequences. Cancer of the colon or rectum is one of the most common cancers, particularly among men. Treatment consists of surgical removal of portions of the colon or rectum; radiation therapy may be given before or after the surgery; and chemotherapy sometimes is used as an adjunct therapy. Surgical techniques vary. The most common operations are abdominoperineal resection and anterior resection with or without creation of an anatomic pouch (Schmidt, Bestmann, Kuchler, & Kremer, 2005). Patients may have a permanent colostomy, or a temporary colostomy may be created while the anastomosis in the colon heals. The standard surgical procedure for cancer in the lower part of the rectum is total mesorectal excision, which removes the rectum and lymphatics and may cause extensive nerve damage and sexual dysfunction, particularly for men (Schmidt, Bestmann, Kuchler, Longo, & Kremer, 2005c). The damage to nerves in the area appears to significantly interfere with a range of sexual responses and causes a number of dysfunctions, including erectile difficulties and absent or retrograde ejaculation in men and dyspareunia and diminished orgasm in women. More modern techniques allow for preservation of nerves with less damage to sexual function (Bonnel et al., 2002).

The Effect of Colorectal Cancer on Sexuality

Colorectal cancer more commonly occurs in individuals older than 60, when age-associated sexual changes already may have begun to appear. However, individuals with familial polyposis coli may have a colectomy to prevent the development of colon cancer. These individuals usually are much younger and may experience distress related to sexual difficulties. Older men diagnosed with colorectal cancer already may be experiencing erectile difficulties, and women may have noticed postmenopausal changes. The type of surgery performed is implicated in sexual side effects, which will add to current sexual difficulties. Abdominoperineal resection and anterior resection with the creation of a pouch appear to have the worst side effects (Schmidt, Bestmann, Kuchler, Longo, & Kremer, 2005b). This most likely is the result of extensive scarring in the pelvis along with damage to nerve plexuses (Schmidt, Bestmann, Kuchler, & Kremer, 2005). Younger patients (< 69 years of age) and men are more likely to report sexual side effects, and men are more likely to be distressed by any changes (Schmidt, Bestmann, Kuchler, Longo, & Kremer, 2005a). Radiation and chemotherapy also have sexual side effects, which are dependent on the dose and extent of radiation or the specific chemotherapeutic agents prescribed (Jenks, Morin, & Tomaselli, 1997). Preoperative radiation therapy is posited as making surgical dissection more difficult, resulting in more damage to nerves and vascular damage, thus causing fibrosis of blood vessels supplying the nerves (Bonnel et al., 2002).

Treatment of Colorectal Cancer

After the extensive surgery required to excise malignant tissue and create a stoma, a lack of desire for sex is common (Weerakoon, 2001). Erectile and ejaculatory problems are also reported, which can affect frequency of sexual activity as well as satisfaction. For women, the most frequently reported sexual side effect is painful intercourse, or dyspareunia, and changes to the frequency and quality of orgasm (Sprangers, Taal, Aaronson, & te Velde, 1995). This often results in decreased sexual activity. The dyspareunia may be caused by scarring around the vagina (Platell, Thompson, & Makin, 2004), particularly in the upper third of the vagina, which is the area that usually expands during arousal. For men, disruption of two specific nerve plexuses affects sexual functioning. The hypogastric nerve plexus is associated with normal erectile functioning, and the sacral plexus is associated with ejaculation. Surgery or adjunctive radiation treatment may damage these nerves (Bonnel et al., 2002). This damage affects the man's ability to achieve an erection and also may result in absence of ejaculation or retrograde ejaculation (where emission enters the bladder rather than flowing out of the urethra) (Sprunk & Alteneder, 2000). Retrograde ejaculation interferes with fertility. Orgasmic changes also may be noted, including diminution or altered sensation.

For couples or individuals who enjoy anal sex, surgical removal of the rectum can present a unique challenge. It often is assumed that all gay men include anal intercourse as part of their sexual repertoire. This is not the case, and nurses must ask a gay patient whether the loss of a functioning rectum will pose a challenge beyond that which it would for anyone else. Nurses should approach the patient about finding alternatives to anal intercourse, if that is a usual part of the patient's sexual activity, in the same nonjudgmental and caring manner as they would use while helping any patient to explore alternative sexual positions or activities.

Body Image Issues

Certainly the most far-reaching sexual consequences are those associated with the creation of a stoma. One major factor in sexuality for the ostomate is the change in body image because of both the stoma and the appliance worn to collect feces. Ostomates often will react with shock and disgust soon after surgery and report feeling sexually unattractive. Fear of the sexual partner's reaction to the stoma/appliance further complicates this reaction. Some partners may have a negative response to the stoma, others are cautious in their response, and some will be positive (Gloeckner, 1991). Common fears related to the stoma itself concern the appearance of the stoma and anxiety about harming the stoma or causing pain if it is touched during sexual activity. Ostomates also may be concerned about odor, leakage, gas, or noises emitted by the appliance (Golis, 1996).

Both men and women appear to experience distress related to body image changes, and the speed with which cancer surgery is carried out might have something to do with this. Too little time may be spent in preparing patients for these changes, and patients may be more concerned with surviving than anticipating what the stoma may look like and how it will affect body image (Golis, 1996; Shell, 1992).

A colostomy is associated with feces and defecation, a topic that carries strong cultural and social taboos and aversion. Ostomates must find a way of controlling their own disgust and fear of others' reactions to their stoma's function, odor, noises, and appearance (Manderson, 2005). This compounds the initial fear of death with a cancer diagnosis, the continued fear of recurrence, and the uncertainty that accompanies the cancer experience for many. Other reported reactions of patients with stomas include feeling vulnerable, a sense of mutilation, depression, despair, and violation (Shell, 1992). The stoma always looks red and moist, and manipulation often causes some superficial bleeding. This can provoke anxiety in many patients and their partners (Weerakoon, 2001). Some ostomates report that they feel baby-like: There is focus on elimination of waste, which is visible and no longer private, and they have to carry additional supplies wherever they go, much like a mother has to carry supplies for a baby. This feeling conflicts with an adult sense of self and self-control and can be a significant psychological barrier to the adult role of sexual partner and equal (Manderson).

Relationship issues may surface in the months following the acute phase of the surgery and recovery. In this phase, the partner often provides a great deal of physical and intimate care and essentially takes on the role of nurse and care provider rather than that of sexual partner. Making the transition from care provider to lover can be difficult, and some relationships falter in the face of both the acute and long-term stress. Because many people with colorectal cancer are older, the challenges brought on by the cancer and associated sexual problems often signal the end of sexual activity in the relationship, which does not mean that the couple welcomes this. Feelings of grief and loss with cessation of sexual activity are common for both men and women.

Nursing Interventions in the Care of Individuals With Colorectal Cancer

Preparation for stoma surgery and anticipation of sexual problems ideally should begin in the preoperative period. Strategies to help patients in coping with the resultant changes in their sexual lives include providing written information with explicit pictures of the stoma and ostomy appliances, as well as encouraging counseling with both professionals and ostomates who have lived the experience. Involvement of the partners is vital, and they should be offered the opportunity for individual counseling. In joint sessions, partners often tend to subjugate their needs and fears in the act of being supportive.

Information Sharing

Information sharing after ostomy is an important aspect of care (MacArthur, 1996). Stoma care nurses provide much of the ongoing care of patients with ostomies, and they usually do not discuss sexuality unless the patient asks a question. These nurses report that young men are counseled about sexuality more often than women. Barriers to including this content in regular patient interaction were stated as cultural limitations, discomfort in dealing with older patients, and difficulty in expressing sexual language (Borwell, 1997).

Interventions for Treatment-Related Side Effects

Problems with lack of interest in sex are not easily treated. Fatigue and emotional consequences resulting from diagnosis and surgery play a major role in sexual interest, and many patients report a total absence of sexual interest for a significant period of time during and after treatment. When this is compounded by the feelings associated with adapting to a stoma, interest in sex may not return for a long time. Counseling the couple together and encouraging them to verbalize their feelings and thoughts can help to promote constructive communication about sexual wants and needs. After extensive surgical and adjunct therapy, sexual functioning and activity may never return to preoperative levels. Depending on the age of the couple, this may be acceptable. However, other couples may find this hard to accept and may want to try medical and psychosocial interventions to maintain sexual activity.

Specific suggestions for patients experiencing sexual difficulties depend on the major issue identified. Medical treatments similar to those suggested for men with prostate cancer can help problems with erectile functioning. A graduated trial of therapy beginning with phosphodiesterase-5 inhibitors (sildenafil, tadalafil, and vardenafil) and then the vacuum pump, intraurethral alprostadil, intracorporeal injections, and surgical implants may be useful until the man finds a therapy that is effective and acceptable to him and his partner.

Retrograde ejaculation generally is not a major problem for older men to whom fertility is not of significance. Receiving an explanation of why this occurs usually is sufficient for patients to accept this change. Men may notice a qualitative difference in the sensation of orgasm in the absence of the propulsion of ejaculate in the urethra, but this usually is not identified as a major sexual problem. For younger men who want to have children, postcoital collection of urine and extraction of sperm may be an option. Referral to a fertility specialist is necessary in these circumstances.

For women experiencing painful intercourse, trying alternative positions for penetrative intercourse and vaginal dilatation may prevent further scar tissue development and stretch existing tissue. Using positions for intercourse where the woman can control the depth of thrusting can be helpful in controlling dyspareunia. The woman-on-top and side-by-side positions can be helpful. Some women prefer to avoid penetrative intercourse altogether, and nurses or counselors can encourage non-penetrative sexual activity such as oral sex, mutual or solitary masturbation, massage, hugging and kissing, or "outercourse," where the man places his erect penis between the thighs of the female partner and initiates thrusting in that position. Acceptance of alternatives to penetrative intercourse can be challenging for older couples whose sexual scripts and activities have remained the same for many years and who are not highly motivated to make significant changes in this area of their lives. Women can insert a clean, well-lubricated finger into their vagina to gently stretch the tissue. Over time they can do this with two or three fingers to maintain patency of the vagina and prevent further fibrosis and pain. Women also can learn to use a dilator in the same manner as women with gynecologic cancer treated with radiation therapy.

A variety of strategies exist to address aesthetic challenges posed by the stoma and appliance. These include using a belt or cummerbund to stabilize the appliance, emptying the appliance prior to any sexual activity, and using an opaque cover over the pouch. Some people may be able to use a stoma cap during sexual activity, which removes the challenge of having a bag attached to the abdomen. Using a smaller, closed pouch during sex also might be a good strategy, as there is less chance of leakage and it is less bulky than the usual pouches. Some women find that using crotchless underwear to conceal the stoma and appliance allows access to the genitalia and also reduces the visual impact of the stoma/appliance. Wearing a teddy or peignoir also can help women to feel more attractive; however, a comfortable T-shirt or men's cotton shirt also can serve the same purpose, as long as the woman is comfortable and confident. Men may find that wearing boxer shorts stabilizes the appliance, and the opening allows for access to the genitals.

Bathing/showering before sexual activity and using perfumes or deodorizers to minimize odor might be helpful. Some people are able to irrigate their colostomy and thus avoid the collection of feces in the bag. Irrigating just before sexual activity will allow for the use of a stoma cover, which may reduce anxiety and make sex feel more "normal." Avoiding foods and drinks that cause gas or odor also can help to prevent leakage or inflation of the bag.

Using alternative sexual positions also may help to reduce discomfort or anxiety related to pain. The woman-on-top position prevents pressure from being applied to the stoma or pouch. The side-lying position on the side of the stoma allows the pouch to fall away toward the surface and thus not come between the partners. The rear-entry position, performed either kneeling or lying down, where the ostomate lies in front of the partner, also prevents pressure on the stoma or appliance. These positions may be challenging for couples who have impaired mobility or other disabilities. They also may be challenging for couples who for many years have had sex in only the missionary position and who do not want to change their usual way of interacting. It is essential to allow the couple to explore options that are acceptable to them, their values, and their previous activities.

As with other cancers, it often is a challenge to bring up the topic of sexuality in the face of life-threatening disease. Figure 8-1 shows an example of how to use the BETTER model (see Figure 3-3) to initiate this conversation with patients with colorectal cancer (Mick, Hughes, & Cohen, 2003).

Case Study

J.H. recently had surgery for colorectal cancer, and she is scheduled to begin chemotherapy next week. She and her husband have come to the clinic for pretreatment teaching related to the chemotherapy and for insertion of a central line. J.H. needs to get up frequently to check her stoma and appliance, and while she is in the washroom, her husband hints that things are stressful at home. On further questioning, he states that she seems to be pushing him away, and he is no longer able to kiss or hug her. The couple does not have children, and he describes feeling very alone.

Questions to consider:
- How should the nurse integrate this information into the discussion with the patient?
- What should the nurse regard as essential for this couple to know at this stage of the patient's therapy?
- What questions would the nurse need to ask to get a deeper understanding of what this couple is facing?

See Appendix B for answers to the case study questions.

Figure 8-1. Example of the BETTER Model in Patients With Colorectal Cancer

- **Bringing up the topic:** Nurses are encouraged to raise the issue of sexuality with patients.

  "Women who have a colostomy often have questions about what this will mean for their sex life in the future. What concerns do you have at the present time?"

- **Explaining that sex is a part of quality of life:** This helps to normalize the discussion and may help patients to feel less embarrassed or alone in having a problem.

  "It may feel like sex is the last thing on your mind right now; however, as you recover over the next few months, you will probably find yourself once again becoming interested in that aspect of your life."

- **Telling patients that resources will be found to address their concerns:** This step suggests to patients that even if the nurse does not have the immediate solution to the problem or question, others are available who can help.

  "We refer all our patients with colorectal cancer to the Ostomy Foundation for information, education, and support. The stoma nurses are very skilled in addressing sexual concerns, and I hope that you will discuss any concerns you have with them."

- **Timing the intervention:** Patients may not be ready to deal with sexual issues at the time a problem is identified, but they can ask for information at any time in the future.

  "Much of your energy in the next few weeks will most likely be directed at recovery and getting used to dealing with your stoma. When you are ready to talk about sexual concerns, help is available through the Ostomy Foundation or the nurses in the outpatient clinic where you will receive your follow-up care."

- **Educating patients about the sexual side effects of treatment:** Educating patients about potential side effects from treatments does not mean that they will occur. However, informing patients about sexual side effects is as important as informing them about any other side effects.

  "Over time you may notice that your vagina feels smaller or tighter. This is a result of scar tissue formation in your pelvis after the surgery. You may need to stretch that area to make penetrative intercourse more comfortable. Conversely, some couples focus on alternatives to penetrative intercourse."

(Continued on next page)

Figure 8-1. Example of the BETTER Model in Patients With Colorectal Cancer
(Continued)

- **Recording:** A brief notation that a discussion about sexuality or sexual side effects occurred is important.

  "Potential side effects related to the planned surgery were discussed. Patient was given reading material as well as contact information for the Ostomy Foundation."

Conclusion

Treatment for colorectal cancer has significant potential for sexual consequences. Patients either will have a permanent ostomy or will undergo sphincter-preserving surgery that obviates the need for a permanent ostomy. The damage to nerves in the area appears to significantly interfere with a range of sexual responses and causes a number of dysfunctions, including erectile difficulties, absent or retrograde ejaculation, dyspareunia, and diminished orgasm. For those with a stoma and external device, body image issues have a profound effect on sexual self-schema.

References

Bonnel, C., Parc, Y.R., Pocard, M., Dehni, N., Caplin, S., Parc, R., et al. (2002). Effects of preoperative radiotherapy for primary resectable rectal adenocarcinoma on male sexual and urinary function. *Diseases of the Colon and Rectum, 45,* 934–939.

Borwell, B. (1997). Psychological considerations of stoma care nursing. *Nursing Standard, 11,* 49–53.

Gloeckner, M. (1991). Perceptions of sexuality after ostomy surgery. *Journal of Enterostomal Therapy, 18,* 36–38.

Golis, A. (1996). Sexual issues for the person with an ostomy. *Journal of Wound, Ostomy, and Continence Nursing, 23,* 33–37.

Jenks, J., Morin, K., & Tomaselli, N. (1997). The influence of ostomy surgery on body image in patients with cancer. *Applied Nursing Research, 10,* 174–180.

MacArthur, A. (1996). Sexuality and the stoma: Helping patients to cope. *Nursing Times, 92*(39), 34–35.

Manderson, L. (2005). Boundary breaches: The body, sex and sexuality after stoma surgery. *Social Science and Medicine, 61,* 405–415.

Mick, J., Hughes, M., & Cohen, M. (2003). Sexuality and cancer: How oncology nurses can address it BETTER. *Oncology Nursing Forum, 30*(Suppl. 2), 152–153.

Platell, C.F., Thompson, P.J., & Makin, G.B. (2004). Sexual health in women following pelvic surgery for rectal cancer. *British Journal of Surgery, 91,* 465–468.

Schmidt, C.E., Bestmann, B., Kuchler, T., & Kremer, B. (2005). Factors influencing sexual function in patients with rectal cancer. *International Journal of Impotence Research, 17,* 231–238.

Schmidt, C.E., Bestmann, B., Kuchler, T., Longo, W.E., & Kremer, B. (2005a). Impact of age on quality of life in patients with rectal cancer. *World Journal of Surgery, 29,* 190–197.

Schmidt, C.E., Bestmann, B., Kuchler, T., Longo, W.E., & Kremer, B. (2005b). Prospective evaluation of quality of life of patients receiving either abdominoperineal resection or sphincter-preserving procedure for rectal cancer. *Annals of Surgical Oncology, 12,* 117–123.

Schmidt, C.E., Bestmann, B., Kuchler, T., Longo, W.E., & Kremer, B. (2005c). Ten-year historic cohort of quality of life and sexuality in patients with rectal cancer. *Diseases of the Colon and Rectum, 48,* 483–492.

Shell, J.A. (1992). The psychosexual impact of ostomy surgery. *Progressions: Developments in Ostomy and Wound Care, 4,* 3–15.

Sprangers, M.A., Taal, B.G., Aaronson, N.K., & te Velde, A. (1995). Quality of life in colorectal cancer. Stoma vs. nonstoma patients. *Diseases of the Colon and Rectum, 38,* 361–369.

Sprunk, E., & Alteneder, R. (2000). The impact of ostomy on sexuality. *Clinical Journal of Oncology Nursing, 4,* 85–89.

Weerakoon, P. (2001). Sexuality and the person with a stoma. *Sexuality and Disability, 19,* 121–129.

CHAPTER 9

Hematologic Cancer

Leukemia commonly occurs in children or middle-aged adults. Leukemia presents in either acute or chronic forms, and the treatments for this disease, commonly chemotherapy with or without bone marrow transplantation, are potentially responsible for sexual difficulties in both the short and long term. Hodgkin lymphoma typically occurs in older adults but also is seen in young adults. Non-Hodgkin lymphoma occurs across the life span from adolescence into old age. As with leukemia, treatment usually involves chemotherapy; however, radiation alone or in combination with chemotherapy may be offered depending on the stage. Late-stage Hodgkin lymphoma also may be treated with bone marrow transplantation.

Patients with leukemia may present with fatigue, malaise, and decreased tolerance for exercise and activities of daily living. Bruising and bleeding may occur, and weight loss is not unusual. For those diagnosed with an acute form of the disease, the life-threatening aspect of the diagnosis may override concerns for sexual functioning. Chronic leukemia, however, also takes its toll, and both forms of the disease are noted as having a high degree of uncertainty (McGrath, 1999). Patients with Hodgkin lymphoma generally present with one or more enlarged lymph nodes, whereas patients with non-Hodgkin lymphoma generally have a more diverse presentation depending on the tissues or organs involved (Pastorek, 1998; Ziegfeld & Shelton, 1998).

The Effect of Hematologic Cancer on Sexuality

Chemotherapy for leukemia is given based on the type of disease (acute or chronic, myeloid or lymphocytic), and all chemotherapeutic agents have the potential to affect sexual functioning. Alkylating agents (busulfan, cyclophosphamide, ifosfamide, nitrogen mustard) are implicated in causing loss of fertility in addition to significant nausea and vomiting. Antimetabolites (cladribine, cytarabine, hydroxyurea, methotrexate) also are used frequently, and they can cause general malaise, mucositis, and nausea and vomiting, all of which will affect sexual functioning. Antitumor antibiotics (daunorubicin, doxorubicin, mitoxantrone) also cause nausea and vomiting and mucositis. Plant alkaloids (vincristine) are known to cause peripheral neuropathy, which may affect sensation. All these agents are used in various combinations, and the side effects may be global (Lubejko & Ashley, 1998). The chemotherapeutic agents used in the treatment of Hodgkin lymphoma include alkylating agents (carmustine, cyclophosphamide, dacarbazine, nitrogen mustard, thiotepa), antitumor antibiotics (bleomycin, doxorubicin), and plant alkaloids (etoposide, vincristine). Non-Hodgkin lymphoma is treated with alkylating agents (carmustine, ifosfamide, thiotepa), antimetabolites (cytarabine, methotrexate), antitumor antibiotics (bleomycin, doxorubicin), and plant alkaloids (vinblastine, vincristine) (Lubejko & Ashley).

When radiation therapy is given for lymphoma, the side effects are dictated by site (chest, abdomen, brain, or spine) and the amount of radiation given (low or high dose). Side effects are dependent on these and other factors. Generally, the ovaries or testicles are shielded if radiation is given to the abdomen. Cranial-spinal radiation is used as prophylaxis for patients with leukemia and non-Hodgkin lymphoma. This has a direct effect on the hypothalamus, thus directly affecting production of gonadotropin-releasing hormone (Byrne et al., 2004) and leading to ovarian failure. This will affect long-term fertility as well as predispose the woman to early menopause and its attendant symptoms, which may have an impact on sexuality.

Treatment of Hematologic Cancer

Treatment of sexual difficulties for individuals with leukemia and lymphoma should begin with a detailed assessment of sexual functioning to identify any problems and clear up any misinformation. This is particularly important for patients who will be undergoing bone marrow transplantation (Molassiotis et al., 1995; Wingard et al., 1992). Treatment of preexisting problems can prevent these from becoming worse or intractable (Watson et al., 1999). A frank discussion about the sexual side effects of the treatment will allow individuals or couples to prepare for potential difficulties (Molassiotis et al.).

Treatment-Related Side Effects

The sexual consequences of leukemia and lymphoma affect all aspects of sexual functioning and are quite common. Men with lymphoma report diminished desire, arousal, erections, and orgasm (Jonker-Pool et al., 2004; Kornblith et al., 1992). Men treated for either leukemia or lymphoma in childhood have noted shrinkage of the testicles; however, many function normally in the sexual domain as adults (Relander, Cavallin-Stahl, Garwicz, Olsson, & Willen, 2000). Interferon-alpha sometimes is used to treat chronic myeloid leukemia and has been shown to cause decreased sexual interest, arousal, and pleasure, which is worse for patients older than 50 (Homewood, Watson, Richards, Halsey, & Shepherd, 2003). Women who survive childhood leukemia appear to experience some alteration in their sexual self-schema, with later initiation of sexual intercourse and more negative body image (Puukko et al., 1997). Women also report decreased desire for sex and decreased satisfaction; this seems to resolve over time and therefore may be related to fatigue from the cancer or treatment (Mumma, Mashberg, & Lesko, 1992).

Bone marrow transplantation frequently is used as curative therapy for leukemia. High-dose chemotherapy with total body irradiation usually is performed before the transplantation of either the patient's own marrow (autologous) or donor marrow (allogeneic). This combination has demonstrated the greatest impact on sexual and reproductive functioning (Davis, 2006). However, many patients report experiencing extensive sexual difficulties before transplantation. These difficulties are assumed to arise because of the cancer diagnosis itself and the emotional consequences of facing the diagnosis and future treatment (Marks, Crilley, Nezu, & Nezu, 1996).

In the year following transplantation, sexual difficulties are very common. Patients often experience profound fatigue and still feel the effects of high-dose chemotherapy and total body irradiation (Marks, Friedman, Carpini, Nezu, & Nezu, 1997). In addition, the effects of graft-versus-host disease may manifest at this time, and skin changes commonly occur as a result. Patients may feel unattractive because of alopecia and surgical scars (Wingard, Curbow, Baker, Zbora, & Piantadosi, 1992). Women seem to fare particularly poorly in this regard (Heinonen et al., 2001).

Many transplant recipients experience a decline in sexual functioning most acutely in the first year following transplant, and these difficulties tend to persist in the long term. For men, erectile difficulties are common, and many will experience ejaculatory problems, which include delayed and/or dry ejaculation. The erectile difficulties may be caused by damage to the cavernosal tissues of the penis as a result of radiation therapy. Dry ejaculation may occur because of testicular damage, also caused by radiation (Chatterjee et al., 2000). For women, vaginal atrophy causes pain resulting from decreased lubrication, and both sexes go through body image changes (Neitzert et al., 1998). Women also experience diminished orgasm. Both sexes report difficulty in reestablishing sexual relationships after long periods of having to limit physical contact because of isolation and precautions to prevent infection (Syrjala et al., 1998). The symptoms of premature menopause often are harsher than with normal menopause, and most women who have had total body irradiation will experience total ovarian failure. Depression and fatigue tend to exacerbate these symptoms (Watson et al., 1999). Prolactinemia also is fairly common in transplant recipients, and this is known to cause decreased libido in men (Molassiotis, van den Akker, Milligan, & Boughton, 1995).

The psychological effects of the disease and transplantation also may affect sexual functioning, with women and older patients experiencing more problems (Molassiotis & Morris, 1999). For adolescents receiving bone marrow transplantation, damage to gonadal function varies with the recipient's age. Prepubertal boys may recover sufficient hormonal function to develop secondary sex characteristics; however, testicular volume may be reduced. Prepubertal girls seem to recover gonadal function better than those treated during and after puberty (Bakker et al., 2000).

Graft-versus-host disease is one of the potential side effects of bone marrow trans-plantation and may affect multiple organs and systems, including the skin and vagina. Patients report that skin changes have an impact on self-image, which is intimately connected to sexuality and sexual self-schema. There are reports of vulvovaginal symptoms caused by graft-versus-host disease: sticky leukorrhea, denuded areas of vulval mucosa, and a subjective experience of burning and pain. If left untreated, this may result in vaginal or vulval stenosis, causing dyspareunia (Spinelli et al., 2003) and even total occlusion of the vaginal canal (Lee et al., 2000).

Stem cell transplantation is a common treatment for chronic myeloid leukemia, especially for younger patients. These individuals also experience sexual consequences years after treatment, with decreases in the amount of sexual activity, level of sexual interest and pleasure, and ability to have sex being reported (Hayden et al., 2004).

Nursing Interventions in the Care of Individuals With Hematologic Cancer

Informing patients about sexual side effects should be part of the informed consent process just as other potential side effects are (Heinonen et al., 2001). An important aspect of preparation for bone marrow transplantation is assessment of the individuals' and partners' expectations in relation to sexual changes, which enables them to be realistic in their expectations and helps to avoid problems related to misconceptions (Tierney, 2004). Figure 9-1 lists examples of questions to ask as part of a sexual assessment using the PLISSIT model (Annon, 1974).

Hormone therapy may be prescribed to alleviate menopausal symptoms for women (Neitzert et al., 1998). However, these should be used with caution, given the findings of increased risk for cardiovascular events and breast cancer for women on this therapy. Little evidence exists as to whether these same risks apply to women

---

Figure 9-1. Example of the PLISSIT Model in Patients With Hematologic Cancer

- **Permission:** An example of this level would be to include a general statement that normalizes the topic.

  "Most of my patients are about the same age as you, and many have questions about sexuality and sexual functioning. I would be happy to answer any questions you have now or at any other time during and after your treatment."

- **Limited information:** In the case of a couple where one person has had a bone marrow transplant, the nurse should be able to give general information about resuming intercourse.

  "Many bone marrow recipients and their partners wonder when it is safe to resume intercourse. When you have the interest and energy, it is fine to go ahead."

- **Specific suggestion:** Information at this level includes anticipatory guidance related to possible sexual consequences of medications and other treatments.

  "You may want to take a little extra time for sexual stimulation, as it can take a little longer to become aroused. After avoiding intimate contact for so long while preparing for the transplant, many people report that they are anxious, and this can affect your ability to become aroused."

- **Intensive therapy:** Nurses should know where to refer patients when problems or issues are disclosed that are beyond the scope of practice or expertise of the nurse.

  "It sounds to me like you would benefit from talking to a sexual medicine expert who will be able to help you with the erectile difficulties you have described. Some medications have been shown to be helpful. With your permission, I will make that referral."

---

experiencing premature menopause as a result of treatment (Chao et al., 1992; Tierney, 2004). Prevention of vaginal stenosis includes having regular penetrative intercourse if the woman has a partner. If the woman does not have a partner or is not desirous of penetrative intercourse, using vaginal dilators can help to maintain patency of the vagina, particularly for women with graft-versus-host disease. Applying local estrogen cream also might help to alleviate symptoms of vaginal atrophy. Using vaginal moisturizers such as Replens® (Lil' Drug Store Products, Cedar Rapids, IA) also can provide local relief. For more severe stenosis, steroidal creams applied to the vagina may be of use (Spinelli et al., 2003).

Hormone therapy for men in the form of testosterone is controversial and may not improve erectile functioning. Hyperprolactinemia may be treated with bromocriptine (Tierney, 2004). The use of erectile aids such as sildenafil, vardenafil, or tadalafil may be helpful for men who are experiencing erectile dysfunction. However, a thorough exploration of the psychogenic components of this condition may prove to be beneficial, and a referral to a sex therapist should be made.

The role of fatigue, depression, and anxiety should not be underestimated in this population, and the impact of these on sexual interest and ability should be acknowledged.

Patients may need to carefully plan sexual activity to occur at times when they are less fatigued. They also might want to consider alternatives to penetrative intercourse if this is too energy depleting. As with all other kinds of cancer, penetrative intercourse may not be possible, and patients and their partners may benefit from guidance and validation that although intercourse is not possible at this time, their sex life is not over. Patients who are depressed or anxious will benefit from referral to a mental health expert, who may prescribe an antidepressant or anxiolytic. The patient needs to know that these medications often have a negative effect on libido, arousal, or orgasm (Ferguson, 2001).

Case Study

P.B. is 43 years old and was recently diagnosed with acute leukemia. He is on the list to have an autologous bone marrow transplant and is expected to begin induction chemotherapy in one month. He mentions to you that he is getting married this summer and has some concerns about the total body irradiation he will have and whether this will affect his wife if they are sexually active.

Questions to consider:
- What additional questions should the nurse ask this man?
- What anticipatory guidance can be given to him at this time?

See Appendix B for answers to the case study questions.

Conclusion

Many of the drugs used to treat hematologic malignancies have significant side effects that may interfere with the normal sexual response cycle. Increasing evidence has shown that both bone marrow and stem cell transplants also have an effect on sexual functioning and fertility. Many of the patients with these conditions are young and at a stage in the life cycle where these issues are a very real part of quality of life and an important part of relationship satisfaction.

References

Annon, J. (1974). *The behavioral treatment of sexual problems.* Honolulu, HI: Enabling Systems.
Bakker, B., Massa, G., Oostdijk, W., Van Weel-Sipman, M., Vossen, J., & Wit, J. (2000). Pubertal development and growth after total-body irradiation and bone marrow transplantation for haematological malignancies. *European Journal of Pediatrics, 159,* 31–37.

Byrne, J., Fears, T., Mills, J., Zeltzer, L., Sklar, C., & Nicholson, H. (2004). Fertility in women treated with cranial radiotherapy for childhood acute lymphoblastic leukemia. *Pediatric Blood and Cancer, 4,* 589–597.

Chao, N.J., Tierney, D.K., Bloom, J.R., Long, G.D., Barr, T.A., Stallbaum, B.A., et al. (1992). Dynamic assessment of quality of life after autologous bone marrow transplantation. *Blood, 80,* 825–830.

Chatterjee, R., Andrews, H., McGarrigle, H., Kottaridis, P., Lees, W., Mackinnon, S., et al. (2000). Cavernosal arterial insufficiency is a major component of erectile dysfunction in some recipients of high-dose chemotherapy/chemoradiotherapy for haematological malignancies. *Bone Marrow Transplantation, 25,* 1185–1189.

Davis, M. (2006). Fertility considerations for female adolescent and young adult patients following cancer therapy: A guide for counseling patients and their families. *Clinical Journal of Oncology Nursing, 10,* 213–219.

Ferguson, J.M. (2001). The effects of antidepressants on sexual functioning in depressed patients: A review. *Journal of Clinical Psychiatry, 62*(Suppl. 3), 22–34.

Hayden, P.J., Keogh, F., Ni, C.M., Carroll, M., Crowley, M., Fitzsimon, N., et al. (2004). A single-centre assessment of long-term quality-of-life status after sibling allogeneic stem cell transplantation for chronic myeloid leukaemia in first chronic phase. *Bone Marrow Transplantation, 34,* 545–556.

Heinonen, H., Volin, L., Uutela, A., Zevon, M., Barrick, C., & Ruutu, T. (2001). Gender-associated differences in the quality of life after allogenic BMT. *Bone Marrow Transplantation, 28,* 503–509.

Homewood, J., Watson, M., Richards, S.M., Halsey, J., & Shepherd, P.C. (2003). Treatment of CML using IFN-alpha: Impact on quality of life. *Hematology Journal, 4,* 253–262.

Jonker-Pool, G., Hoekstra, H.J., van Imhoff, G.W., Sonneveld, D.J., Sleijfer, D.T., Van Driel, M.F., et al. (2004). Male sexuality after cancer treatment—needs for information and support: Testicular cancer compared to malignant lymphoma. *Patient Education and Counseling, 52,* 143–150.

Kornblith, A.B., Anderson, J., Cella, D.F., Tross, S., Zuckerman, E., Cherin, E., et al. (1992). Hodgkin disease survivors at increased risk for problems in psychosocial adaptation. The Cancer and Leukemia Group B. *Cancer, 70,* 2214–2224.

Lee, W.L., Yuan, C.C., Chao, H.T., Chen, P.M., Lin, H.D., & Wang, P.H. (2000). Vaginal obliteration after total body irradiation and chemotherapy as treatment for acute myeloid leukemia. *European Journal of Obstetrics, Gynecology, and Reproductive Biology, 90,* 77–79.

Lubejko, B., & Ashley, B. (1998). Chemotherapy. In C. Ziegfeld, B. Lubejko, & B. Shelton (Eds.), *Oncology fact finder: Manual of cancer care* (2nd ed., pp. 30–47). Philadelphia: Lippincott Williams & Wilkins.

Marks, D., Crilley, P., Nezu, C., & Nezu, A. (1996). Sexual dysfunction prior to high-dose chemotherapy and bone marrow transplantation. *Bone Marrow Transplantation, 17,* 595–599.

Marks, D., Friedman, S., Carpini, L., Nezu, C., & Nezu, A. (1997). A prospective study of the effects of high-dose chemotherapy and bone marrow transplantation on sexual function in the first year after transplant. *Bone Marrow Transplantation, 19,* 819–822.

McGrath, P. (1999). Update on psychosocial research on leukaemia for social work practitioners. *Social Work in Health Care, 29,* 1–20.

Molassiotis, A., & Morris, P. (1999). Quality of life in patients with chronic myeloid leukemia after unrelated donor bone marrow transplantation. *Cancer Nursing, 22,* 340–349.

Molassiotis, A., van den Akker, O., Milligan, D., & Boughton, B. (1995). Gonadal function and psychosexual adjustment in male long-term survivors of bone marrow transplantation. *Bone Marrow Transplantation, 16,* 253–259.

Mumma, G.H., Mashberg, D., & Lesko, L.M. (1992). Long-term psychosexual adjustment of acute leukemia survivors: Impact of marrow transplantation versus conventional chemotherapy. *General Hospital Psychiatry, 14,* 43–55.

Neitzert, C., Ritvo, P., Dancey, J., Weiser, K., Murray, C., & Avery, J. (1998). The psychosocial impact of bone marrow transplantation: A review of the literature. *Bone Marrow Transplantation, 22,* 409–422.

Pastorek, M. (1998). Leukemia. In C. Ziegfeld, B. Lubejko, & B. Shelton (Eds.), *Oncology fact finder: Manual of cancer care* (2nd ed., pp. 195–205). Philadelphia: Lippincott Williams & Wilkins.

Puukko, L.R., Hirvonen, E., Aalberg, V., Hovi, L., Rautonen, J., & Siimes, M.A. (1997). Sexuality of young women surviving leukaemia. *Archives of Disease in Childhood, 76,* 197–202.

Relander, T., Cavallin-Stahl, E., Garwicz, S., Olsson, A.M., & Willen, M. (2000). Gonadal and sexual function in men treated for childhood cancer. *Medical and Pediatric Oncology, 35,* 52–63.

Spinelli, S., Chiodi, S., Costantini, S., Van Lint, M.T., Raiola, A.M., Ravera, G.B., et al. (2003). Female genital tract graft-versus-host disease following allogeneic bone marrow transplantation. *Haematologica, 88,* 1163–1168.

Syrjala, K., Roth-Roemer, S., Abrams, J., Scanlan, J., Chapko, M., Visser, S., et al. (1998). Prevalence and predictors of sexual dysfunction in long-term survivors of marrow transplantation. *Journal of Clinical Oncology, 16,* 3148–3157.

Tierney, D.K. (2004). Sexuality following hematopoietic cell transplantation. *Clinical Journal of Oncology Nursing, 8,* 43–47.

Watson, M., Wheatley, K., Harrison, G., Zittoun, R., Gray, R., Goldstone, A., et al. (1999). Severe adverse impact on sexual functioning and fertility of bone marrow transplantation, either allogeneic or autologous, compared with consolidation chemotherapy alone. *Cancer, 86,* 1231–1239.

Wingard, J., Curbow, B., Baker, F., Zbora, J., & Piantadosi, S. (1992). Sexual satisfaction in survivors of bone marrow transplantation. *Bone Marrow Transplantation, 9,* 185–190.

Ziegfeld, C., & Shelton, B. (1998). Malignant lymphomas. In C. Ziegfeld, B. Lubejko, & B. Shelton (Eds.), *Oncology fact finder: Manual of cancer care* (2nd ed., pp. 206–215). Philadelphia: Lippincott Williams & Wilkins.

CHAPTER 10

Cancer of the Head, Neck, and Brain

Cancer of the head and neck is described as cancer of either soft tissue or bone that lies above the clavicle but excludes the brain, spinal cord, axial skeleton, and vertebrae (Dropkin, 1999). The development of head and neck cancer is strongly associated with the use of alcohol and tobacco (Metcalfe & Fischman, 1985). It has been suggested that the personality traits that contribute to substance abuse also are associated with poor coping skills, which influence the way these individuals cope with both the diagnosis and the treatment-related side effects of the cancer (Burgess, 1994). Cancer of the brain can affect different areas of functioning depending on the location of the cancer. Tumors of the pituitary gland have specific endocrine effects.

Treatment of head and neck cancer usually involves surgery, radiation, and, increasingly, chemotherapy, depending on the site of the cancer (Hanna et al., 2004). What is common to all people diagnosed with these forms of cancer is that some degree of disfigurement will occur, which causes long-standing consequences both emotionally and functionally. This disfigurement not only is highly visible but also can have an impact on communication with others and may impair how individuals express themselves in the social and sexual realms (Dropkin, 1989).

The Effect of Head and Neck Cancer on Sexuality

For individuals who are treated with surgery, loss of skin, muscle, and bone leaves some degree of disfigurement and functional deficit. For those treated with radiation, the tattoo marks made for the treatment itself serve as visible markers of the disease and treatment. Women cannot wear makeup during the active phase of radiation treatment, and this precludes the hiding of scars and skin discoloration (Burgess, 1994).

Treatment-Related Side Effects

Direct effects of treatment result in both short- and long-term side effects, such as pain, mucositis, dry mouth, altered taste sensations, drooling, problems chewing, difficulty swallowing, dental problems, and limitations in how the lips, tongue, and jaw move (Epstein, Robertson, Emerton, Phillips, & Stevenson-Moore, 2001). Problems with pain, dry mouth, and dentition persist over time (Hammerlid, Silander, Hornestam, & Sullivan, 2001), and even long-term survivors experience problems in these domains more than 10 years after completion of treatment (Bjordal & Kaasa, 1995). These side effects have been shown to cause long-term psychological distress, including depression, and women appear to be more distressed than men (Hammerlid, Bjordal, et al., 2001), which may reflect society's attitudes about female physical attractiveness.

Disfigurement has a direct effect on sexuality. The face is an important aspect of body image, which, in turn, is intimately linked to how people see themselves as sexual beings. People use their face to express feelings and communicate what they are thinking and feeling, and components of the face are involved in all aspects of sexual expression and function. People use the mouth and nose as part of sexual expression in activities such as talking, kissing, and subconscious stimulation via pheromones. The mouth and tongue are used extensively in oral stimulation of the entire body and also in oral stimulation of the genitalia. Any alterations to the normal functioning of facial components will affect one's sexual expression.

The greater the disfigurement, the greater the sexual problems experienced by the individual (Hanna et al., 2004). The individual with cancer can perceive any form of facial disfigurement as a barrier, and it may, in reality, be a challenge to sexual partners also (Monga, Tan, Ostermann, & Monga, 1997). Altered self-image is tied to self-esteem. People with substance abuse problems, often an underlying factor in head and neck cancer, already may have significant self-esteem issues that affect their intimate relationships. In addition, alcohol and tobacco use are associated with a wide range of sexual dysfunctions, including loss of libido, erectile dysfunction, orgasmic dysfunction, and vaginal atrophy (Metcalfe & Fischman, 1985).

Individuals with cancer of the larynx, tongue, floor of the mouth, hypopharynx, or salivary glands report decreased interest in sex. Those with cancer of the sinus or nose report decreased enjoyment. These effects on sexual life are likely underreported, as these patients often are not asked about sexual changes (Hammerlid, Silander, et al., 2001), or because this type of cancer is assumed to not have sexual side effects, as it does not directly affect sexual organs (Monga et al., 1997).

The challenges for patients who are not in a partnered relationship also are significant. Difficulties with chewing and swallowing make eating in public a challenge. They may be reluctant to date, as one of the avenues for social interaction, having coffee or a meal with a potential partner, is fraught with the potential for embarrassment.

Laryngectomy patients are unable to talk normally, and even when they learn to use a speech aid, verbal communication remains altered. This affects the person's ability to call to ask someone out on a date, to flirt, or to have emotional and intimate conversations. Facial disfigurement is so visible that social isolation is a real possibility. The patient may perceive that no one ever could find him or her attractive and so may not be open to signals from others that a flirtation or relationship is possible.

Even within long-standing partnered relationships, at times, the partner may be reluctant to be sexually active with the patient because of fear of hurting them or because of the nature of the physical disfigurement (Monga et al., 1997). The disfigurement may become a barrier between the couple, which inevitably will affect the sexual relationship (Gamba et al., 1992). Sexual functioning may deteriorate after treatment, and if no assistance is sought, long-term problems may occur (Gritz et al., 1989).

Nursing Interventions in the Care of Individuals With Head and Neck Cancer

Counseling for patients with head and neck cancer must include a thorough exploration of the meaning of any disfigurement to the body and self-image. If the patient has a partner, including this person is vital so that the couple can talk to each other about what this means. Strategies to reduce symptoms related to sexuality, such as dry mouth, can be discussed with patients individually as the need arises.

An important part of integrating changes to body image takes place on the cognitive level. Patients need to recognize the changes that have occurred and also must integrate these on an emotional level. By experiencing these changes on both a cognitive and emotional level, a set of behavioral responses will be elicited that are either adaptive or not. Gentle guidance and support can help patients in developing a response that is constructive and helps in the formation of a new or altered body image (Dropkin, 1989).

Couples Counseling

Many couples have a restricted set of sexual activities that have brought them pleasure and satisfaction over the years. Having to do things differently may be a challenge, particularly for older couples who may lack knowledge of or experience with alternatives to penetrative intercourse. An open and honest discussion directed by a knowledgeable nurse can help couples to identify what their needs are in relation to sexual expression and how these can be modified because of limitations caused by surgery or radiation.

Assisting single patients to negotiate the often anxiety-provoking situation of dating and finding a partner is challenging. There is no perfect time to disclose to a potential partner a history that includes cancer. However, for someone who has a facial disfigurement, dating is even more challenging. Many patients often assume that no one will want to become close to them or even look at them. Finding strategies to cope with these fears and the responses of others to facial disfigurement is part of rehabilitation for these patients, and nurses should obtain as much professional expertise as possible to help them.

Nurses must include other members of the multidisciplinary team, such as physical therapists and speech and language pathologists. They bring a unique set of solutions to symptom management, and although they may not be immediately connected to sexual functioning, they will have solutions to issues affecting sexuality and sexual expression. These experts can give valuable advice related to treatment. For example, they can recommend products that are available to both prevent and alleviate dry mouth, maintain oral hygiene, and prevent oral and dental infections. The timely use of these products may make oral contact more comfortable for both patients and their partners.

As with other cancers, it often is a challenge to bring up the topic of sexuality in the face of life-altering disease. Figure 10-1 provides an example for using the BETTER model (Mick, Hughes, & Cohen, 2003) to initiate this conversation.

Figure 10-1. Example of the BETTER Model in Patients With Head and Neck Cancer

- **Bringing up the topic:** Nurses are encouraged to raise the issue of sexuality with patients. In teaching a preoperative patient with cancer of the tongue, the nurse should include information about the potential for sexual difficulties.

  "Many people who are about to have this kind of surgery have questions about how the treatment will affect their sexual lives. If you have questions, please do not hesitate to ask me at any time during your hospital stay."

- **Explaining that sex is a part of quality of life:** This helps to normalize the discussion and may help patients to feel less embarrassed or alone in having a problem. This is particularly important with older patients who may feel embarrassed about asking questions or who think that they should not be sexual at their age.

  "I ask all my patients if they have any concerns about sexual functioning because it is an important part of life for most people, and age has nothing to do with it."

- **Telling patients that resources will be found to address their concerns:** This step suggests to patients that even if the nurse does not have the immediate solution to the problem or question, others are available who can help.

  "Patients often describe having difficulty opening their mouths after treatment, and this makes it difficult to talk, eat, or kiss. It may be helpful for you to meet with a physiotherapist at the same time that you meet with the speech and language pathologist. Together they will find ways to help you with this problem."

(Continued on next page)

Figure 10-1. Example of the BETTER Model in Patients With Head and Neck Cancer (Continued)

- **Timing the intervention:** Patients may not be ready to deal with sexual issues at the time a problem is identified. However, patients can ask for information at any time in the future. Although studies suggest that the most important time for patients to come to terms with a facial defect is between days four and six after surgery, this may be too early for concerns about sexuality to be articulated (Dropkin, 1989).

    "I realize that you have a lot to deal with right now, and sex is probably not high on your list of priorities. But as you recover, you may have questions about this, and we are available at any time to talk about this with you and your partner."

- **Educating patients about the sexual side effects of treatment:** Educating patients about the potential side effects from treatments does not mean that they will occur. However, informing them about sexual side effects is as important as informing them about any other side effects.

    "You may find that both during and after your radiation treatment your mouth is very dry, and your saliva may feel sticky. This may interfere with eating and talking but also with kissing and other sexual activities. There are some things you can do to help with this, and I have a list of suggestions for you that you can read at your convenience."

- **Recording:** A brief notation that a discussion about sexuality or sexual side effects occurred is important.

    "The potential for sexual side effects related to radiation therapy was discussed with patient and partner. They had no questions at the present time but are aware that they can ask questions at any time."

Case Study

J.H. is a 44-year-old man who recently has completed radiation therapy for cancer of the tonsil. He is divorced and has not dated since his diagnosis. He states that he is reluctant to interact with women as he has lost his confidence and is certain that no one will be interested in him because of his health history. He is wearing a turtleneck sweater even though it is a warm day, and he seems reluctant to talk about his treatment and any side effects he has experienced.

Questions to consider:

- What questions could the nurse ask this patient to gain more information about his fears?
- How can the nurse help him to come to terms with the physical changes brought about by his treatment?

See Appendix B for answers to the case study questions.

The Effect of Brain Cancer on Sexuality

Cancer of the brain manifests in many different ways with a multitude of symptoms. The cancer itself and the treatment may result in cognitive, emotional, and functional deficits that all have the potential to affect sexual functioning. The pituitary gland is involved in the signaling pathway for the release of hormones that influence sexual function (see Chapter 2). The hypothalamus and pituitary gland regulate secretion of hormones by the ovaries and testes through feedback loops involving luteinizing and follicle-stimulating hormone. Prolactin also is released in the brain and is thought to have a direct effect on libido (Regan, 1999).

Sudden loss of libido in men or amenorrhea in women may be the first symptom of a pituitary tumor and resulting hyperprolactinemia (Kadioglu et al., 2005), but this may be ignored for extended periods of time because other more common causes exist for both these symptoms. Women with hyperprolactinemia also may suffer from anxiety, which might be attributed to other causes (Reavley, Fisher, Owen, Creed, & Davis, 1997), and global sexual dysfunction is a common experience for these women (Hulter & Lundberg, 1994). Loss of libido, decreased arousal, and anorgasmia are common manifestations.

Individuals with brain lesions might exhibit changes related to the location of the tumor and associated structures. For example, alterations in fine or gross motor coordination and sensory or cognitive impairment will have direct and indirect effects on sexual functioning. Disinhibition commonly occurs as a result of brain tumors, and this may manifest as an increased interest in sex, inappropriate sexual demands on a partner, or inappropriate sexual behavior. Treatment can result in additional changes to cognitive, emotional, and sexual functioning. The patient's partner may find it difficult to maintain a sexual relationship with someone whose personality is different, and to them it feels as though they are being sexual with someone else.

Nursing Interventions in the Care of Individuals With Brain Cancer

Often, counseling about the sexual side effects of brain cancer is directed primarily at the partner, who must learn to accommodate changes in the patient's functioning. A multidisciplinary team approach often is helpful, as sexual problems tend to be symptomatic of problems in social and emotional spheres. Opening up the discussion may be difficult. Figure 10-2 shows an example of statements/questions using the PLISSIT model (Annon, 1974), which nurses can use to initiate the discussion with patients and their partners.

Figure 10-2. Example of the PLISSIT Model in Patients With Brain Cancer

- **Permission:** An example of this level would be to include a general statement that normalizes the topic.

  "I hear from many patients' husbands that they feel that their spouse is a different person since the tumor started to grow. This can cause changes in all aspects of a couple's life together, including their sex life. If you want to talk about this, please know that I am willing to listen."

- **Limited information:** In the case of a couple where one person is being treated for a brain tumor, the nurse should be able to give general information about what the couple may expect.

  "It is not uncommon for individuals with brain tumors to notice changes in sensation or coordination. This may interfere with your wife's ability to feel it when you touch her."

- **Specific suggestion:** This level of the model requires a deeper level of expertise on the part of the nurse. Information at this level includes anticipatory guidance related to possible sexual consequences of medications and other treatments.

  "Your wife may gain weight and her face may appear puffy as a result of the steroids she is taking to reduce swelling in her brain. It also may affect her mood. She may not feel attractive, which may make her less interested in being sexual."

- **Intensive therapy:** Nurses should know where to refer patients when problems or issues are disclosed that are beyond their scope of practice or expertise.

  "The behavior you describe on the part of your husband is something we call 'disinhibition.' It can be very stressful for you and your family. We will try to find a medication that will help him, and in addition, I am going to suggest that you see our social worker, who can help you to find strategies to cope with this behavior."

Case Study

J.S. and R.S. are a young couple who have been married for three years. Six months ago, R.S. began to notice some muscle weakness in his right arm. Over three months, this became worse, and one month ago, he had a seizure at the dinner table. He was diagnosed with a frontal lobe tumor. This has been devastating for his wife. She says that he also has become quite aggressive with her and demands sex once or twice a day. She states that she is frightened of him at these times and generally agrees because she is fearful of what might happen if she refuses him. But, she also states that she feels as though she is making love to another man because he does not behave like the man she fell in love with.

Questions to consider:
- What questions should the nurse ask this young woman?
- What strategies might the patient's wife use to control the situation, which is very distressing to her?
- What referral or other services may be useful for the couple at this time?
See Appendix B for answers to the case study questions.

Conclusion

Cancer of the head and neck causes disfigurement that potentially can affect intimacy and sexual functioning. The treatment for this cancer does not affect sexual organs or hormonal status; however, the residual scarring and loss of function have the potential to cause long-lasting sequelae. Cancer of the brain is commonly associated with sensory, cognitive, or personality changes that can negatively affect the sexual and emotional relationships of the patient.

References

Annon, J. (1974). *The behavioral treatment of sexual problems.* Honolulu, HI: Enabling Systems.

Bjordal, K., & Kaasa, S. (1995). Psychological distress in head and neck cancer patients 7–11 years after curative treatment. *British Journal of Cancer, 71,* 592–597.

Burgess, L. (1994). Oncology focus. Facing the reality of head and neck cancer. *Nursing Standard, 8,* 30–34.

Dropkin, M.J. (1989). Coping with disfigurement and dysfunction after head and neck cancer surgery: A conceptual framework. *Seminars in Oncology Nursing, 5,* 213–219.

Dropkin, M.J. (1999). Body image and quality of life after head and neck cancer surgery. *Cancer Practice, 7,* 309–313.

Epstein, J.B., Robertson, M., Emerton, S., Phillips, N., & Stevenson-Moore, P. (2001). Quality of life and oral function in patients treated with radiation therapy for head and neck cancer. *Head and Neck, 23,* 389–398.

Gamba, A., Romano, M., Grosso, I.M., Tamburini, M., Cantu, G., Molinari, R., et al. (1992). Psychosocial adjustment of patients surgically treated for head and neck cancer. *Head and Neck, 14,* 218–223.

Gritz, E.R., Wellisch, D.K., Wang, H.J., Siau, J., Landsverk, J.A., & Cosgrove, M.D. (1989). Long-term effects of testicular cancer on sexual functioning in married couples. *Cancer, 64,* 1560–1567.

Hammerlid, E., Bjordal, K., Ahlner-Elmqvist, M., Boysen, M., Evensen, J.F., Biorklund, A., et al. (2001). A prospective study of quality of life in head and neck cancer patients. Part I: At diagnosis. *Laryngoscope, 111,* 669–680.

Hammerlid, E., Silander, E., Hornestam, L., & Sullivan, M. (2001). Health-related quality of life three years after diagnosis of head and neck cancer—a longitudinal study. *Head and Neck, 23,* 113–125.

Hanna, E., Sherman, A., Cash, D., Adams, D., Vural, E., Fan, C.Y., et al. (2004). Quality of life for patients following total laryngectomy vs. chemoradiation for laryngeal preservation. *Archives of Otolaryngology—Head and Neck Surgery, 130,* 875–879.

Hulter, B., & Lundberg, P.O. (1994). Sexual function in women with hypothalamo-pituitary disorders. *Archives of Sexual Behavior, 23,* 171–183.

Kadioglu, P., Yalin, A.S., Tiryakioglu, O., Gazioglu, N., Oral, G., Sanli, O., et al. (2005). Sexual dysfunction in women with hyperprolactinemia: A pilot study report. *Journal of Urology, 174,* 1921–1925.

Metcalfe, M.C., & Fischman, S.H. (1985). Factors affecting the sexuality of patients with head and neck cancer. *Oncology Nursing Forum, 12,* 21–25.

Mick, J., Hughes, M., & Cohen, M. (2003). Sexuality and cancer: How oncology nurses can address it BETTER. *Oncology Nursing Forum, 30*(Suppl. 2), 152–153.

Monga, U., Tan, G., Ostermann, H.J., & Monga, T.N. (1997). Sexuality in head and neck cancer patients. *Archives of Physical Medicine and Rehabilitation, 78,* 298–304.

Reavley, A., Fisher, A.D., Owen, D., Creed, F.H., & Davis, J.R. (1997). Psychological distress in patients with hyperprolactinemia. *Clinical Endocrinology, 47,* 343–348.

Regan, P. (1999). Hormonal correlates and causes of sexual desire: A review. *Canadian Journal of Human Sexuality, 8,* 1–16.

CHAPTER 11

Cancer of the Bladder

Bladder cancer is treated according to the stage of disease, but most patients with this cancer require some type of surgery. Because of the location of the bladder, surgery puts patients at risk for sexual difficulties. Radiation therapy may be added either pre- or postoperatively, and some patients also require chemotherapy in the perioperative period. Removal of the bladder remains central to the treatment of bladder cancer. Patients will be left with a urinary diversion, often through a urostomy, which requires an external pouch. More modern techniques create an internal reservoir, which may require intermittent catheterization, or an orthoptic neobladder, which is connected to the urethra and thus allows for almost normal passage of urine.

The Effect of Bladder Cancer on Sexuality

Radical cystectomy in men traditionally is accompanied by removal of the prostate gland and the seminal vesicles, as well as the proximal urethra. This results in profound erectile dysfunction and dry orgasm (Zippe, Raina, Massanyi, et al., 2004). These persist in the long term and have a significant impact on quality of life (Matsuda, Aptel, Exbrayat, & Grosclaude, 2003). Pelvic lymph nodes are removed, as well as adipose tissue and fascia in both men and women (Herr, 2005). For women, cystectomy also involves removal of the anterior vaginal wall, the uterus, uterine tubes, ovaries, and urethra, with the associated sexual difficulties as described for women with gynecologic cancer. This results in major sexual difficulties for most women, with reduced clitoral sensation, diminished ability to achieve orgasm, decreased libido, and painful intercourse. Some women are unable to have intercourse at all because of the extensive excision of tissue and resultant scar tissue formation (Zippe, Raina, Shah, et al., 2004). The presence of a stoma increases sexual difficulties because of both body image issues and the technical difficulties that some patients experience with the appliance during sexual activity (Caffo, Fellin, Graffer, & Luciani, 1996).

Treatment-Related Side Effects

More modern surgical techniques attempt to preserve function by not removing the prostate gland, vas deferens, and seminal vesicles in men and by reconstructing the bladder using a section of bowel. Erectile function and normal ejaculation may be preserved; however, most studies have been performed in a highly select population and may not be applicable to all (Botto et al., 2004; Nieuwenhuijzen, Meinhardt, & Horenblas, 2005; Tal & Baniel, 2005). Modified surgery in women involves removal of the bladder only and the creation of a neobladder and spares the uterus, uterine tubes, and ovaries (Horenblas, Meinhardt, Ijzerman, & Moonen, 2001). Decreased desire and arousal and difficulty achieving orgasm are reported by women even after modified surgery (Hart et al., 1999).

Patients treated with only radiation therapy also experience alterations in sexual functioning. Men report poorer quality of erections, decreased frequency of morning erections, less intense orgasms, and smaller volume of ejaculate (Little & Howard, 1998). Women report little or no desire for sex, but sexual outcomes remain better than for women treated with radical cystectomy (Henningsohn, Wijkstrom, Dickman, Bergmark, & Steineck, 2002). Overall, patients treated with radiation therapy tend to experience fewer sexual side effects compared to those treated with surgery (Caffo et al., 1996).

Nursing Interventions in the Care of Individuals With Bladder Cancer

Counseling of patients who have had surgical treatment for bladder cancer should begin before the surgery with a discussion of what the surgery will entail, whether patients will be left with a stoma, and what type of care will be needed to maximize continence and prevent complications. Nurses should explore what expectations patients and their partners have and whether these are realistic. At the time of diagnosis, many patients and partners do not consider what effect the treatment may have on sexuality, as the threat to survival is deemed most important. In the weeks and months following treatment, this threat to life usually diminishes, and then sexual issues may become more pressing. The couple may not recall any information that they were given in this regard, and they must be informed of who to contact to get information. Nurses also should offer this information even if it was previously given, because recall may be poor.

Body Image

The sexual issues for people with bladder cancer who have a urostomy are similar to those experienced by patients with colon cancer (see Chapter 8). A challenge to sexuality for these patients is the change in body image related to both the stoma and the appliance worn to collect urine. A common reaction is shock and disgust soon after surgery, and many ostomates report feeling sexually unattractive. Fear of the sexual partner's reaction to the stoma and appliance further complicates this reaction (Gloeckner, 1991). Marital breakdown has been reported following treatment for bladder cancer (Mansson & Mansson, 1999); however, most relationships continue with a high degree of satisfaction despite challenges to sexual functioning (Bjerre, Johansen, & Steven, 1995). Common fears related to the stoma have to do with the appearance of the stoma and anxiety about harming the stoma or causing pain if it is touched during sexual activity. Ostomates also may be concerned about odor and leakage (Golis, 1996). For women, changes to body image because of scarring or the presence of a stoma and appliance are common and especially distressing.

Some individuals choose to have a neobladder rather than a urostomy because the idea of having a stoma and wearing an appliance is distressing. Even with a neobladder, life is not as it was before, and patients need to self-catheterize on a regular basis. Men still may experience erectile dysfunction after this kind of surgery and will not ejaculate normally. Some men report being disappointed with their sexual functioning after the surgery because they expected better results with the newer surgical techniques (Beitz & Zuzelo, 2003). Even with a neobladder, some urine leakage may occur during sexual activity, which can be distressing to patients and their partners, and the fear or anticipation of this also can provoke anxiety.

Information Sharing

Providing strategies to cope with the threat of involuntary urine loss may help the couple to return to sexual functioning if that is desired. Explaining to the couple that urine is sterile and will not harm the partner may be the starting point. Fear of odor can be dealt with by suggesting the use of a favorite perfume or body lotion. Incorporating sexual play in the shower or bathtub removes the fear of leakage and also is relaxing. Using a protective cover on the bed can prevent damage to the mattress. Self-catheterizing before sexual activity and restricting fluids also can help to minimize the risk of leakage, as can using different positions for sexual intercourse. The side-lying position prevents pressure on the neobladder or urostomy appliance, and the woman-on-top position has the same effect.

Treatment of erectile dysfunction following surgery is essentially the same as for men who are experiencing erectile dysfunction after prostatectomy (see

Chapter 5). Oral therapies (phosphodiesterase-5 inhibitors), vacuum devices, intraurethral pellets (MUSE® [Vivus, Inc., Mountain View, CA]), intracorporeal injections (Caverject® [Pfizer Inc., New York, NY], Trimix), and penile implants may be used to treat this condition. Success may be affected by pretreatment erectile functioning, and this issue often contains a significant psychological component.

Women with bladder cancer often experience sexual difficulties similar to those experienced by women with gynecologic cancer who are treated surgically (see Chapter 6). Treatment of sexual symptoms depends on the extent of the surgery. Pain with intercourse can result from vaginal dryness, muscle tension, scar tissue, or anxiety. The experience of pain can start a cycle of vaginismus, in which the muscles at the vaginal introitus contract in anticipation of pain with penetration. This has implications not only for the woman's sexual life but also for pelvic examinations in the future. Women can learn to relax the vaginal muscles in much the same way that they learn to do Kegel exercises, which deliberately contract the same pubococcygeal muscle.

Hormone therapy may be helpful if the ovaries have been removed and vaginal dryness is a problem. Local estrogen cream or pessaries can be used to alleviate vaginal dryness. If hormones are not used, a vaginal moisturizer such as Replens® (Lil' Drug Store Products, Cedar Rapids, IA) may help to alleviate burning and itching of vaginal tissues. A number of lubricants are available to help women to feel more comfortable with sexual activity, and silicone-based products seem to be the most helpful in making intercourse more comfortable.

If the vagina is shortened by scar tissue, women may need to use a dilator on a regular basis to maintain patency and allow for intercourse. Initially, women should be advised to use a dilator with a narrow diameter (0.5–1 inch) and gradually increase the diameter up to a maximum of 1.5 inches. Women should be encouraged to use the dilator daily in the hopes that they will use it at least three times a week. They should use a lubricant to ease insertion.

Some couples may prefer to not attempt intercourse and can meet their intimate needs by nonpenetrative activity. However, some couples may cease all forms of physical touching. This is acceptable as long as it does not cause distress for either of them. Asking the couple about their needs and desires is important in establishing whether a problem exists and helps to identify how motivated the couple is to work on the issue. For some couples, cessation of sexual activity is not seen as a major problem, and they do not need further assistance or referral.

The BETTER model (Mick, Hughes, & Cohen, 2003) can provide a useful framework for initiating the discussion and providing patients with anticipatory guidance and information (see Figure 11-1).

Figure 11-1. Example of the BETTER Model in Patients With Bladder Cancer

- **Bringing up the topic:** Nurses are encouraged to raise the issue of sexuality with patients.

  "Many of our patients ask questions about how this surgery will impact their sexual life. Is this a good time to talk?"

- **Explaining that sex is a part of quality of life:** This helps to normalize the discussion and may help patients to feel less embarrassed or alone in having a problem.

  "After surgery for bladder cancer, many couples have questions about resuming sexual activity. How can I help you in this regard?"

- **Telling patients that resources will be found to address their concerns:** This step suggests to patients that even if the nurse does not have the immediate solution to the problem or question, others are available who can help.

  "There is a specialized physical therapist who deals with problems related to urine leakage. She has a clinic not far from here, and I can send in a referral for her to see you."

- **Timing the intervention:** Patients may not be ready to deal with sexual issues at the time a problem is identified. However, patients can ask for information at any time in the future.

  "I realize that we have given you a lot of information in a short period of time today. You probably need some time to think about it all. However, we are just a phone call away, and you can contact us at any time once you are at home and have managed to find some time alone to discuss this."

- **Educating patients about the sexual side effects of treatment:** Educating patients about potential side effects from treatments does not mean that they will occur, but informing them about sexual side effects is as important as informing them about any other side effects.

  "It is not uncommon for some urine to leak when you are sexually excited. Urine is sterile and will not harm either of you. However, some people find it a little distasteful, and I have some suggestions to help you overcome this."

- **Recording:** A brief notation that a discussion about sexuality or sexual side effects occurred is important.

  "Potential side effects related to the planned surgery were discussed. Patient was given reading material as well as contact information for the Resource Center."

Case Study

G.T. is 63 years old and was recently diagnosed with bladder cancer. He is scheduled for surgery in two weeks. At his preoperative assessment appointment, he asks the nurse what is going to happen to his sex life. His wife is with him, and she appears embarrassed when he raises the topic. She rolls her eyes and tells him to be quiet and not bother the "nice" nurse with these sorts of questions.

Questions to consider:
- How should the nurse respond to the patient's question?
- How should the nurse respond to the wife's obvious discomfort?

The nurse sees G.T. three months after his surgery. He had a neobladder procedure and appears to have recovered quite well. His wound is healed, and he states that he is back to his usual self. His wife is not with him at this appointment.
- What are some questions the nurse would want to ask regarding sexual functioning?
- Should the patient's wife be present for this conversation?

See Appendix B for answers to the case study questions.

Conclusion

Cancer of the bladder, similar to colorectal cancer, has the significant potential to affect sexuality because of nerve and vascular damage resulting from treatment along with the presence of a stoma and external appliance after some surgical procedures. It also has psychological consequences, as individuals have to adapt to an altered body image and a conscious focus on elimination.

References

Beitz, J.M., & Zuzelo, P.R. (2003). The lived experience of having a neobladder. *Western Journal of Nursing Research, 25,* 294–316.

Bjerre, B., Johansen, C., & Steven, K. (1995). Health-related quality of life after cystectomy: Bladder substitution compared with ileal conduit diversion. A questionnaire study. *British Journal of Urology, 75,* 200–205.

Botto, H., Sebe, P., Molinie, V., Herve, J.M., Yonneau, L., & Lebret, T. (2004). Prostatic capsule- and seminal-sparing cystectomy for bladder carcinoma: Initial results for selected patients. *BJU International, 94,* 1021–1025.

Caffo, O., Fellin, G., Graffer, U., & Luciani, L. (1996). Assessment of quality of life after cystectomy or conservative therapy for patients with infiltrating bladder carcinoma. A survey by a self-administered questionnaire. *Cancer, 78,* 1089–1097.

Gloeckner, M. (1991). Perceptions of sexuality after ostomy surgery. *Journal of Enterostomal Therapy, 18,* 36–38.

Golis, A. (1996). Sexual issues for the person with an ostomy. *Journal of Wound, Ostomy, and Continence Nursing, 23,* 33–37.

Hart, S., Skinner, E.C., Meyerowitz, B.E., Boyd, S., Lieskovsky, G., & Skinner, D.G. (1999). Quality of life after radical cystectomy for bladder cancer in patients with an ileal conduit, cutaneous or urethral kock pouch. *Journal of Urology, 162,* 77–81.

Henningsohn, L., Wijkstrom, H., Dickman, P., Bergmark, K., & Steineck, G. (2002). Distressful symptoms after radical radiotherapy for urinary bladder cancer. *Radiotherapy and Oncology, 62,* 215–225.

Herr, H.W. (2005). Is less radical cystectomy better, and how can we be sure? *Journal of Urology, 173,* 1063.

Horenblas, S., Meinhardt, W., Ijzerman, W., & Moonen, L.F. (2001). Sexuality preserving cystectomy and neobladder: Initial results. *Journal of Urology, 166,* 837–840.

Little, F.A., & Howard, G.C. (1998). Sexual function following radical radiotherapy for bladder cancer. *Radiotherapy and Oncology, 49,* 157–161.

Mansson, A., & Mansson, W. (1999). When the bladder is gone: Quality of life following different types of urinary diversion. *World Journal of Urology, 17,* 211–218.

Matsuda, T., Aptel, I., Exbrayat, C., & Grosclaude, P. (2003). Determinants of quality of life of bladder cancer survivors five years after treatment in France. *International Journal of Urology, 10,* 423–429.

Mick, J., Hughes, M., & Cohen, M. (2003). Sexuality and cancer: How oncology nurses can address it BETTER. *Oncology Nursing Forum, 30*(Suppl. 2), 152–153.

Nieuwenhuijzen, J.A., Meinhardt, W., & Horenblas, S. (2005). Clinical outcomes after sexuality preserving cystectomy and neobladder (prostate sparing cystectomy) in 44 patients. *Journal of Urology, 173,* 1314–1317.

Tal, R., & Baniel, J. (2005). Sexual function-preserving cystectomy. *Urology, 66,* 235–241.

Zippe, C., Raina, R., Massanyi, E.Z., Agarwal, A., Jones, J., Ulchaker, J., et al. (2004). Sexual function after male radical cystectomy in a sexually active population. *Urology, 64,* 682–686.

Zippe, C.D., Raina, R., Shah, A.D., Massanyi, E.Z., Agarwal, A., Ulchaker, J., et al. (2004). Female sexual dysfunction after radical cystectomy: A new outcome measure. *Urology, 63,* 1153–1157.

CHAPTER 12

Cancer of the Penis

Penile cancer is rare in North America and developed countries. However, this cancer is devastating for men because of the significant psychological impact of the diagnosis, body image issues, and the sexual consequences of treatment (Romero et al., 2005). Diagnosis may be delayed because men may either ignore a penile lesion or might not recognize a small skin lesion as something that requires medical attention. Some men may be so fearful that they avoid seeking medical attention and present for care with advanced cancer that already has spread to lymph nodes. Very little exists in the research or sex therapy literature on this form of cancer.

Treatment for penile cancer traditionally has been surgical removal of the entire penis (penectomy) or partial removal. Treatment is based on staging, with early-stage cancer treated with the least-mutilating surgery possible. Recurrence is common with penile cancer, and every attempt is made to excise enough tissue to obtain a cure. Laser therapy is increasingly being used (Windahl, Skeppner, Andersson, & Fugl-Meyer, 2004), and radiation and chemotherapy sometimes are used in the adjunct setting.

The Effect of Penile Cancer on Sexuality

The glans of the penis is theorized to serve a protective function as a shock absorber during penetrative intercourse. The glans does not contain the fibrous tunica albuginea that surrounds the erectile tissue in the shaft of the penis. The glans protects the tissue of the shaft by limiting the pressure inside the corpora cavernosa during the thrusting of intercourse. Absence of the glans as a consequence of partial penectomy has been shown to increase the pressure inside the corpora during intercourse. Female partners of men with no glans report experiencing pain during thrusting, particularly in the anterior vaginal wall, which is known to be sensitive (Hatzichristou et al., 2003).

Sexual consequences of surgery include significant impacts on body image and masculinity. Men who have undergone total penectomy obviously will be unable to have penetrative intercourse, although their capacity for genital sensation remains intact if the scrotum, upper thighs, and penile stub are stimulated. Physical shortening of the penis in the case of partial penectomy may still allow for penetrative intercourse to occur, and many men are as satisfied with their sex life after this surgery as they were before (D'Ancona et al., 1997; Romero et al., 2005). Men may have a perineal urethrostomy created after total penectomy, which allows them to urinate while sitting. Some men might still be able to stand to urinate following a partial penectomy.

Men may find the period of diagnosis to be particularly stressful, and lack of libido and erectile dysfunction may occur during this time. Many men find that with a supportive partner, they can regain sexual interest and functioning. Some men may assume that their sex life will cease after treatment; however, although the frequency of penetrative intercourse usually decreases, most men continue to engage in some level of sexual activity.

Laser surgery is suggested to have the best cosmetic and functional results for treatment of penile cancer because the structure of the penis is maintained (Opjordsmoen, Waehre, Aass, & Fossa, 1994). Painful intercourse has been reported after laser surgery, but this is rare (Windahl et al., 2004).

Psychological consequences of treatment for penile cancer include feelings of shame and embarrassment about the reduced penis size. The threat to masculinity from this is substantial. However, over time, most men become adjusted to the physical alteration and report normal or only slightly reduced levels of sexual interest, activity, orgasm, and satisfaction with both their sex life and their relationship with their partner (D'Ancona et al., 1997; Romero et al., 2005; Windahl et al., 2004). Some men might struggle with the decision they made related to surgical treatment and have reported regretting it in hindsight, instead preferring less radical treatment with lower long-term survival in favor of remaining sexually active (Opjordsmoen & Fossa, 1994).

Treatment-Related Side Effects

Treatment of sexual difficulties related to penile cancer focuses on helping men and their partners to understand the extent of the surgery and possible consequences in both the preoperative and postoperative period. Educating the couple—or the man alone if he is single—that sexual activity is possible after treatment will prevent much of the anxiety that most men experience when faced with this diagnosis. Education can correct erroneous assumptions, and men may attempt sexual activity instead of assuming that this part of their life is over. Involvement of partners in all education and counseling is necessary because they may be reluctant to resume sexual activity out of fear of contagion, fear of causing pain, or general lack of interest in sex.

Postoperative erectile difficulties can be dealt with in the same manner as with any man experiencing erectile dysfunction. Some older men already may have noticed some changes in their ability to achieve or maintain an erection. Some may want to seek treatment for this, whereas others will see it as a part of aging and may not wish to pursue medical therapy.

For men who have had a total penectomy, it is useful to explain that although there is no penis to become erect, nerves in the genital area generally remain intact and responsive to touch and stimulation. Alternatives to penetrative intercourse are possible, and men can still provide pleasure to their partners and, in turn, receive pleasure. Men can experience orgasm from stimulation of the genital area alone. Many patients are not aware of this, and explaining it can serve a significant therapeutic purpose and give hope where previously the situation was perceived as hopeless. Instructing the couple on the use of sensate focus exercises may open an entirely new repertoire for them, which will encourage the continuation of a meaningful, though altered, range of sexual activities.

The PLISSIT model (Annon, 1974) provides a useful framework to start the conversation with patients and partners, and Figure 12-1 provides examples of how to talk to patients with penile cancer.

Figure 12-1. Example of the PLISSIT Model in Patients With Penile Cancer

- **Permission:** An example of this level would be to include a general statement that normalizes the topic.

  "You may think that your sex life is over. However, many men with penile cancer recover from the surgery and have a satisfying sex life with their partner. What are the most important concerns that you have at the present time?"

- **Limited information:** In the case of a couple where the man is having a partial penectomy, the nurse should be able to give general information about resuming intercourse.

  "After surgical removal of part of the penis, penetration is still possible. You should wait for the surgical wound to heal before attempting penetration."

- **Specific suggestion:** Information at this level includes anticipatory guidance related to possible sexual consequences of medications and other treatments.

  "Laser surgery has the best cosmetic results of any of the treatments for penile cancer. In a few weeks, the redness and pain will have gone away, and you will see that erections feel pleasurable again. Once healing is complete, it is fine to attempt intercourse again."

- **Intensive therapy:** Nurses should know where to refer patients when problems or issues are disclosed that are beyond the scope of their practice or expertise.

  "It sounds as if your diagnosis and treatment have raised all sorts of issues for you that go back to your childhood. I am going to suggest that you see a therapist who specializes in treating people who have experienced childhood trauma."

Case Study

J.G. is a 67-year-old man who presented to his family physician with a nine-month history of a white lesion on the shaft of his penis. He thought that this was just dry skin and had ignored it. He mentioned it to a family friend who is an internist, who then encouraged him to seek medical attention. A biopsy confirmed the presence of penile cancer, and J.G. was offered the options of partial penectomy or laser surgery. He chose partial penectomy because he was concerned that laser therapy might not "catch it all." At a follow-up visit three months after surgery, he tells the nurse that he has not attempted intercourse yet because he is not sure that it will not be harmful.

Questions to consider:
- What questions should the nurse ask to understand what he means by "harmful"?
- Why is it important to involve the partner in this discussion?
- What would be helpful to know about his previous level of sexual functioning?

See Appendix B for answers to the case study questions.

Conclusion

Cancer of the penis, although rare in North America, has devastating psychosexual effects. Partial or complete surgical removal of the penis is the treatment of choice. However, laser surgery is showing promise with good cosmetic and sexual outcomes. Men and their partners may need extensive counseling to assist them in coping with the physical and psychological effects of both the cancer and its treatment.

References

Annon, J. (1974). *The behavioral treatment of sexual problems.* Honolulu, HI: Enabling Systems.

D'Ancona, C.A., Botega, N.J., DeMoraes, C., Lavoura, N.S., Jr., Santos, J.K., & Rodrigues, N.N., Jr. (1997). Quality of life after partial penectomy for penile carcinoma. *Urology, 50,* 593–596.

Hatzichristou, D.G., Tzortzis, V., Hatzimouratidis, K., Apostolidis, A., Moysidis, K., & Panteliou, S. (2003). Protective role of the glans penis during coitus. *International Journal of Impotence Research, 15,* 337–342.

Opjordsmoen, S., & Fossa, S.D. (1994). Quality of life in patients treated for penile cancer. A follow-up study. *British Journal of Urology, 74,* 652–657.

Opjordsmoen, S., Waehre, H., Aass, N., & Fossa, S.D. (1994). Sexuality in patients treated for penile cancer: Patients' experience and doctors' judgement. *British Journal of Urology, 73,* 554–560.

Romero, F.R., Romero, K.R., Mattos, M.A., Garcia, C.R., Fernandes, R.C., & Perez, M.D. (2005). Sexual function after partial penectomy for penile cancer. *Urology, 66,* 1292–1295.

Windahl, T., Skeppner, E., Andersson, S.O., & Fugl-Meyer, K.S. (2004). Sexual function and satisfaction in men after laser treatment for penile carcinoma. *Journal of Urology, 172,* 648–651.

Section III

The Impact of Cancer on the Individual and Family

CHAPTER 13

The Adolescent With Cancer

Adolescence is the time between the onset of puberty and adulthood and generally is thought of as occurring between the ages of 13 and 19. It is a time of physical, emotional, and social growth and is characterized by psychosexual changes.

Psychosexual Changes of Adolescence

Puberty begins with the development of secondary sex characteristics. In girls, these changes generally begin between the ages of 8 and 11. Breast bud development often is the first sign of change, and then pubic hair begins to grow. The labia enlarge, and the internal reproductive organs also begin to grow. Sometime after the 10th year, menarche occurs, and changes to body shape begin. The breasts begin to fully develop, pubic hair covers the mons pubis, and underarm hair is present. The menstrual cycle becomes more regular over time, and the young woman is capable of becoming pregnant.

In boys, the changes usually occur about a year later than in girls. Starting at about age nine in some boys, the testicles begin to grow and the skin of the scrotum becomes darker and coarser. A few pubic hairs appear, and the boy becomes taller and more muscular. Over the next two years, genital growth continues. The shoulders broaden and the hips become narrower. The voice begins to deepen in response to the larynx enlarging, which is caused by increased testosterone levels. Fine facial hair also begins to grow, as does underarm hair. Gradually, the pubic hair becomes coarser, and penile growth starts to slow down, but the testicles may continue to grow larger until they reach full size. Many boys start to shave sometime between the ages of 15 and 19 and will have experienced ejaculation, either spontaneously at night (nocturnal emission) or through masturbation. By the end of puberty, young men are close to their adult height and have the adult distribution of chest and pubic hair, but further growth can occur into their 20s.

During adolescence, social and emotional changes also are significant. Peer group attachments grow stronger, and sexual attraction to members of the peer group are common. Often the emotional and social changes do not quite keep up with the physical changes, and the result is an adolescent who looks like an adult but still acts and thinks like a child. Body image preoccupation is a central event throughout this stage. Adolescents often are very unhappy with the way they look and constantly compare themselves to peers or media images with great dissatisfaction. Self-esteem can be negatively affected, and low self-esteem may result in risky social and sexual behaviors. Cognitive changes during adolescence comprise the ability to think in an abstract manner and to envision potential consequences (Duncan, Dixon, & Carlson, 2003).

All these changes occur in the context of the family of origin and the larger society and culture. Families in which parents are loving, supportive, and affectionate to one another and to their children usually produce adolescents who are well equipped to meet the challenges of adulthood. Societal attitudes and norms may conflict with the values of the family, and this may cause dissonance for adolescents who must find a way of negotiating the balance between what they see in the home and what the media and other groups in society regard as acceptable (Brown, 2000).

The major developmental tasks to be completed by the end of adolescence are to separate from the family and achieve independence, to identify and pursue a vocational goal, to achieve a mature level of sexuality, and to achieve a realistic and positive self-image (Brown, 2000). Other tasks of adolescents are to learn to control impulses, to deal with frustration, and to delay gratification. These play out in psychosexual challenges such as delaying or initiating sexual activity (Westheimer & Lopater, 2005).

Adolescents commonly begin exploring their sexual feelings at some time during these years. This is the time when attraction to members of the opposite or same sex becomes apparent, and some adolescents are confused about their sexual identity and feel pressured to identify themselves as heterosexual, bisexual, or homosexual. It often is difficult for adolescents who are attracted to same-sex peers to talk about this, and feelings of exclusion are common.

Masturbation is a common activity, although boys report practicing it more frequently than girls. It most often is a solitary activity, but some adolescents engage in mutual masturbation as an alternative to sexual intercourse. Masturbation may be accompanied by feelings of guilt, as it is an activity that continues to carry with it some elements of taboo. In recent years, oral-genital stimulation has become more common as an alternative to sexual intercourse, and many adolescents regard themselves as virgins if they have not had intercourse, even though they are participating in what many adults regard as sexual activity.

Adolescents link sexual activity and intimacy or emotional connection, and many place a great deal of importance on the relationship in which sexual activity takes place and the need for a sexually exclusive relationship (McCabe & Cummins, 1998). Although this may be a positive thing for many adolescents, when one of the partners goes outside the relationship for sexual activity, the result may be a great deal of hurt on the part of the person who feels betrayed. Adolescents may lack the emotional skills to deal effectively with a break-up. Challenges such as this may have long-lasting and significant effects on self-esteem and self-worth. Also, sexual activity is not always completely consensual. Young women, in particular, may feel pressured to become sexually active in the hopes of attracting or keeping a boyfriend. Peer pressure to do what everyone else seems to be doing is another factor in the initiation of sexual activity (Blythe & Rosenthal, 2000).

Society tends to view adolescence as a time of risk taking and sexual experimentation. Adolescents are seen as believing that they are immortal, invulnerable, and immune to many of the consequences of risky behaviors. Concerns about adolescent pregnancy and sexually transmitted infections predominate in the literature on adolescent sexuality, with little attention focused on raising sexually healthy individuals with the communication skills necessary for a full and satisfying sexual life. Adolescents regard the media as important sources of sexual information, along with parents and peers. They may prefer the depictions of sexuality in the media, which largely focus on passion and present sex in a positive light rather than the negative and fear-based messages about pregnancy and disease that many parents offer in the hope of preventing sexual activity (Brown & Keller, 2000).

Adolescents With Cancer

The challenges for adolescents diagnosed with cancer are complex. Management of cancer in adolescents frequently involves multimodality treatment with multi-agent chemotherapy, high-dose radiation, and aggressive surgery (Pentheroudakis & Pavlidis, 2005). Cancer and its treatment have direct effects on the four major tasks of adolescence, namely to separate from the family and achieve independence, to identify and pursue a vocational goal, to achieve a mature level of sexuality, and to achieve a realistic and positive self-image (Brown, 2000). The cancer experience directly affects self-image, which relates to self-esteem, peer relationships, and psychosocial development, as well as sexual maturation and activity (Chambas, 1991; Heiney, 1989).

When cancer is diagnosed, adolescents are forced to face issues of mortality (Roberts, Turney, & Knowles, 1998), which directly conflicts with the usual attitude of adolescents, who see themselves as immortal and invulnerable. Fear of recurrence may be a life-long consequence of experiencing cancer in adolescence and may alter life choices such as whether to get married. Although treatments have improved and most adolescents survive their cancer, the treatments themselves and the short- and long-term side effects cause significant distress and suffering.

Short-Term Side Effects

Short-term side effects of treatment that affect adolescents may interfere with the attainment of normal developmental tasks. These include alopecia, nausea and vomiting, skin changes, and weight gain or loss caused by medications or the disease itself. These side effects alter patients' body image, which is a central aspect of the adolescent experience and leads the individuals to feel different from the peer group at a time when sameness is important (Davis, 2006). Adolescents report that pain and nausea and vomiting are the worst parts of having cancer (Roberts et al., 1998). However, alopecia also is described as being the most devastating side effect. For young men, hair is seen as a symbol of virility and sex appeal; for girls, it is a symbol of attractiveness and femininity (Klopovich & Clancy, 1985). Adolescents generally are quite preoccupied with their appearance, and the gradual loss of hair that accompanies treatment leads to a feeling of otherness and may lead to social isolation. Weight gain and the typical moon-face from steroids are other physical manifestations that have an impact on adolescents' self-image. Pallor and skin changes such as the appearance of acne also will affect body image and self-esteem.

Radiation to the head and total body irradiation may damage the pituitary gland, thus resulting in decreased production of growth hormone and stunted physical growth. Surgical amputation of a limb results in permanent alteration in both appearance and function. These effects will profoundly influence patients' body image and self-esteem.

The need for hospitalization and absences from school and sports have an impact on developing and maintaining peer relationships, one of the central tasks of adolescence. The need for parents to assist with activities of daily living, treatments, and attendance at medical appointments may prevent young people from developing the communication and life skills consistent with their chronologic age (Finnegan, 2004). It also may delay the development of independence, another sentinel task of this developmental stage. Adolescent patients may feel different from their peers and so may perceive themselves as being socially isolated. Extended absences from social activities because of treatments, complications of treatments, and the need to avoid crowds if they are neutropenic decrease the time that patients spend with friends and peers. This may affect the acquisition of skills in interacting with members of the opposite sex, which can have far-reaching effects on sexual maturation (Ropponen, Aalberg, Rautonen, Kalmari, & Siimes, 1990).

Some adolescents may respond to social isolation by being sexually active in an attempt to gain popularity. This behavior is a compensatory mechanism to gain acceptance and inclusion and to achieve status within the peer group (Haka-Ikse, 1997). The physical and emotional risks of this response are significant, but it should be seen as an attempt at coping and not as deviant or pathologic.

Long-Term Side Effects

Long-term side effects of treatment include alterations to fertility and sexual functioning. Achieving sexual maturation is one of the tasks of adolescence, and this is anatomic and physiologic as well as psychosocial and psychosexual. Alkylating agents are gonadotoxic and cause permanent DNA damage to ovarian tissue. Other chemotherapeutic agents are less toxic to the ovaries or do not cause permanent damage. The prepubertal ovary is less susceptible to permanent damage; however, women treated in childhood and adolescence may experience premature ovarian failure many years later. Essentially, the damage to the ovaries is dose and drug dependent and is related to the patient's age at the time of treatment (Beerendonk & Braat, 2005). The production of follicle-stimulating hormone, luteinizing hormone, and testosterone also might be affected by radiation damage to the pituitary gland, which will have an impact on patients' reproductive capacity (Relander, Cavallin-Stahl, Garwicz, Olsson, & Willen, 2000). This also may delay the development of secondary sex characteristics, which will make the adolescents look different from their peers, and sexual and/or menstrual functioning also might be delayed or halted.

Radiation therapy to the pelvis may lead to impaired uterine growth if the treatment was given before puberty. In young women who are postpubertal, damage caused by radiation to the uterus may manifest as an inability to expand with the growing fetus during pregnancy, leading to miscarriage or premature birth (Beerendonk & Braat, 2005). Radiation to the spine can damage the epiphyseal plates between the vertebrae and limit spinal growth.

Individuals treated in adolescence may be infertile. Assuming this to be true, adolescents may believe that if they cannot get pregnant or cannot impregnate a woman, then protection is not necessary during sexual intercourse. They are then at increased risk for acquiring a sexually transmitted infection if they do not use condoms (Finnegan, 2004) or may become pregnant or impregnate someone. Some young men may assume that because of their particular cancer or treatment, they are not only infertile but also impotent and thus not capable of sexual intercourse. This may affect normal sexual experimentation such as masturbation, which is seen as an essential aspect of attaining mature sexuality (Ropponen et al., 1990).

Counseling Adolescents With Cancer

Addressing sexual issues is an essential part of providing care to adolescents with cancer and their families. Unfortunately, although most nurses acknowledge that information about sexuality is an important aspect of care for these patients, many do not include this topic as part of treatment for essentially the same reasons as discussed in Chapter 3. Nurses are more inclined to wait for the adolescent to raise the topic than to initiate the discussion with the patient (Williams & Wilson, 1989). At times, this discussion with adolescent patients may be difficult, as the question of whether their parents should be present is a sensitive one. Some parents do not want their child to be given information about sexuality because they fear that this will lead to early sexual activity (Finnegan, 2004). This view ignores the evidence that providing sexual education and information does not lead to early sexual experimentation. Giving information to adolescents is important because most adolescents, unlike adults, may not have had prior sexual experience to even know what changes may occur. However, their natural curiosity, assumptions based on what their peers are doing, and messages from the media give them a sense of what is normal and how they may be different. Adolescents with cancer want information on sexuality and fertility (Zebrack, Oeffinger, Hou, & Kaplan, 2006). Anticipatory guidance is an important part of the care that nurses provide in other aspects of cancer treatment, so this should be a part of routine care. The cancer itself or its treatments may lead to altered sexual functioning, and adolescents may experience sexual dysfunction (e.g., painful intercourse, inability to achieve an erection, ejaculation dysfunction). Without help, these problems will not resolve spontaneously and will persist into adulthood (Greydanus, Rimsza, & Newhouse, 2002).

Collaborating with the parents of the adolescent in all aspects of care is a useful strategy. The patient should be a central part of the care team and should be included in all aspects of care and treatment as an equal partner in decision making. When rapport is established and trust has been developed, adolescents are more likely to ask questions; the parents also are more likely to allow them to attend appointments without their supervision, which will allow for an assessment of sexual knowledge and information needs.

Assessment of Sexual Knowledge

An assessment of the adolescent's sexual knowledge and attitudes should be performed before giving any specific information (Klopovich & Clancy, 1985). This should be done in private with an accompanying discussion about confidentiality. Terminology should be used that is comfortable for the adolescent and to normalize the topic. While putting patients at ease, it is not appropriate to attempt to seem cool or hip; adolescents do not want their healthcare provider to act like a friend. However, empathy and professionalism will help to minimize embarrassment (Christie & Viner, 2005). Assessing sexual knowledge allows for the correction of misinformation and myths and offers the opportunity for patients to ask questions. Examples of introductory statements are given using the PLISSIT (Annon, 1974) and BETTER (Mick, Hughes, & Cohen, 2003) models as in previous chapters (see Figures 13-1 and 13-2).

Dealing With Changes to Body Image

Interventions to deal with changes to the body and resultant body image concerns can be addressed in a number of ways. Nurses should show patients what may happen

---

Figure 13-1. Example of the PLISSIT Model in Adolescent Patients With Cancer

- **Permission:** An example of this level would be to include a general statement that normalizes the topic.

  "Kids your age often have concerns about dating and interacting with people of the opposite sex. Perhaps we can spend a couple of minutes talking about this before your mom comes back."

- **Limited information:** Adolescents need information provided at the appropriate age level when they ask for it; however, anticipatory guidance also is necessary because adolescent patients may not know what they need to know or may be too shy to ask.

  "Can you tell me what has happened to your periods since staring chemotherapy? They may be irregular or they may have gone away completely; however, it is possible to get pregnant if you are having sex."

- **Specific suggestion:** Information at this level includes anticipatory guidance related to possible sexual consequences of medications and other treatments.

  "There is a risk that the treatment you have had means that your testicles will no longer produce sperm that can make a baby. Even though it seems like a million years away, at some point in the future you may be thinking about starting a family. When that time comes, you will need to see a specialist (usually a urologist) who will test you to see if you have active sperm. In the meantime, you still need to use condoms to protect both yourself and your sexual partner from infection."

- **Intensive therapy:** Nurses should know where to refer patients when problems or issues are disclosed that are beyond their scope of practice or expertise.

  "It sounds as if you are having a really hard time at school with some of those kids who are mean to you. With your permission, I would like to talk to the guidance counselor at your school to see if we can get you some help with dealing with them."

**Figure 13-2. Example of the BETTER Model in Adolescent Patients
With Cancer**

- **Bringing up the topic:** Nurses are encouraged to raise the issue of sexuality with patients at any age.

  "I would like to spend some time talking to you about how cancer and its treatments can affect your body and the way it feels."

- **Explaining that sex is a part of quality of life:** This helps to normalize the discussion and may help patients to feel less embarrassed or alone in having a problem.

  "At your age, we expect kids to be interested in dating and relationships and figuring out what feels good about your body. Cancer and chemo can change that. If you have any questions, any one of the nurses can help you to find the answers, so please ask if there is anything you want to know about."

- **Telling patients that resources will be found to address their concerns:** This step suggests to patients that even if the nurse does not have the immediate solution to the problem or question, others are available who can help.

  "I know a psychologist who does a lot of work with teenagers who have the same sorts of concerns as you do about dating and relationships. We can stop by his office and see if he can see you today."

- **Timing the intervention:** Patients may not be ready to deal with sexual issues at the time a problem is identified. However, patients can ask for information at any time in the future.

  "It is common for your periods to stop while you are having chemo. We can do tests after your treatment is over to see if your hormones are back at normal levels, and we also can arrange for you to see a fertility specialist if and when you are thinking about having a baby."

- **Educating patients about the sexual side effects of treatment:** Educating patients about potential side effects from treatments does not mean that they will occur. However, informing them about sexual side effects is as important as informing them about any other side effects.

  "You may find that you have some dryness in your vagina after the radiation treatments. This is usually temporary, but if it causes you pain, we can give you some gel that helps to keep that area well lubricated."

- **Recording:** A brief notation that a discussion about sexuality or sexual side effects occurred is important.

  "Anticipatory guidance about vaginal changes discussed with patient. Patient informed about the usefulness of vaginal moisturizers."

---

to them through the use of pictures or by arranging for contact with other adolescents with a similar diagnosis. The imagination is a powerful influence, and many patients are fearful because they have no idea about the reality of what to expect and instead imagine something far worse. Some adolescents may feel pressured into wearing a wig or head covering by parents or healthcare professionals and actually may prefer to shave their head at the early signs of hair loss and keep their head uncovered. Many role models exist in the world of sports and entertainment who are bald or shave their head and who can be positive influences for self-acceptance. Nurses should emphasize to adolescents that these changes are temporary—their hair will grow back, their skin will return to its normal tone, and, when treatment is complete, many of the other changes will resolve themselves. Although scars are permanent, their appearance will change over time, and they will be less noticeable. Adolescents with amputations tend to adapt well over time and actually may mature in the face of the challenges of living with altered appearance and function. Participating in a support group can be very beneficial, as can attending special events such as a summer camp for other adolescents with cancer (Zebrack et al., 2006). However, healthcare professionals should be empathetic and not unrealistically positive because this may further alienate a sensitive adolescent who already feels misunderstood. The use of hormone therapy can alleviate the symptoms of premature menopause that result from ovarian failure, and hormone therapy also can mimic normal menstrual cycles, thus helping adolescent females to feel more like their peers (Davis, 2006).

Impact on Fertility and Sexuality

The type of treatment administered may affect sexual maturation, and treatment decisions often are made by the parents under stressful circumstances in which the primary goal is to treat patients successfully and prevent the disease from causing death. Thoughts of future fertility and alterations to sexual functioning may seem of minor importance during diagnosis. Unfortunately, it is at precisely this time that a discussion of interventions such as sperm banking needs to be initiated. Nurses should have information about sperm banking on hand and should be willing to discuss this with adolescent patients and their parents, recognizing that this is a difficult decision to make in the face of life-threatening illness. The family should have the opportunity to think and talk about this. Depending on the chronologic and developmental age of the adolescent, the patient's parents may make this decision for him.

The general principle of both chemotherapy and radiation therapy in preserving or protecting fertility for young women is to offer treatment that has the lowest potential for affecting fertility. However, many families will choose a treatment that has the greatest potential for saving the patient's life, regardless of what the effect on future fertility may be. If pelvic irradiation is necessary, healthcare providers should consider surgically transposing the ovaries to a position above the iliac crests or shielding the ovaries with lead slabs during treatment (Beerendonk & Braat, 2005).

Families often assume that with advances in assisted reproductive technologies, future pregnancy is possible using a variety of in vitro fertilization techniques. The success rates of these techniques are low, currently in the 10% range, and this refers to embryo transfer only. An adolescent female is unlikely to have a partner whose sperm can be used to fertilize her ova. These procedures also require time for hyperstimulation of the ovaries and oocyte extraction, which often is not possible because of the need to start chemotherapy in a timely manner. Cryopreservation of ovarian tissue and oocytes is still experimental and may be precluded in certain types of cancer that carry a risk of reintroducing malignant tissue (Beerendonk & Braat, 2005). Timely referral to a geneticist, endocrinologist, urologist, or gynecologist also may be necessary to more fully explore reproductive potential (Kelton, 1999).

Contraception

Contraception is a topic that many regard as sensitive when dealing with adolescents in general and with adolescents with cancer in particular. As discussed previously, having knowledge about contraception does not lead to earlier sexual activity. Although many adolescents with cancer are told about the risks to fertility, a discussion about contraception often does not occur, and these patients are just as likely to be sexually active as their healthy peers (Laurence, Gbolade, Morgan, & Glaser, 2004). Sexual activity can occur in the spur of the moment, and adolescents must be prepared to protect themselves or their partner from pregnancy. This is particularly important for female adolescents with cancer, in whom pregnancy can be physically and emotionally dangerous.

The options for contraception are the same as for any other adolescent, but some cautions apply. Abstinence, if practiced perfectly, appears to offer the lowest risk of pregnancy. However, some adolescents with cancer may perceive that with a limited life span, they are not willing to forgo a sexual relationship. Periodic abstinence (avoiding intercourse around the time of ovulation) is risky, as female adolescents may have irregular cycles.

Oral contraceptives are the most effective method of contraception but are contraindicated for women with breast cancer. For patients with severe and/or prolonged thrombocytopenia from chemotherapy, continuous use of monophasic oral contraceptives will stop withdrawal bleeding and may be a good option. Women who experience vomiting with chemotherapy should be cautious because vomiting will affect absorption of oral contraceptives. Drug interactions also are possible for women on oral contraceptives, especially with cyclosporin and prednisolone; this applies in particular to women who have had an allogeneic bone marrow transplant. Progestin-only pills are not highly effective as a method of contraception and are not recommended for adolescents because they require a high degree of compliance. The availability of emergency contraception should be discussed with all adolescents, including those with cancer, as this is an effective method of preventing pregnancy when intercourse is unplanned or if another method of contraception fails.

The injectable contraceptive depot medroxyprogesterone acetate (known as DMPA) may be suitable for some adolescents with cancer because it induces amenorrhea and requires little in the way of compliance, as it is given every 12 weeks. However, it is a deep intramuscular injection and can cause a hematoma or infection in patients undergoing chemotherapy. Furthermore, long-term use of this contraceptive method is associated with decreased bone mass, which is a concern for patients who are on chemotherapy.

Intrauterine contraceptive devices are not recommended for adolescents because the presence of a foreign body in the uterus increases the risk for pelvic infection. This is particularly concerning in adolescents, who tend to practice serial monogamy and are thus at greater risk of acquiring a sexually transmitted infection. For adolescents at risk for infection because of chemotherapy, this is an additional caution. Thrombocytopenia increases the risk of heavy bleeding, which is common in women using this type of contraceptive method.

Barrier methods include the diaphragm, the cervical cap, the vaginal sponge, and the female and male condom. Although female-controlled methods of contraception appear to be a good idea, the failure rate with these contraceptive devices is high because they require planning and can be expensive. Adolescents generally regard them as preventing spontaneity and often are not comfortable touching their bodies when they have to insert the devices. The male condom is relatively inexpensive and easily available and provides protection against infection as well as pregnancy. Compliance can be a problem with any form of contraception that requires planning. Barrier devices, especially male condoms, may be a good choice for adolescents with cancer because they also prevent exposure to cytotoxics in vaginal or ejaculatory fluids and prevent transmission of sexually transmitted infections, including the human papillomavirus and HIV. The ideal method of contraception includes the use of oral contraceptives with consistent use of condoms.

Peer Relationships

Adolescents with cancer should be asked about their friendships with peers and their feelings of isolation and being different. Parents may be either overpermissive or overprotective, which will affect social functioning. Talking about what it feels like to be an adolescent in the context of the family is an important aspect of identifying concerns and facilitating a discussion within the family. For adolescents, being cut off from their peers is regarded as the ultimate form of alienation (Van Roosmalen, 2000), and every attempt should be made to encourage contact with friends, whether in person, on the phone, or via the Internet. This is particularly important for adolescents who are having stem cell or bone marrow transplantation, for which long periods of isolation are usual because of the risk of infection.

A social worker, psychologist, or child development specialist may be needed to assist if problems are identified or to provide anticipatory guidance. Participation in peer support groups helps to meet the needs of both parents and patients. Other adolescents with cancer will be able to normalize many of the feelings that the individual is experiencing and serve as positive role models, as having dealt with the same issues and concerns (Roberts et al., 1998). When the adolescent has completed treatment, he or she can become involved as a peer counselor or experienced group member, which aids in establishing self-esteem.

The Parents' Relationship

The needs and adaptation of the parents also are important considerations when caring for the family when a child has cancer. The bond between the parents may become threatened over time, and couples commonly struggle to cope with some aspect of their life while meeting the needs of the ill adolescent and also of other children in the family. Although the cancer experience often draws couples closer, other aspects of their life may suffer. For example, couples report that a health crisis strengthened trust and communication, whereas their sexual life tended to deteriorate significantly (Lavee & Mey-Dan, 2003).

Case Study

S.K. is 17 years old and was diagnosed and treated at the age of two for rhabdomyosarcoma of the pelvis. His treatment included surgical removal of the prostate, bladder, and part of the colon. He now has a girlfriend and mentions at one of his annual follow-up appointments that he is thinking about becoming sexually active and is not sure that he will be able to perform.

Questions to consider:
- What factors are important in the assessment of this young man?
- What anticipatory guidance should he receive?
- Should the nurse's advice be influenced by the fact that he is legally still a minor?

See Appendix B for answers to the case study questions.

Conclusion

Adolescence is a time of significant physical, emotional, and psychosexual development. Normal maturation is challenged by the diagnosis and treatment of cancer, and consequences may persist well into adulthood. Nurses must provide advice and guidance regarding sexual changes with tact, rapport, and sensitivity to the values and attitudes of the family and also must recognize the normal developmental needs of adolescents.

References

Annon, J. (1974). *The behavioral treatment of sexual problems.* Honolulu, HI: Enabling Systems.

Beerendonk, C.C., & Braat, D.D. (2005). Present and future options for the preservation of fertility in female adolescents with cancer. *Endocrine Development, 8,* 166–175.

Blythe, M., & Rosenthal, S. (2000). Female adolescent sexuality. *Obstetrics and Gynecology Clinics of North America, 27,* 125–141.

Brown, J., & Keller, S. (2000). Can the mass media be healthy sex educators? *Family Planning Perspectives, 32,* 255–256.

Brown, R. (2000). Adolescent sexuality at the dawn of the 21st century. *Adolescent Medicine, 11,* 19–34.

Chambas, K. (1991). Sexual concerns of adolescents with cancer. *Journal of Pediatric Oncology Nursing, 8,* 165–172.

Christie, D., & Viner, R. (2005). Adolescent development. *BMJ, 330,* 301–304.

Davis, M. (2006). Fertility considerations for female adolescent and young adult patients following cancer therapy: A guide for counseling patients and their families. *Clinical Journal of Oncology Nursing, 10,* 213–219.

Duncan, P., Dixon, R.R., & Carlson, J. (2003). Childhood and adolescent sexuality. *Pediatric Clinics of North America, 50,* 765–780.

Finnegan, A. (2004). Sexual health and chronic illness in childhood. *Paediatric Nursing, 16*(7), 32–36.

Greydanus, D.E., Rimsza, M.E., & Newhouse, P.A. (2002). Adolescent sexuality and disability. *Adolescent Medicine, 13,* 223–247.

Haka-Ikse, K. (1997). Female adolescent sexuality. The risks and management. *Annals of the New York Academy of Sciences, 816,* 466–470.

Heiney, S.P. (1989). Adolescents with cancer. Sexual and reproductive issues. *Cancer Nursing, 12,* 95–101.

Kelton, S. (1999). Sexuality education for youth with chronic conditions. *Pediatric Nursing, 25,* 491–495.

Klopovich, P.M., & Clancy, B.J. (1985). Sexuality and the adolescent with cancer. *Seminars in Oncology Nursing, 1,* 42–48.

Laurence, V., Gbolade, B.A., Morgan, S.J., & Glaser, A. (2004). Contraception for teenagers and young adults with cancer. *European Journal of Cancer, 40,* 2705–2716.

Lavee, Y., & Mey-Dan, M. (2003). Patterns of change in marital relationships among parents of children with cancer. *Health and Social Work, 28,* 255–263.

McCabe, M., & Cummins, R. (1998). Sexuality and quality of life among young people. *Adolescence, 33,* 761–773.

Mick, J., Hughes, M., & Cohen, M. (2003). Sexuality and cancer: How oncology nurses can address it BETTER. *Oncology Nursing Forum, 30*(Suppl. 2), 152–153.

Pentheroudakis, G., & Pavlidis, N. (2005). Juvenile cancer: Improving care for adolescents and young adults within the frame of medical oncology. *Annals of Oncology, 16,* 181–188.

Relander, T., Cavallin-Stahl, E., Garwicz, S., Olsson, A.M., & Willen, M. (2000). Gonadal and sexual function in men treated for childhood cancer. *Medical and Pediatric Oncology, 35,* 52–63.

Roberts, C.S., Turney, M.E., & Knowles, A.M. (1998). Psychosocial issues of adolescents with cancer. *Social Work in Health Care, 27*(4), 3–18.

Ropponen, P., Aalberg, V., Rautonen, J., Kalmari, H., & Siimes, M.A. (1990). Psychosexual development of adolescent males after malignancies in childhood. *Acta Psychiatrica Scandinavica, 82,* 213–218.

Van Roosmalen, E. (2000). Forces of patriarchy: Adolescent experiences of sexuality and conceptions of relationships. *Youth and Society, 32,* 202–208.

Westheimer, R., & Lopater, S. (2005). Sexuality in childhood and adolescence. In R. Westheimer & S. Lopater (Eds.), *Human sexuality: A psychosocial perspective* (2nd ed., pp. 421–457). Baltimore: Lippincott Williams & Wilkins.

Williams, H.A., & Wilson, M.E. (1989). Sexuality in children and adolescents with cancer: Pediatric oncology nurses' attitudes and behaviors. *Journal of Pediatric Oncology Nursing, 6,* 127–132.

Zebrack, B.J., Oeffinger, K.C., Hou, P., & Kaplan, S. (2006). Advocacy skills training for young adult cancer survivors: The Young Adult Survivors Conference at Camp Mak-a-Dream. *Supportive Care in Cancer, 14,* 779–782.

CHAPTER 14

The Adult With Cancer

Little to no change occurs in anatomic and physiologic functioning related to sexuality in early adulthood (ages 20–40); however, this is a developmental stage in which many people choose a mate, decide whether to have children, and then act on these decisions. A diagnosis of cancer in early adulthood may delay these life cycle events or may prevent individuals from ever committing to a partner, having children, and creating their own nuclear family. Cancer in this stage of life is unexpected, and often few other examples are available of how to cope (Bakewell & Volker, 2005).

Cancer in mid-adulthood also presents challenges. This usually is a time of stable intimate relationships; however, this sometimes is a period when divorce and separation occur, and the newly single adult must face many of the same challenges of establishing new relationships while also dealing with physical aging.

Psychosexual Challenges of Cancer in Young Adulthood

Young adults with cancer face a number of challenges in relation to healthy sexual functioning. This is the time when long-term primary relationships generally are established. Young adults with cancer may struggle with many issues in this regard. When does one tell a potential romantic or sexual partner that he or she has cancer and is undergoing treatment or that one has had cancer in the recent or distant past? In previous chapters, the physical changes resulting from cancer treatment have been described, but exactly how and when one should disclose these changes remains one of the biggest challenges for adults with cancer. There is no perfect time to inform a potential partner about a cancer diagnosis, missing or altered body parts, or ongoing treatment and monitoring. If this disclosure happens very soon after meeting someone, it may seem preemptive and may confuse the issue when the relationship does not progress. The individual with cancer may be left wondering if it was the disclosure, the cancer, or just the way things were going that caused the lack of progress. On the other hand, waiting to disclose this information may result in shock and a negative reaction by the partner, who may feel that the individual with cancer has not been honest.

Young adults with cancer and survivors also face other challenges. Fear of recurrence of a treated cancer and anxiety about the reality of cancer treatment are described as the most important aspects of recovery. Young adults with cancer also describe feeling different from their peers (Elad, Yagil, Cohen, & Meller, 2003). The usual tasks of young adulthood—establishing a career, having hopes and dreams for the future—are threatened by the illness. Progress through this developmental stage may be hampered by the need to depend on parents for physical and financial support. Parents may be reluctant to see their adult child move on after the years of fear and hands-on caring that have continued beyond the usual adolescent period.

Fertility Issues

Fertility issues often dominate the lives of young adults with cancer and survivors when they have found a mate. Having children is one of the hallmarks of young adulthood, and well-meaning friends and relatives may apply pressure to the couple by asking when they will start a family. Up to 30% of healthy couples experience some difficulties in achieving a pregnancy, and this figure is higher for adults with cancer.

For young women with breast cancer, treatment often is aggressive, with surgery, radiation, and chemotherapy being the usual regimen. Each of these modalities presents challenges to sexuality and normal sexual functioning. As discussed in Chapter 4, any surgical procedures on the breast can cause body image changes and altered sexuality. Radiation also affects patients, with altered sensations and fatigue as possible side effects. Chemotherapy affects body image and perception of physical attractiveness by causing hair loss and weight gain (Taylor et al., 2002). Younger women appear to experience greater psychosocial distress (Wenzel et al., 1999).

Chemotherapy also has the most direct effect on fertility. However, this depends on the agent used and the total dose administered. Menstruation may cease during the active phase of treatment, although younger women will experience amenorrhea to a lesser extent than their older counterparts (Simon, Lee, Partridge, & Runowicz, 2005). Pregnancy is possible, and patients should be cautioned that they may be fertile. Patients should avoid pregnancy for two to three years after completion of treatment, as this is the time when recurrence is most common (Simon et al.). Hormonal therapy often is used for years after other treatment to prevent a recurrence of breast cancer, and this too can affect fertility in addition to causing menopausal side effects that threaten everyday quality of life.

Deciding what treatment to have and whether to use adjuvant treatment is difficult for women who have completed their family, and it is that much more difficult for younger women who have either not started their family or who have fewer children than they desire (Partridge et al., 2004). Younger women often plan to have more children when treatment is over (Ganz, Greendale, Petersen, Kahn, & Bower, 2003) and may assume that pregnancy will be possible or that assisted reproductive technologies will be available and successful for them. Although many women report being bombarded with information at the time of diagnosis (Thewes, Meiser, Rickard, & Friedlander, 2003), others report that they cannot recall this discussion, which may reflect their inability to process information rather than the lack of discussion (Duffy, Allen, & Clark, 2005). Fertility-related information is seen as very important at the time of diagnosis, more so than menopause-related information (Thewes et al., 2005). When a breast cancer survivor becomes pregnant, the couple may have increased anxiety about the effect of the pregnancy on the woman and the potential effects on the fetus (Braun, Hasson-Ohayon, Perry, Kaufman, & Uziely, 2005). Younger women with breast cancer are known to experience higher levels of distress than their older counterparts, as well as fatigue and sexual dysfunction. All of these may persist for years after completion of treatment (Bakewell & Volker, 2005; Ganz et al.).

Cervical cancer is commonly diagnosed in women in young adulthood. As described in Chapter 6, radiation and surgery are the most common treatments and have far-reaching consequences for sexual functioning and fertility. In recent years, more conservative therapy such as trachelectomy (cervicectomy) has been attempted, especially for microinvasive disease. Variable results related to fertility have been achieved, and an increased risk for spontaneous abortion and preterm delivery has been seen (Simon et al., 2005).

Women diagnosed with ovarian cancer are treated with unilateral removal of the affected ovary whenever possible to preserve fertility. This cancer commonly is diagnosed at a later stage of disease, and more extensive surgery with removal of the uterus is common. Chemotherapy for ovarian cancer is used in selected cases, and regimens containing bleomycin, etoposide, and platinum are reported to not have an effect on long-term fertility (Simon et al., 2005).

Women with leukemia and lymphoma commonly are treated with chemotherapy regimens that cause amenorrhea and premature ovarian failure. Radiation therapy to the abdomen also may affect ovarian and uterine anatomy, and translocation of the ovaries is recommended to minimize damage. Fertility-related side effects are highly correlated with specific chemotherapeutic agents, and the newer regimens that do not include alkylating agents are less gonadotoxic. Men treated for these types of cancer also are at risk. Bone marrow transplantation frequently is used to treat leukemia. High-dose chemotherapy with total body irradiation usually is performed before the transplantation of either the patient's own marrow or donor marrow. This combination is noted to have the greatest impact on reproductive functioning (Davis, 2006).

The sexual effects of testicular cancer are discussed in great detail in Chapter 7. Subfertility is an important issue for men with testicular cancer; 75% of men with this cancer will have decreased sperm production at the time of diagnosis. This is thought to be associated with cryptorchidism (undescended testicle[s]) among other factors. Radiation and chemotherapy further degrade spermatogenesis in a dose-related manner, and for those who have lymph node dissection or tumor resection, ejaculatory disturbances have a further impact on fertility (Spermon et al., 2003). Some men may be able to impregnate their partners naturally (Brydoy et al., 2005); however, most will require some form of fertility assistance.

Preservation of fertility needs to be discussed and considered when establishing a treatment plan. Although it may be very difficult for newly diagnosed patients with cancer to make a decision about childbearing in the future while overwhelmed with a life-threatening diagnosis, young adults often are ill-prepared for the reality of reduced or absent fertility after treatment. They may assume that new reproductive technologies will be available and successful for them, but this may not be the case. Although cryopreservation of sperm is an efficient way of protecting the future fertility of males, women have far fewer options. This is particularly important for young women who have not yet chosen a life partner. All men should be offered the opportunity to bank sperm before starting treatment for any malignancy in which the gonads may be affected (Nalesnik, Sabanegh, Eng, & Buchholz, 2004). Men with cancer may have low sperm counts or high numbers of defective sperm. However, modern fertility treatments can maximize the potential for impregnation of a partner in the future by bypassing the normal physiologic barriers that sperm have to overcome (Sweet, Servy, & Karow, 1996).

Sperm must be collected according to very strict criteria and transported to a storage facility within certain time limits. Three days should elapse between each collection of ejaculate, and in some instances, even a short delay of 10 days (to allow for three ejaculations) may be too long to wait before starting treatment. Healthcare professionals at the storage facility should conduct a post-thaw analysis of the semen sample to establish whether the sperm contained in the ejaculate is viable (Sweet et al., 1996). There is no point in storing nonviable sperm for a long period of time. The cost of transporting and storing sperm is significant and usually is not covered by insurance. Access to laboratories and storage facilities also may be limited for men who live at a distance from larger cities. Although storing sperm for future use has clear advantages, the option is not always discussed with young adult patients with cancer. Many reasons for this exist, including lack of time, uncertainty of where the sperm can be stored, and a poor prognosis or the need for rapid initiation of treatment (Schover, 2005). In men who have not banked sperm, performing a testicular biopsy can assess whether some pools of sperm are present that can then be extracted and stored. However, this approach is not optimal (Tremelin & Petrucco, 2003).

Options for young women are more limited. Attempts to freeze oocytes have not met with great success, and the genetic integrity of these is questionable. For a young woman in an established relationship, the best option is to harvest multiple ova with subsequent in vitro fertilization with the partner's sperm and cryopreservation of the embryos for future implantation in her uterus or that of a surrogate (Schover, 2005). For a young woman who does not have a partner, this obviously is not an option. Attempts have been made to surgically remove ovarian tissue and freeze it with the intent of transplanting the stored tissue back into the woman in the future, but concerns exist that ovarian tissue could harbor malignant cells (Schover). There also is some hope that shutting down ovarian function with luteinizing hormone-releasing hormone–agonists during treatment may be protective and allow for normal ovarian function after completion of treatment; however, this remains controversial (Agarwal & Said, 2004). An organization called Fertile Hope has many resources for individuals with cancer who are concerned about fertility issues, and its Web site (www.fertilehope.org) provides information and support.

Although many young adult patients with cancer find that they experience reduced or absent fertility, this is not something that should be assumed, and the need for contraception should remain an issue while undergoing treatment and afterward. A more detailed discussion about the need for contraception is contained in Chapter 13, and the same cautions and advice pertain to young adults.

Psychosexual Challenges of Cancer in Mid-Adulthood

A cancer diagnosis in mid-adulthood (ages 41–65) also may change life goals and affect choices. This is a time when many individuals are secure in their primary relationships, have raised their children to near adulthood, and may be making plans for retirement. Most adults achieve some measure of comfort and acceptance of their sexual selves by this stage. During this period, the physiologic changes of aging appear. Women enter the menopausal trajectory, and men may notice that their sexual functioning begins to decrease. This may lead to fears of loss of sexual attractiveness and capacity (Finan, 1997). This also is a period when illness and death may occur among peers, family members, and friends.

The assumption often is made that mid-life relationships are stable, are based on open and honest communication, and are satisfying for both partners. Some relationships in mid-life are indeed like that; however, many individuals at this stage find themselves newly separated, divorced, or widowed. The same concerns about dating and establishing new relationships in the context of cancer arise for these individuals in mid-life as they do for younger adults. Mid-life adults who are in new relationships often find that the passions and energy that had left their old relationship are rekindled, and the physical and emotional changes brought on by a cancer diagnosis and treatment can be frustrating.

The normal physiologic signs of aging (e.g., graying hair, wrinkles) are interpreted differently by people and are heavily influenced by societal messages. A woman who is saddened by the changes that she sees in the mirror may find that her sense of self is altered, and with that, her sensuality and sexuality also are changed. When this is combined with scars from cancer surgery, radiation damage to skin, and alopecia from cancer treatment, the end result for the woman may be a significant lack of desire and the cessation of a sexual life. The same may be said for men. As men age, they may find that their desire for sex lessens and that their erections are less firm and less frequent. When challenged with a prostate cancer diagnosis, they may give up on attempting any sexual activity at all. Although no preferred way to be sexual exists, many couples in mid-life find that when sex is absent, they begin to drift apart, as the activity that promoted connectedness and intimacy between them is lost. The strongest predictor of sexual health for mid-life adults is the presence of a partner who is willing and able to participate in sexual activities. Poor health in a partner is commonly cited as the main reason that sexual activity has ceased.

As people age, their risk of being diagnosed with any type of cancer increases. Therefore, this diagnosis commonly occurs when individuals are in mid-life or beyond. The specifics of the sexual consequences of different cancer types are highlighted in Section II of this book. These chapters contain suggestions for counseling and advice; however, nurses should be able to introduce the topic of sexuality and aging in a general way. Figures 14-1 and 14-2 provide examples of the PLISSIT (Annon, 1974) and BETTER (Mick, Hughes, & Cohen, 2003) models, which may be helpful.

Figure 14-1. Example of the PLISSIT Model in Adult Patients With Cancer

- **Permission:** An example of this level would be to include a general statement that normalizes the topic.

  "At your age, many women wonder what effect the treatment may have on future fertility. Is there anything that you would like to ask me?"

- **Limited information:** In the case of a young couple where the woman has had surgery, the nurse should be able to give general information about resuming inter-course.

  "We generally advise couples to wait for the six-week checkup before having penetra-tive intercourse, but you may have intercourse sooner than that if you are feeling well and the mood is right. That way you can tell the surgeon if you noticed any changes at your follow-up appointment."

- **Specific suggestion:** Information at this level includes anticipatory guidance related to possible sexual consequences of medications and other treatments.

  "You need to use a condom every time you have intercourse while you are having chemotherapy. This is to protect you from infection and your partner from the toxicity of the chemo drugs that may be in your vaginal fluids."

- **Intensive therapy:** Nurses should know where to refer patients when problems or issues are disclosed that are beyond their scope of practice or expertise.

  "It sounds like you are really concerned about a future pregnancy and the potential for genetic defects because of the treatments you have had. It may be prudent for you to see the genetics counselor who works with us, and he/she can explain what, if any, risks apply in your case."

Case Study

T.B. is 28 years old and was recently diagnosed with testicular cancer. He is eager to begin chemotherapy as soon as possible after having a left-sided orchiectomy earlier in the week. He currently is not in a relationship and seems reluctant to discuss sperm banking with anyone.

Questions to consider:
- What specific suggestions or advice can the nurse give him to further encourage his participation in this procedure?
- What might be causing the patient's reluctance?
- How should the nurse deal with this?

See Appendix B for answers to the case study questions.

Figure 14-2. Example of the BETTER Model in Adult Patients With Cancer

- **Bringing up the topic:** Nurses are encouraged to raise the issue of sexuality with patients.

  "I always like to have some time to talk about the sexual side effects of the treatments patients have been prescribed. Can we take a few minutes to do that now?"

- **Explaining that sex is a part of quality of life:** This helps to normalize the discussion and may help patients to feel less embarrassed or alone in having a problem.

  "It is common for young women to wonder how they will ever meet a man after they have been diagnosed and treated for cancer. Let me share with you some of what I have heard from other young women like you."

- **Telling patients that resources will be found to address their concerns:** This step suggests to the patient that even if the nurse does not have the immediate solution to the problem or question, others are available who can help.

  "Although I am not an expert on this, other young women have told me that the second date is the time to tell a prospective partner that you have had cancer. The first date may seem too early, and the third date may seem too late. You may find that attending the support group for young adults with cancer will provide you with some helpful strategies, as there are many others who have gone through a similar experience."

- **Timing the intervention:** Patients may not be ready to deal with sexual issues at the time a problem is identified. However, patients can ask for information at any time in the future.

  "It is often difficult to imagine that you will feel better and that one day you will be thinking about starting a family of your own. A number of fertility specialists work with young survivors of cancer, and we can arrange for you to see one of them when you are ready."

- **Educating patients about the sexual side effects of treatment:** Educating patients about potential side effects from treatments does not mean that they will occur. However, informing them about sexual side effects is as important as informing them about any other side effects.

  "In the past, chemotherapy shut down all ovarian functioning, and many women stopped menstruating and were not able to conceive. The medication we are giving you has a much lower risk of doing that, and you should continue to menstruate and one day can have a baby."

- **Recording:** A brief notation that a discussion about sexuality or sexual side effects occurred is important.

  "Risks of premature ovarian failure discussed with patient and partner."

Conclusion

Cancer in people in this developmental stage provides some unique challenges to individuals and their partners. Young adults with cancer face issues related to fertility in addition to the usual demands of establishing and maintaining intimate relationships. Middle-aged adults begin to experience changes in physiologic functioning, which may lead to fears of loss of sexual attractiveness. Although some people are able to deal with these challenges with anticipatory guidance and good information, others will need a great deal of support to help them to cope with the changes they experience.

References

Agarwal, A., & Said, T.M. (2004). Implications of systemic malignancies on human fertility. *Reproductive Biomedicine Online, 9,* 673–679.

Annon, J. (1974). *The behavioral treatment of sexual problems.* Honolulu, HI: Enabling Systems.

Bakewell, R.T., & Volker, D.L. (2005). Sexual dysfunction related to the treatment of young women with breast cancer. *Clinical Journal of Oncology Nursing, 9,* 697–702.

Braun, M., Hasson-Ohayon, I., Perry, S., Kaufman, B., & Uziely, B. (2005). Motivation for giving birth after breast cancer. *Psycho-Oncology, 14,* 282–296.

Brydoy, M., Fossa, S.D., Klepp, O., Bremnes, R.M., Wist, E.A., Wentzel-Larsen, T., et al. (2005). Paternity following treatment for testicular cancer. *Journal of the National Cancer Institute, 97,* 1580–1588.

Davis, M. (2006). Fertility considerations for female adolescent and young adult patients following cancer therapy: A guide for counseling patients and their families. *Clinical Journal of Oncology Nursing, 10,* 213–219.

Duffy, C., Allen, S., & Clark, M. (2005). Discussions regarding reproductive health for young women with breast cancer undergoing chemotherapy. *Journal of Clinical Oncology, 23,* 766–773.

Elad, P., Yagil, Y., Cohen, L., & Meller, I. (2003). A jeep trip with young adult cancer survivors: Lessons to be learned. *Supportive Care in Cancer, 11,* 201–206.

Finan, S.L. (1997). Promoting healthy sexuality: Guidelines for early through older adulthood. *Nurse Practitioner, 22*(12), 54–64.

Ganz, P.A., Greendale, G.A., Petersen, L., Kahn, B., & Bower, J.E. (2003). Breast cancer in younger women: Reproductive and late health effects of treatment. *Journal of Clinical Oncology, 21,* 4184–4193.

Mick, J., Hughes, M., & Cohen, M. (2003). Sexuality and cancer: How oncology nurses can address it BETTER. *Oncology Nursing Forum, 30*(Suppl. 2), 152–153.

Nalesnik, J.G., Sabanegh, E.S., Jr., Eng, T.Y., & Buchholz, T.A. (2004). Fertility in men after treatment for stage 1 and 2A seminoma. *American Journal of Clinical Oncology, 27,* 584–588.

Partridge, A., Gelber, S., Peppercorn, J., Sampson, E., Knudsen, K., Laufer, M., et al. (2004). Web-based survey of fertility issues in young women with breast cancer. *Journal of Clinical Oncology, 22,* 4174–4183.

Schover, L.R. (2005). Sexuality and fertility after cancer. *Hematology: The American Society of Hematology Education Program Book* (pp. 523–527). Washington, DC: American Society of Hematology.

Simon, B., Lee, S., Partridge, A., & Runowicz, C.D. (2005). Preserving fertility after cancer. *CA: A Cancer Journal for Clinicians, 55,* 211–228.

Spermon, J.R., Kiemeney, L.A., Meuleman, E.J., Ramos, L., Wetzels, A.M., & Witjes, J.A. (2003). Fertility in men with testicular germ cell tumors. *Fertility and Sterility, 7*(Suppl. 9), 1543–1549.

Sweet, V., Servy, E.J., & Karow, A.M. (1996). Reproductive issues for men with cancer: Technology and nursing management. *Oncology Nursing Forum, 23,* 51–58.

Taylor, K.L., Lamdan, R.M., Siegel, J.E., Shelby, R., Hrywna, M., & Moran-Klimi, K. (2002). Treatment regimen, sexual attractiveness concerns and psychological adjustment among African American breast cancer patients. *Psycho-Oncology, 11,* 505–517.

Thewes, B., Meiser, B., Rickard, J., & Friedlander, M. (2003). The fertility- and menopause-related information needs of younger women with a diagnosis of breast cancer: A qualitative study. *Psycho-Oncology, 12,* 500–511.

Thewes, B., Meiser, B., Taylor, A., Phillips, K.A., Pendlebury, S., Capp, A., et al. (2005). Fertility- and menopause-related information needs of younger women with a diagnosis of early breast cancer. *Journal of Clinical Oncology, 23,* 5155–5165.

Tremelin, K., & Petrucco, O.M. (2003). Management of fertility issues in cancer survivors. *Australian Family Physician, 32,* 15–18.

Wenzel, L.B., Fairclough, D.L., Brady, M.J., Cella, D., Garrett, K.M., Kluhsman, B.C., et al. (1999). Age-related differences in the quality of life of breast carcinoma patients after treatment. *Cancer, 86,* 1768–1774.

CHAPTER 15

The Older Adult With Cancer

Societal attitudes toward sexuality in older adults contribute a significant number of myths to our knowledge and attitudes about this topic. Foremost among those is that older adults are not sexual and that romantic, passionate love disappears from the lives of older adults. Another is that older adults are too frail to enjoy sexual activity and that their sexual anatomy deteriorates to the point where sexual activity is no longer possible. Many assume that feelings of sexual arousal are based on physical attractiveness; older adults are not perceived to be sexually attractive and, thus, are thought to not be sexual at all. These myths are perpetuated by the media and often go unchallenged, so many healthcare providers believe them and find it difficult to deal with sexuality in their older adult patients.

Psychosexual Challenges of Cancer in Older Adulthood

As adults move through the life span, physical changes are inevitable. For older adults, the physical changes brought on by aging place individuals at increased risk for disease and chronic ill health; included in this is an increased risk for developing all kinds of cancers. Despite this risk, many older adults continue to experience an active and satisfying sexual life well into the seventh and eighth decades of life. Although anatomy and physiology change and illness and disability challenge many, human beings continue to have a fundamental need for affection and touch.

In both men and women, levels of sex hormones decline beginning as early as their 40s. By age 55, most women will have passed through menopause. After menopause, women no longer menstruate and are at risk for osteoporosis and heart disease, as they no longer have the protective effects of estrogen. Many men of this age note some changes related to lowered testosterone levels; they may lose muscle mass and experience a decline in interest in sexual intercourse. Both sexes experience a change in skin elasticity, leading to wrinkles and sagging of the breasts and loss of muscle mass. Pubic hair tends to turn gray and become sparser.

After menopause, women experience physical changes in the sexual organs, including thinning of the vaginal walls and loss of fatty tissue in the labia majora. Other changes occur that directly relate to sexual response. Women may experience reduced vaginal lubrication because of reduced levels of estrogen, which may result in pain with penetration and intercourse. The vaginal walls also may be less elastic. During arousal, the breasts do not increase in size to the same extent as they did in earlier years, and the muscle spasms felt during orgasm tend to be weaker.

Older adult men are still capable of achieving erections, but they may require more direct stimulation to achieve an erection, and these erections may be less firm than they once were. Erectile dysfunction increases in incidence with each decade (Dhar, 2001). However, since the advent of drugs such as sildenafil, tadalafil, and vardenafil, erections may be maintained for men well into their 80s, and sexual decline is not inevitable (Potts, Grace, Vares, & Gavey, 2006). During the arousal phase, the testicles may not elevate as high into the scrotum as they once did. Also, the testes may decrease in size. During orgasm, less ejaculate is emitted, and the force of ejaculation may be significantly less than before. As in women, orgasmic contractions may be lessened. The refractory period is lengthened—it will take the man a much longer period after orgasm before he can have another erection.

Although interest in sexual activity and frequency of activity tend to wane with aging, sexual satisfaction remains high among the older adult population. Men's interest remains primarily focused on sexual intercourse, whereas older women report that they are more interested in kissing and cuddling and hearing loving words from their spouse (Johnson, 1996). The emotional aspects of sexuality are enhanced for many older adults. With maturation and experience comes an ability to be emotionally intimate, and, in turn, this leads to greater levels of sexual intimacy (Kingsberg, 2002). Older individuals are intellectually and emotionally more capable of focusing on the relational characteristics of love and sometimes describe their sexual experiences as having a deep spiritual aspect (Ogden, 2001).

The most salient factor related to lack of sexual activity in older adults is either ill health in themselves or in their partners or the absence of a partner (DeLameter & Sill, 2005; Levy, 1994). Factors commonly associated with age such as ill health in one or both partners or loss of a partner can lead individuals to see sex as being less important. Conversely, being older is seen as helping individuals to cope with the loss of sex in a relationship (Gott & Hinchliff, 2003). Similarly, one's perception of personal health and adaptation to challenges to health status are important in the development of attitudes toward sexuality and sexual functioning (Johnson, 1998).

Comorbid disease and, specifically, the medications used to treat these conditions also can play a major role in altered sexuality (Gelfand, 2000). Drugs used to treat hypertension, including diuretics and alpha- and beta-blockers, cause erectile dysfunction and ejaculatory inhibition. Antidepressants, especially the selective serotonin reuptake inhibitors, cause decreased libido and inhibition of orgasm. Anticholinergic agents, histamine-H_2 receptor agonists, and digoxin also bring about adverse sexual side effects (Schiavi, 1994).

Disease tends to decrease mobility and tolerance for physical activity, which affects not only the perception that sexual activity is possible but also the ability to engage in sexual activity. The body image changes brought on by illness and disability also can have an effect. Cardiovascular disease, arthritis, and diabetes commonly occur in older adults, and these three conditions have a significant impact on sexual functioning (Camacho & Reyes-Ortiz, 2005).

Cancer in the Older Adult

The incidence of many cancers peaks in the sixth decade of life or later, and detailed descriptions of the effects of breast, prostate, gynecologic, colon, hematologic, head and neck, bladder, and penile cancers on sexual functioning are discussed in Section II of this text. Older individuals have already faced many challenges to health and family life over the years and therefore may be able to respond to a cancer diagnosis with more stability and less distress. This is the case for older women with breast cancer, who report that they get over the shock of the diagnosis quite quickly and then face the reality of living with the disease and facing the treatment. They state that they are grateful for an early diagnosis and hope for a good response to treatment. The experience of supporting others in their peer group through traumatic life events is seen as a form of preparation for the cancer experience and acceptance of the diagnosis (Ghizzani, Pirtoli, Bellezza, & Velicogna, 1995). However, the fatigue that often accompanies cancer treatment may have a greater impact on global physical functioning for older patients with cancer than their younger counterparts (Schmidt, Bestmann, Kuchler, Longo, & Kremer, 2005). If older men are not prepared for the possibility of sexual dysfunction related to treatment, their sense of loss and disappointment may be greater than if they had been prepared. This is particularly important information for care providers who might assume that a man is not sexually active because of advanced age and thus might not discuss this issue with the patient (Pinnock, O'Brien, & Marshall, 1998).

Information Sharing

Communicating about sexual issues is an area where healthcare providers often have some difficulty, and this is especially pertinent in the case of older adults. As discussed at length in Chapter 3, some healthcare providers may presume that because of the stage of life of the patient, sexuality is not an important issue (Huang, 1999). Healthcare providers are subject to the same influences as the general population, and ageist attitudes are common. Nurses who are more permissive in their own attitudes toward sexuality may be more open to discussing sexuality with older adult patients (Smook, 1992).

Older adults often feel that they are viewed differently than younger members of society and report that they do not feel validated in their interactions with healthcare providers (Tannenbaum, Nasmith, & Mayo, 2003). Older women have reported that they feel that physicians are not interested in talking with them about sexuality and that they are willing to be asked about their sexual functioning if they are given an explanation about why the questions are being asked (Loehr, Verma, & Seguin, 1997). This is an important reminder that certain norms and values exist that may be influenced by one's generation. Questioning about sexuality may be more acceptable to younger people, and although healthcare providers should explain or give a rationale for everything they do with patients, including explaining why they are asking certain questions, this is perhaps more important with older adult patients who may be more conservative.

Providing anticipatory guidance for older adult patients who are being treated for cancer always should include information on sexual side effects or changes. Older patients may assume that changes they experience are related to aging rather than the disease or its treatment and might not volunteer information about changes if they are not asked. Giving information about sexual side effects may help to allay patients' fears and also may allow for prompt treatment and prevention of further problems. Changes that patients experience should be placed in the context of the normal anatomic and physiologic processes of aging. Patients make the decision regarding medications for erectile dysfunction or urogenital aging. Healthcare providers should not be making suggestions or denying the patient access to treatment because of their assumptions about the patient based on his or her age.

One of the interventions for altered sexual functioning that often is suggested in the context of illness- or treatment-related changes is finding alternatives to penetrative intercourse. This may be especially challenging for older couples, who may have a limited sexual repertoire and may not consider alternatives to genital sex as acceptable. Older women (and men, for that matter) may never have masturbated and may not even know what this means (Szwabo, 2003). Choice of language and sensitivity to the cultural and/or religious background of patients and their partners are essential to keeping communication open. Older patients often are very appreciative of information and education about sexuality, as many did not have the information available to them when they were younger and thus may have limited choices because of lack of knowledge

(Tannenbaum et al., 2003). However, many couples have learned by trial and error and have established a satisfactory sex life within their relationship that has grown over the years. For many couples, the focus has moved away from penetrative intercourse and into activities that focus on giving and receiving pleasure from touch, words, and the sharing of emotions (Potts et al., 2006). Examples of how to introduce the topic of sexuality to older adult patients are given in Figures 15-1 and 15-2 using the PLISSIT model (Annon, 1974) and the BETTER model (Mick, Hughes, & Cohen, 2003), which may help to bring up the topic and discuss it in a more structured manner.

Figure 15-1. Example of the PLISSIT Model in Older Adult Patients With Cancer

- **Permission:** An example of this level would be to include a general statement that normalizes the topic.

  "Many people find that sexual functioning changes as they grow older. Can you tell me how things may have changed for you over the years?"

- **Limited information:** In the case of a couple where the man has had prostate surgery, the following statement will help to explain the onset of erectile dysfunction.

  "After removal of the prostate gland, men often find that they cannot have an erection or that their erection is less firm than it was before."

- **Specific suggestion:** Information at this level includes anticipatory guidance related to possible sexual consequences of medications and other treatments.

  "It is very common that men who take blood pressure medication have some difficulty with having erections. I would like to review all your medications with you, and this may help us identify what else may be contributing to this problem."

- **Intensive therapy:** Nurses should know where to refer patients when problems or issues are disclosed that are beyond the scope of practice or expertise of the nurse.

  "It sounds to me like you may be depressed since your surgery. We have a social worker on staff who works with patients to find ways to help cope with these feelings. I can check to see if she is available to see you now."

Figure 15-2. Example of the BETTER Model in Older Adult Patients With Cancer

- **Bringing up the topic:** Nurses are encouraged to raise the issue of sexuality with patients.

  "As we get older, we experience all sorts of changes in our bodies. Many of these alter the way we function as sexual beings. I would like to spend a little bit of time asking you some questions about this."

(Continued on next page)

**Figure 15-2. Example of the BETTER Model in Older Adult Patients
With Cancer *(Continued)***

- **Explaining that sex is a part of quality of life:** This helps to normalize the discussion and may help patients to feel less embarrassed or alone in having a problem.

   "Sex is a normal part of life and is something that we all do. I ask all my patients about how they are doing in this regard as we know that sex is an important part of overall quality of life and is important to many if not all of us."

- **Telling patients that resources will be found to address their concerns:** This step suggests to patients that even if the nurse does not have the immediate solution to the problem or question, others are available who can help.

   "If I am not able to answer any question you may have, I will ask one of my colleagues if she has the answer. There are also books that I can consult for the answers to your questions."

- **Timing the intervention:** Patients may not be ready to deal with sexual issues at the time a problem is identified. However, patients can ask for information at any time in the future.

   "You seem a little tired after being here for most of the afternoon. If this is not a good time for you, I can make another appointment for you to come back and talk about this."

- **Educating patients about the sexual side effects of treatment:** Educating patients about potential side effects from treatments does not mean that they will occur. However, informing them about sexual side effects is as important as informing them about any other side effects.

   "It is not uncommon for couples to think that their sex life is over after one has been treated for cancer. This is not always the case, but there are some things that you may need to do differently when you go home, and I have a book about this that you can read. However, if you have some questions now, I can answer them."

- **Recording:** A brief notation that a discussion about sexuality or sexual side effects occurred is important.

   "Short discussion with patient about resuming intercourse after discharge. Reading material given."

Case Study

Mr. and Mrs. M are an older adult couple who came to see the nurse when Mr. M completed his treatment for lung cancer. He had surgery to remove one lobe of his left lung followed by radiation and chemotherapy. When the nurse asks them about any changes to their sexual life, Mrs. M gets tearful. She states that she feels very alone and does not know how to help her husband. He seems embarrassed that she is even talking about this and says forcefully that there is no problem.

Questions to consider:
- The patient does not want to talk about it, but this is an issue for his wife. What should the nurse do in this instance?
- What are some of the factors that may be contributing to this situation?
- What are some of the factors that need to be considered when dealing with an older adult couple that may not be applicable to a younger couple?
See Appendix B for answers to the case study questions.

Conclusion

Older adults with cancer face the disease in the context of the unique developmental milestones of this stage and within the competing context of comorbidities of self and significant others. Although sexual changes are normal with aging and may be exacerbated with the treatment of cancer, this does not mean that older adult patients do not want to continue having a satisfying sex life or that healthcare providers should not ask about this or provide anticipatory guidance in this regard.

References

Annon, J. (1974). *The behavioral treatment of sexual problems.* Honolulu, HI: Enabling Systems.

Camacho, M.E., & Reyes-Ortiz, C.A. (2005). Sexual dysfunction in the elderly: Age or disease? *International Journal of Impotence Research, 17*(Suppl. 1), S52–S56.

DeLameter, J.D., & Sill, M. (2005). Sexual desire in later life. *Journal of Sex Research, 42,* 138–149.

Dhar, H.L. (2001). Gender, aging, health and society. *Journal of the Association of Physicians of India, 49,* 1012–1020.

Gelfand, M.M. (2000). Sexuality among older women. *Journal of Women's Health and Gender-Based Medicine, 9,* S15–S20.

Ghizzani, A., Pirtoli, L., Bellezza, A., & Velicogna, F. (1995). The evaluation of some factors influencing the sexual life of women affected by breast cancer. *Journal of Sex and Marital Therapy, 21,* 57–63.

Gott, M., & Hinchliff, S. (2003). How important is sex in later life? The views of older people. *Social Science and Medicine, 56,* 1617–1628.

Huang, C. (1999). Discussing sex with disabled patients. *Western Journal of Medicine, 171,* 76–77.

Johnson, B.K. (1996). Older adults and sexuality: A multidimensional perspective. *Journal of Gerontological Nursing, 22*(2), 6–15.

Johnson, B.K. (1998). A correlational framework for understanding sexuality in women age 50 and older. *Health Care for Women International, 19,* 553–564.

Kingsberg, S.A. (2002). The impact of aging on sexual function in women and their partners. *Archives of Sexual Behavior, 31,* 431–437.

Levy, J.A. (1994). Sex and sexuality in later life stages. In A.S. Rossi (Ed.), *Sexuality across the lifespan* (pp. 287–309). Chicago: University of Chicago Press.

Loehr, J., Verma, S., & Seguin, R. (1997). Issues of sexuality in older women. *Journal of Women's Health, 6,* 451–457.

Mick, J., Hughes, M., & Cohen, M. (2003). Sexuality and cancer: How oncology nurses can address it BETTER. *Oncology Nursing Forum, 30*(Suppl. 2), 152–153.

Ogden, G. (2001). Spiritual passion and compassion in late-life sexual relationships. *Electronic Journal of Human Sexuality, 4*. Retrieved January 3, 2007, from http://www.ejhs.org/volume4/Ogden.htm

Pinnock, C., O'Brien, B., & Marshall, V.R. (1998). Older men's concerns about their urological health: A qualitative study. *Australian and New Zealand Journal of Public Health, 22*, 368–373.

Potts, A., Grace, V., Vares, T., & Gavey, N. (2006). "Sex for life"? Men's counter-stories on "erectile dysfunction," male sexuality and aging. *Sociology of Health and Illness, 28*, 306–329.

Schiavi, R.C. (1994). Effect of chronic disease and medication on sexual functioning. In A.S. Rossi (Ed.), *Sexuality across the lifespan* (pp. 313–339). Chicago: University of Chicago Press.

Schmidt, C.E., Bestmann, B., Kuchler, T., Longo, W.E., & Kremer, B. (2005). Impact of age on quality of life in patients with rectal cancer. *World Journal of Surgery, 29*, 190–197.

Smook, K. (1992). Nurses' attitudes towards the sexuality of older people: An investigative study. *Nursing Practice, 6*, 15–17.

Szwabo, P. (2003). Counseling about sexuality in the older person. *Clinics in Geriatric Medicine, 19*, 595–604.

Tannenbaum, C., Nasmith, L., & Mayo, N. (2003). Understanding older women's health care concerns: A qualitative study. *Journal of Women and Aging, 15*, 3–16.

CHAPTER 16

The Terminally Ill

In the terminal stages of the cancer trajectory, sexuality often is not regarded as important by healthcare providers. They often assume that when life nears its end, individuals and couples are not concerned about sexual issues, so these issues are not talked about. This attitude is borne out by the paucity of research into the topic. However, sexuality is much more than sexual activity, as discussed in Chapter 1 of this book.

Sexual functioning is but one aspect of sexuality. Other aspects include the need for intimacy and touch, emotional and physical closeness, and self-image as male or female. People express sexuality through thoughts, fantasies, and dreams, as well as through communication and social interaction with others. But it also is a personal and private experience that never may be openly expressed. Sexuality is part of being a whole person and thus is a part of one's sense of self.

Although the need or ability to participate in sexual activity may wane in the terminal stages of illness, the need for touch and intimacy and how one views oneself do not necessarily wane in tandem. Individuals may, in fact, suffer from the absence of loving and intimate touch in the final months, weeks, or days of life, and if healthcare providers do not recognize and deal with this, they are doing their patients a disservice and are not providing holistic care.

Communicating About Sexuality With the Terminally Ill

Attitudes of healthcare professionals act as a barrier to the discussion and assessment of sexuality at the end of life. As previously discussed, healthcare providers bring a set of attitudes, beliefs, and knowledge to their practice that they assume applies equally to their patients. Their experience during their training and practice may lead them to believe that patients at the end of life are not interested in things that are commonly perceived as sexual. How often are a patient and his or her partner seen in bed together or in an intimate embrace? Healthcare professionals may have never seen this type of affection because the circumstances of hospitals and even hospice may be such that privacy for the couple can never be assured, so couples do not attempt to lie together. The bed may be too small, and another patient may be in the room. Staff may insist that the door to the room remain open at all times, and staff may enter the room frequently and without knocking. Patients may avoid expressing physical affection to their partner/spouse if they perceive that this is something that is not allowed or considered "proper" in the hospital or hospice setting.

For patients who remain at home during the final stages of illness, the scenario is not that different. Often they are moved to a central location in the house, such as a family or living room, and no longer have privacy. Although this may be more convenient for providing care, it precludes the expression of sexuality as patients are always in view. Professional and volunteer helpers frequently are in the house, and patients may never be alone or alone with their partner to afford an opportunity for sexual expression.

Healthcare providers may not include an assessment of patients' sexual functioning at the end of life, assuming that this does not matter at this stage of the illness trajectory. This sends a very clear message to patients and their partners that it is either taboo or of no importance. In turn, patients and/or their partners may find it difficult to ask questions or bring up the topic if they think that the subject is not to be discussed. All patients should be offered the opportunity to discuss sexual concerns or questions regardless of their stage of illness (Ananth, Jones, King, & Tookman, 2003).

Sexual Functioning at the End of Life

Factors affecting sexual functioning at the end of life are essentially the same as those affecting individuals with cancer at any stage of the disease trajectory. These include psychosocial issues such as change in roles, changes in body- and self-image, depression, anxiety, and poor communication. Side effects of treatment also may alter sexual functioning; fatigue, nausea, pain, scarring, hormonal manipulation, and effects of other medications all play a role in how patients feel and see themselves and how their partners view them. Fear of pain may be a major factor in the cessation of sexual activity, and partners may be equally fearful of hurting the patient.

Sexual health assessment should include questions about how the patients view themselves as sexual beings, the importance of sexuality for the individual now and in former times both as an individual and for the couple, and how the illness has affected this (Stausmire, 2004). These may be difficult questions to ask and answer, so it should be discussed once rapport and trust have been established in the care provider-patient relationship. Ideally this topic should have been broached repeatedly along the disease trajectory and should not be first mentioned at a time when death is near.

The partner must participate in this discussion because this may be the only opportunity that the couple has to openly discuss the subject. Couples commonly avoid this topic, as the partner may feel selfish and demanding if he or she expresses a need for physical contact in the face of end-of-life issues (Cort & Monroe, 2004). Patients may feel that they are not "normal" if they want physical contact when they are supposed to be dying. Gentle, probing questions can facilitate a discussion between the couple and can highlight the normalcy of sexual intimacy, although often in an altered format, for couples when death is drawing near.

The Needs of the Couple

Couples may find that in the final stages of illness, emotional connection to the loved one becomes an important part of sexual expression. Verbal communication and physical touching that is nongenital may take the place of previous sexual activity (Lemieux, Kaiser, Pereira, & Meadows, 2004). Many note the cessation of sexual activity as one of the many losses resulting from the illness, and this has a negative impact on quality of life. Some partners may find it difficult to be sexual when they have taken over much of the day-to-day care of the patient and see their role as caregiver rather than lover. The physical and emotional toll of providing care may be exhausting and may affect the desire for sexual contact. In addition, some partners find that as the end of life nears for the patient, they need to begin to distance themselves, and part of this may include avoiding intimate touch (Cort & Monroe, 2004). This is not wrong, but can make the partners feel guilty and become more likely to avoid physical interactions.

Couples may need to be given permission to touch each other at this stage of the illness, and healthcare providers need to consciously address the physical and attitudinal barriers that prevent this from happening. Privacy issues need to be dealt with, including encouraging patients to close their door when private time is desired and having all levels of staff respect this. A sign on the door indicating that the patient is not to be disturbed should be enough to prevent staff from walking in, and all staff and visitors should abide by this. Partners should be given explicit permission to lie with patients in the bed. In an ideal world, double beds could be provided, but this would present obvious challenges in terms of moving beds into and out of rooms and also for staff who may need to move or turn patients. Kissing, stroking, massaging, and embracing are unlikely to cause physical harm to a patient and actually may facilitate relaxation and decrease pain. Partners also may be encouraged to participate in the routine care of the patient. Having the partner assist with bathing the patient and applying body lotion may be a nonthreatening way of encouraging touch if the partner fears hurting the patient.

Specific strategies for couples who want to continue their usual sexual activities can be suggested depending on what physical or emotional barriers exist. Giving patients permission to think about themselves as sexual in the face of terminal illness is the first step. Offering patients/couples the opportunity to discuss sexual concerns or needs validates their feelings and may normalize their experience, which might bring comfort (Hordern & Currow, 2003).

More specific strategies for symptoms include the following suggestions. The timing of analgesia may need to be altered to maximize pain relief and avoid sedation when couples want to be sexual. Narcotics, however, can interfere with arousal, which may be counterproductive (Lamb, 2001). Fatigue is a common experience in the end stages of cancer, and couples/individuals can be encouraged to set realistic goals for what is possible and try to use the time of day when they are most rested to be sexual either alone or with their partner. Using a bronchodilator or inhaler before sexual activity may be helpful for patients who are short of breath. Using additional pillows or wedges will allow patients to be more upright and breathe more easily. Couples may find information about alternative sexual positions very useful if there is scarring or stenosis in the genital area. The female-on-top position allows the woman to control the depth of penile thrusting, which can allow intercourse to be more comfortable. If intercourse is not desirable or possible, the couple can use a vibrator, either for mutual masturbation or to facilitate orgasm for the woman alone. Incontinence or the presence of an indwelling catheter may represent a loss of control and dignity and may be seen as an insurmountable barrier to genital touching. An indwelling catheter can be removed just before sexual activity, making genital touching still possible, and should not affect pleasurable physical sensations. The potential for leakage of urine or feces can be dealt with by using towels and plastic sheets to protect bedding. The bathtub or shower can provide an alternative venue for sexual activity where the fear of leakage can be controlled and the hot water itself can be relaxing.

Often, permission to talk about or experiment with different forms of sexual play opens the path to a different but satisfying sexual experience for couples whose sexual script has remained the same for many years. Healthcare providers must emphasize that no right or wrong way of being sexual exists in the face of terminal illness; whatever couples or individuals choose to do is appropriate and right for them. Couples commonly find that impending death draws them much closer and that they are able to express themselves in ways that they had not for many years. Using the PLISSIT (Annon, 1974) and BETTER (Mick, Hughes, & Cohen, 2003) models may be helpful in introducing the topic for discussion (see Figures 16-1 and 16-2).

Additional questions healthcare providers can ask patients are

- How important is your sexuality to you?
- How has your sexuality been affected by your illness?
- If there have been changes to your sexual life, what do you miss the most?
- How have you been able to express your sexuality since becoming ill?
- What barriers prevent you and your partner/spouse from expressing yourselves sexually at this time?
- How can these be changed/modified so that you are able to express yourselves at this time?
- What have you tried, and what has worked or not been helpful?
- How has your illness affected your partner's sexuality?
- How have you been able to talk about this?

Figure 16-1. Example of the PLISSIT Model in Terminally Ill Patients With Cancer

- **Permission:** An example of this level would be to include a general statement that normalizes the topic.

  "Many couples facing end-of-life issues find it a little difficult for a variety of reasons to express their love for each other. What, if any, thoughts have you had about this?"

- **Limited information:** In the case of a couple where one person is facing death in the near future, the nurse should be able to provide suggestions for maintaining intimacy.

  "Why don't I put a notice on the door that you are not to be disturbed by anyone for the next hour? That way you can spend some time cuddling and chatting and no one will come through the door."

- **Specific suggestion:** Information at this level includes anticipatory guidance related to possible sexual consequences of medications and other treatments.

  "Taking some additional morphine before sexual activities will make your husband more comfortable, but it also is going to sedate him and make it more difficult for him to experience sexual feelings. This is a delicate balance, and perhaps we should just experiment and see what trade-offs you are prepared to make."

- **Intensive therapy:** Nurses should know where to refer patients when problems or issues are disclosed that are beyond their scope of practice or expertise. However, intensive therapy is not something that is usually initiated in the terminal stages of illness.

Figure 16-2. Example of the BETTER Model in Terminally Ill Patients With Cancer

- **Bringing up the topic:** Nurses are encouraged to raise the issue of sexuality with patients.

  "I always ask my patients about their sexuality and how it has been affected by their illness. Is this a good time to have a chat?"

- **Explaining that sex is a part of quality of life:** This helps to normalize the discussion and may help patients to feel less embarrassed or alone in having a problem.

  "Even though you are in the hospice, you are still the same person you always were. Part of being human is having sexual feelings and seeing yourself as a sexual being. How has that changed for you?"

- **Telling patients that resources will be found to address their concerns:** This step suggests to patients that even if the nurse does not have the immediate solution to the problem or question, others are available who can help.

  "You seem to be having a real struggle finding the words to tell your wife how you feel. Do you think it may be helpful to have one of the social workers come down and see you, and you can talk about this more and perhaps even practice what you want to tell her?"

- **Timing the intervention:** Patients may not be ready to deal with sexual issues at the time a problem is identified. However, patients can ask for information at any time in the future.

  "We can talk to the staff about giving you and your husband some private time. You may not feel like this today, but perhaps tomorrow may be better for you. We even have a sign that we can hang on the doorknob."

- **Educating patients about the sexual side effects of treatment:** Educating patients about potential side effects from treatments does not mean that they will occur. However, informing patients about sexual side effects is as important as informing them about any other side effects.

  "Most of the pain killers you are taking will have an effect on any sexual feelings that you are used to having. We can try to alter the dose or the timing, but there will be a trade-off in terms of pain relief."

- **Recording:** A brief notation that a discussion about sexuality or sexual side effects occurred is important.

  "The patient and his wife would like to have some private, undisturbed time. Staff were informed of this, and a sign is to be placed on the door after lunch every day."

Case Study

B.S. and R.S. are a young couple who have been married for 10 years. They have three children under the age of eight, and B.S. is in the final stages of breast cancer. She was diagnosed when she was pregnant with their youngest child, who is now two and a half years old. The patient has managed to remain at home during the terminal stages of her illness. Her bed is now in the family room, and she spends most of her time surrounded by her young family and the many friends and family members who are supporting them.

At one of her appointments with the pain and symptom management nurse, B.S. breaks down when the nurse asks her about her relationship with her husband. She admits that she misses the physical closeness they once had and feels cheated that so much of their intimate life together has been "taken away," first by the three pregnancies so close together and then the times when she was breastfeeding and caring for infants. She feels as if she has been denied so much pleasure and now that she is facing death, she is full of regrets for what might have been.

Questions to consider:

- What additional questions should the nurse ask this young woman?
- What are some strategies that the nurse could suggest to alleviate some of the patient's distress?
- What other healthcare providers may be helpful in dealing with this situation?
- Could this distress have been prevented? How?

See Appendix B for answers to the case study questions.

Conclusion

Sexuality in terminally ill patients is a subject that has traditionally been avoided. Attitudes of staff, significant others, and patients may need to be examined to fully understand why this is so. However, terminally ill people have continued needs for affection and touch. There is no reason for sexual touch to be precluded in the final stages of a terminal illness, but specific interventions related to pain control and comfort may be necessary.

References

Ananth, H., Jones, L., King, M., & Tookman, A. (2003). The impact of cancer on sexual function: A controlled study. *Palliative Medicine, 17,* 202–206.

Annon, J. (1974). *The behavioral treatment of sexual problems.* Honolulu, HI: Enabling Systems.

Cort, E., & Monroe, B.O.D. (2004). Couples in palliative care. *Sexual and Relationship Therapy, 19,* 337–354.

Hordern, A.J., & Currow, D.C. (2003). A patient-centered approach to sexuality in the face of life-limiting illness. *Medical Journal of Australia, 179*(Suppl. 6), S8–S11.

Lamb, M.A. (2001). Sexuality. In B.R. Ferrell & N. Coyle (Eds.), *Textbook of palliative nursing* (pp. 309–315). New York: Oxford University Press.

Lemieux, L., Kaiser, S., Pereira, J., & Meadows, L.M. (2004). Sexuality in palliative care: Patient perspectives. *Palliative Medicine, 18,* 630–637.

Mick, J., Hughes, M., & Cohen, M. (2003). Sexuality and cancer: How oncology nurses can address it BETTER. *Oncology Nursing Forum, 30*(Suppl. 2), 152–153.

Stausmire, J.M. (2004). Sexuality at the end of life. *American Journal of Hospice and Palliative Care, 21,* 33–39.

The Effect of the Cancer Experience on Couples

Cancer has been described as a couple's experience, in that life-threatening illness in one partner affects all aspects of the other partner's life and their life together. Despite this, little research has been done on the effect of cancer on couple functioning outside of breast and prostate cancers. Most of what healthcare providers know about the cancer experience in couples in which the woman has breast cancer focuses on communication, support, and coping. With prostate cancer, the stronger focus is on erectile functioning; however, the perspective of the partner has had little attention in this regard. The literature also focuses almost exclusively on heterosexual couples.

Prostate Cancer

When a man is diagnosed with prostate cancer, both he and his partner are affected. Initially the focus is on survival, fear that the man will die, and finding some control in what feels like an uncontrollable situation. Couples often will find themselves talking about their relationship and connecting with each other on an emotional level between the time of diagnosis and treatment. Women tend to focus on the survival of their spouse (Harden et al., 2002) and often are more stressed by the diagnosis than their spouse (Crowe & Costello, 2003). At this time, communication between spouses may decrease as the man withdraws and refuses to talk and the female spouse is reluctant to insist on having a discussion as she does not want to make the situation for her husband any worse (Boehmer & Clark, 2001a).

This is a time when rationalization about treatment side effects takes place, with men minimizing the anticipated loss of sexual function in the light of the partner's support and desire for survival above all else (Gray, Fitch, Phillips, Labrecque, &

Klotz, 1999). Anticipating how sexual problems may impact the relationship is different for men and women. Men are aware that erections are more important to them than to their female partners. Women, on the other hand, tend to believe that the importance of penetrative sex in the relationship is less than the emotional aspects of a long-term relationship. In fact, women may overestimate the importance of erections to their husbands (Jacobs et al., 2002; Wilson, Dowling, Abdolell, & Tannock, 2000). Couples might be hopeful that medication will allow them to continue at the same level of sexual functioning after treatment (Boehmer & Babayan, 2004) and may be unable to conceive of a life devoid of sex if these medications do not work.

Later in the disease process, when erectile difficulties are experienced after treatment, the relationship may undergo some profound changes as the partners struggle to find a new role in their intimate relationship. For men, sexual performance often equates to intimacy, but for women, intimacy and sexual intercourse are not synonymous (Heyman & Rosner, 1996). Women also are distressed when their partner is experiencing erectile dysfunction (Wagner, Fugl-Meyer, & Fugl-Meyer, 2000). If the partners do not communicate their feelings, each may be left to suffer in isolation (Soloway, Soloway, Kim, & Kava, 2005). Conflict may arise in the relationship because of feelings of distancing and lack of communication (Butler, Downe-Wamboldt, Marsh, Bell, & Jarvi, 2000). Some couples are able to communicate their feelings verbally, whereas others are able to show love and support without the use of words (Gray et al., 1999). Communication should be constructive and honest and understood by both partners. Couples may attempt to deal with sexual changes through the use of humor and teasing; however, this may be effective for only a brief period, after which communication about sexual difficulties tends to decrease or cease completely (Boehmer & Clark, 2001a). Some couples try to maintain the relationship through affectionate displays, finding hobbies that they can pursue as a couple, or initiating noncoital contact. However, this requires effort and a willingness to do things differently and may not always be successful (Navon & Morag, 2003). When a couple fails to reconnect after a life-challenging event such as a cancer diagnosis, dissonance and unhappiness may result (Gray et al.). Displays of jealousy on the part of the male are common and often are a result of failure to communicate feelings and uncertainty in the context of the illness (Boehmer & Clark, 2001a).

Some men with erectile dysfunction report increased libido after surgery. One man described it as "wanting what you cannot have" (Lavery & Clarke, 1999), but this may abate over time as adjustments to reality are made. But for many couples, particularly those who are older, sex may not be an issue at all (Lavery & Clarke), and the cancer experience may bring them closer emotionally (Phillips et al., 2000). However, for those whose main means of achieving closeness and intimacy was through intercourse, the loss of this activity can threaten the integrity of the relationship in fundamental ways (Navon & Morag, 2003).

Men may not talk about prostate health-related problems with their wives and may not communicate treatment options with them (Boehmer & Clark, 2001a). They may not share their feelings about the physical changes they experience in an attempt to protect their wives. Once treatment is initiated and sexual functioning is affected, communication about sexuality can cease completely, and all physical closeness might end (Boehmer & Clark, 2001b). Men may feel that if penetrative intercourse is impossible because of erectile dysfunction, it is unfair to their wives to be physically affectionate if intercourse will not result. These men may believe that their wives are not upset by a unilateral decision; however, when the wives are interviewed, the loss of this aspect of married life frequently is acknowledged (Jakobsson, Hallberg, & Loven, 2000). Women may experience sexual dysfunction correlating to erectile difficulties in their husbands. Female partners of men who have had radical prostatectomy report more pain with intercourse, which may be related to attempts at penetration with a partially erect penis (Shindel, Quayle, Yan, Husain, & Naughton, 2005). Women may be unsure of how to initiate sexual contact of a different kind following treatment, and if they have been left out of discussions with healthcare providers about treatment side effects, they may not know how sexual functioning will be altered (Mason, 2005).

For some men, the thought of losing the ability to have intercourse may be as disturbing as being diagnosed with cancer. Some men might delay treatment because they are unwilling to give up that part of their lives or they see themselves as being less of a man if they cannot have an erection. They may feel so despondent that they would rather be dead than be unable to function sexually. Men reported that the inability to have an erection, the loss of sexual desire, and the lack of sexual functioning threatened their masculinity (Boehmer & Clark, 2001b). This inability to have an erection, and thus penetrative intercourse, caused them to refrain from any form of sexual interaction with their wives. Others, particularly if older, are not as profoundly affected, as they have been experiencing age-related changes and adjusting to them (Bertero, 2001).

Men who were sexually active before the diagnosis of prostate cancer may find it very difficult to adjust to erectile dysfunction (Moore & Estey, 1999). This symptom is suggested to irreversibly change the marital relationship. Suggestions to find alternative ways of achieving sexual satisfaction and maintaining intimacy are not always helpful, and many couples are unable to change their usual sexual activities in response to the challenges of erectile dysfunction (Heyman & Rosner, 1996). Younger men may have more difficulty with these factors than older men, who may have been experiencing problems with sexual functioning prior to the diagnosis (Steginga et al., 2001). Erectile dysfunction also can interfere with nonsexual aspects of life. A man who is unable to have an erection might see himself as less of a man and can experience role strain (Harden, 2005). This can have far-reaching consequences in his interactions with people other than his sexual partner (Bokhour, Clark, Inui, Silliman, & Talcott, 2001).

Breast Cancer

The relationship that women with breast cancer have with their partner/spouse is important in terms of their adaptation to the disease and any consequences they may experience. Some couples report that the breast cancer experience draws them closer (Dorval et al., 2005); however, there also is the potential for distancing in the relationship (Schultz, Klein, Beck, Stava, & Sellin, 2005). Both partners will have different needs at various points in the disease, treatment, and recovery trajectory, and although the woman usually is thought to have higher needs, at times the needs of her spouse/partner may, in fact, be higher (Hoskins, 1995). Support from significant others is assumed to mitigate the distress that most women experience with a diagnosis of cancer. However, some partners actually withdraw in the face of the high levels of distress experienced by women with breast cancer, and this withdrawal prevents patients from getting the support they need (Bolger, Foster, Vinokur, & Ng, 1996). Women perceive active engagement of the partner in the relationship, even if that means conflict, as a positive sign and prefer it over withdrawal (Giese-Davis, Weibel, & Spiegel, 2000).

The partner's sexual interest in the woman is important for her perception of herself and satisfaction with the relationship. Women who perceive that their partner finds them sexually desirable, who have a positive experience when sexual activity is first attempted after treatment, and who believe that their partner is emotionally invested in the relationship appear to adjust well in the first year after treatment (Wimberly, Carver, Laurenceau, Harris, & Antoni, 2005). However, some men suppress their sexual urges or find that their need for sex decreases in the face of the illness (Holmberg, Scott, Alexy, & Fife, 2001). This, in turn, may make women feel less desirable and unsure of themselves and their attractiveness.

Women who are in a relationship with someone who shares their thoughts and feelings and who perceives these thoughts and feelings as caring and accepting are more likely to describe the relationship as an intimate one (Manne, Ostroff, Rini, et al., 2004). The disclosure of thoughts and feelings is reciprocal; when a woman's disclosure is met with disclosure by the spouse, distress is reduced (Manne, Sherman, et al., 2004). This reciprocity and sharing may be construed as an aspect of emotional support and is one factor in the strengthening and growth of relationships following the trauma of a life-threatening diagnosis (Manne, Ostroff, Winkel, et al., 2004). If the partner appears to understand the feelings of the woman with breast cancer, less disturbance of body image and fewer sexual problems occur (Fobair et al., 2006).

Other Cancers

Women with cervical cancer consider their partner to be an important factor in their healing and also regard the partner as playing an essential role in the integrity of the relationship. Sexual consequences of treatment are complicated by the belief that men need intercourse and will seek it outside of the relationship if their partners are not willing to engage in sexual activity. For women, verbal and nonverbal expressions of intimacy (e.g., reassurance, sensual touching) are satisfying. Women also are likely to misinterpret their partner's reluctance to recommence sexual activity; men often are fearful of hurting the woman with cancer, but the woman may erroneously interpret this as the man not finding her attractive (Juraskova et al., 2003).

Women with cervical cancer and their partners report disruption in their relationship, alteration in sexual and intimate functioning, and problems with instrumental functioning (de Groot et al., 2005). Although both female patients and their partners reported similar concerns, the timing of educational interventions to address these concerns may differ. Men may need more information in the early stages after diagnosis, as their distress levels fall in the year following diagnosis and treatment of their partner. Women appear to have higher levels of concern even one year after treatment and may require ongoing support for an extended period of time.

Most men treated for testicular cancer found that their marital or partner relationships were strengthened by their cancer diagnosis and treatment (Heidenreich & Hofmann, 1999), and support from partners increased during the treatment and then returned to pretreatment levels (Fleer, Hoekstra, Sleijfer, & Hoekstra-Weebers, 2004). However, sexual satisfaction tends to be lower in couples where the man has had testicular cancer, and satisfaction is especially low for men who develop a relationship after completion of treatment (Tuinman, Fleer, Sleijfer, Hoekstra, & Hoekstra-Weebers, 2005).

Counseling for Couples

Healthcare providers can help couples to be more communicative and supportive of one another in the context of cancer. Nurses should assess the couple's needs before initiating educational or supportive interventions. Healthcare providers frequently assume the most pressing needs of the patient and his or her partner and address these perceptions instead of asking the couple. An example of this is the information that is deemed important to couples when the man has prostate cancer. Both physicians and nurses may assume that erectile dysfunction is the most important topic to be addressed; however, patients and their partners have identified fear of the unknown as their priority (Jacobs et al., 2002; Wilson et al., 2000). Nurses should ask the patient with prostate cancer who he wants to be involved in aspects of his care and to explain that providing his wife with information is important in helping her to cope (Manne, Babb, Pinover, Horwitz, & Ebbert, 2004). Ultimately, this will help him, as most men depend on their wives for emotional support (Boehmer & Babayan, 2005). Men may choose not to involve their wives in their decision about prostate cancer treatment and may prefer to seek information from other men, particularly those who have been treated for the disease themselves (Boehmer & Babayan, 2005). This may lead to the wife feeling excluded and isolated. Wives have an important role to play from diagnosis to recovery (Maliski, Heilemann, & McCorkle, 2002). However, couples' established communication and support patterns, particularly with older couples, may not be amenable to change. Women might feel reluctant to be involved in the treatment decision, believing that men have to live with the consequences, so only they can make this decision (Davison, Goldenberg, Gleave, & Degner, 2003). Conversely, though, the wife often is the primary seeker of information (Echlin & Rees, 2002) and may be more active in this than the patient (Feltwell & Rees, 2004).

Support for couples after a cancer diagnosis may include not only factual or treatment-related information but also assistance with coping along the disease trajectory. This may include encouraging patients and their partners to see the event in a positive light, which ultimately may help couples to experience some positive outcomes (Thornton & Perez, 2006). For example, reframing a prostate cancer diagnosis in the context of the indolent natural history of the disease may help couples to avoid panic or the impulse to rush to treatment.

When couples experience sexual difficulties after treatment, interventions to assist them should focus on the couples and not merely on a pharmaceutical or mechanical solution to the problem. Mutuality of the relationship is an important aspect of support and understanding (Manne, Ostroff, Rini, et al., 2004), and for this reason, interventions focusing on the couple are more likely to be effective. An essential part of sexual functioning is communication, and interventions that include communication skills are more likely to be successful (Manne et al., 2005; Scott, Halford, & Ward, 2004). Couples also will benefit from information about how to engage in noncoital activities (Monturo, Rogers, Coleman, Robinson, & Pickett, 2001).

Many couples find it difficult to access help for sexual difficulties, which may, in part, be because they have different needs. Men are more inclined to seek a quick and effective pharmaceutical solution, and women are more inclined to give up and not seek help at all (Neese, Schover, Klein, Zippe, & Kupelian, 2003). The presence of the partner at sexuality counseling sessions is important. However, the evidence is contradictory in men with prostate cancer. A study by Davison, Elliott, Ekland, Griffin, and Wiens (2005) suggested that participation of the partner is necessary, whereas another study found that the presence of a partner did not affect outcomes (Canada, Neese, Sui, & Schover, 2005).

As discussed in previous chapters, most couples are willing to discuss sexual issues if they are afforded the opportunity to do so in a safe and trusting environment. Indicating that this is a topic of concern for many couples in which one partner has cancer allows one or both partners to open up and communicate their questions and concerns either immediately or later. Chapter 22 provides a more detailed discussion of sexuality counseling.

Case Study

S.W. is 62 years old and is recovering in the hospital from surgery for endometrial cancer. She had a total hysterectomy and will receive chemotherapy in five weeks. Her husband is very attentive to her needs; however, she appears cold and distant when he is there and cries quietly when he leaves.

Questions to consider:
- Should the healthcare provider ask what S.W. is feeling?
- What might the issue be?

The patient tells you that her husband is "highly sexed" and she is afraid that he is going to leave her if she cannot be sexually active with him.
- What are the important questions to ask at this time?
- How should the nurse go about correcting any myths or misconceptions the patient has?
- Would a referral for sex therapy be helpful at this point?

See Appendix B for answers to the case study questions.

Conclusion

All aspects of the cancer experience have the potential to affect the role and emotional functioning of couples when one partner is going through the cancer experience. At times of crisis, couples may need assistance to communicate clearly and to involve the partner in various aspects of decision making and ongoing care. Sexual difficulties are common along the disease trajectory, and a couples approach to solving them is more effective than the patient seeing a problem as his or hers alone and attempting to deal with it in isolation.

References

Bertero, C. (2001). Altered sexual patterns after treatment for prostate cancer. *Cancer Practice, 9,* 245–251.

Boehmer, U., & Babayan, R.K. (2004). Facing erectile dysfunction due to prostate cancer treatment: Perspectives of men and their partners. *Cancer Investigation, 22,* 840–848.

Boehmer, U., & Babayan, R.K. (2005). A pilot study to determine the support during the pre-treatment phase of early prostate cancer. *Psycho-Oncology, 14,* 442–449.

Boehmer, U., & Clark, J.A. (2001a). Communication about prostate cancer between men and their wives. *Journal of Family Practice, 50,* 226–231.

Boehmer, U., & Clark, J.A. (2001b). Married couples' perspectives on prostate cancer diagnosis and treatment decision-making. *Psycho-Oncology, 10,* 147–155.

Bokhour, B.G., Clark, J.A., Inui, T.S., Silliman, R.A., & Talcott, J.A. (2001). Sexuality after treatment for early prostate cancer: Exploring the meanings of "erectile dysfunction." *Journal of General Internal Medicine, 16,* 649–655.

Bolger, N., Foster, M., Vinokur, A., & Ng, R. (1996). Close relationships and adjustment to a life crisis: The case of breast cancer. *Journal of Personality and Social Psychology, 70,* 283–294.

Butler, L., Downe-Wamboldt, B., Marsh, S., Bell, D., & Jarvi, K. (2000). Behind the scenes: Partners' perceptions of quality of life post radical prostatectomy. *Urologic Nursing, 20,* 254–258.

Canada, A.L., Neese, L.E., Sui, D., & Schover, L.R. (2005). Pilot intervention to enhance sexual rehabilitation for couples after treatment for localized prostate carcinoma. *Cancer, 104,* 2689–2700.

Crowe, H., & Costello, A.J. (2003). Prostate cancer: Perspectives on quality of life and impact of treatment on patients and their partners. *Urologic Nursing, 23,* 279–285.

Davison, B.J., Elliott, S., Ekland, M., Griffin, S., & Wiens, K. (2005). Development and evaluation of a prostate sexual rehabilitation clinic: A pilot project. *BJU International, 96,* 1360–1364.

Davison, B.J., Goldenberg, S.L., Gleave, M., & Degner, L.F. (2003). Provision of individualized information to men and their partners to facilitate treatment decision making in prostate cancer. *Oncology Nursing Forum, 30,* 107–114.

de Groot, J.M., Mah, K., Fyles, A., Winton, S., Greenwood, S., Depetrillo, A.D., et al. (2005). The psychosocial impact of cervical cancer among affected women and their partners. *International Journal of Gynecological Cancer, 15,* 918–925.

Dorval, M., Guay, S., Mondor, M., Masse, B., Falardeau, M., Robidoux, A., et al. (2005). Couples who get closer after breast cancer: Frequency and predictors in a prospective investigation. *Journal of Clinical Oncology, 23,* 3588–3596.

Echlin, K.N., & Rees, C.E. (2002). Information needs and information-seeking behaviors of men with prostate cancer and their partners: A review of the literature. *Cancer Nursing, 25,* 35–41.

Feltwell, A., & Rees, C.E. (2004). The information-seeking behaviors of partners of men with prostate cancer: A qualitative pilot study. *Patient Education and Counseling, 54,* 179–185.

Fleer, J., Hoekstra, H.J., Sleijfer, D.T., & Hoekstra-Weebers, J.E. (2004). Quality of life of survivors of testicular germ cell cancer: A review of the literature. *Supportive Care in Cancer, 12,* 476–486.

Fobair, P., Stewart, S.L., Chang, S., D'Onofrio, C., Banks, P.J., & Bloom, J.R. (2006). Body image and sexual problems in young women with breast cancer. *Psycho-Oncology, 15,* 579–594.

Giese-Davis, J., Weibel, D., & Spiegel, D. (2000). Quality of couples' relationship and adjustment to metastatic breast cancer. *Journal of Family Psychology, 14,* 251–266.

Gray, R., Fitch, M., Phillips, C., Labrecque, M., & Klotz, L. (1999). Presurgery experiences of prostate cancer patients and their spouses. *Cancer Practice, 7,* 130–135.

Harden, J. (2005). Developmental life stage and couples' experiences with prostate cancer: A review of the literature. *Cancer Nursing, 28*, 85–98.

Harden, J., Schafenacker, A., Northouse, L., Mood, D., Smith, D., Pienta, K., et al. (2002). Couples' experiences with prostate cancer: Focus group research. *Oncology Nursing Forum, 29*, 701–709.

Heidenreich, A., & Hofmann, R. (1999). Quality-of-life issues in the treatment of testicular cancer. *World Journal of Urology, 17*, 230–238.

Heyman, E.N., & Rosner, T.T. (1996). Prostate cancer: An intimate view from patients and wives. *Urologic Nursing, 16*, 37–44.

Holmberg, S.K., Scott, L.L., Alexy, W., & Fife, B.L. (2001). Relationship issues of women with breast cancer. *Cancer Nursing, 24*, 53–60.

Hoskins, C. (1995). Adjustment to breast cancer in couples. *Psychological Reports, 77*, 435–454.

Jacobs, J.R., Banthia, R., Sadler, G.R., Varni, J.W., Malcarne, V.L., Greenbergs, H.L., et al. (2002). Problems associated with prostate cancer: Differences of opinion among health care providers, patients, and spouses. *Journal of Cancer Education, 17*, 33–36.

Jakobsson, L., Hallberg, I.R., & Loven, L. (2000). Experiences of micturition problems, indwelling catheter treatment and sexual life consequences in men with prostate cancer. *Journal of Advanced Nursing, 31*, 59–67.

Juraskova, I., Butow, P., Robertson, R., Sharpe, L., McLeod, C., & Hacker, N. (2003). Post-treatment sexual adjustment following cervical and endometrial cancer: A qualitative insight. *Psycho-Oncology, 12*, 267–279.

Lavery, J., & Clarke, V. (1999). Prostate cancer: Patients' and spouses' coping and marital adjustment. *Psychology, Health and Medicine, 4*, 289–302.

Maliski, S.L., Heilemann, M.V., & McCorkle, R. (2002). From "death sentence" to "good cancer": Couples' transformation of a prostate cancer diagnosis. *Nursing Research, 51*, 391–397.

Manne, S., Babb, J., Pinover, W., Horwitz, E., & Ebbert, J. (2004). Psychoeducation group intervention for wives of men with prostate cancer. *Psycho-Oncology, 13*, 37–46.

Manne, S., Ostroff, J., Rini, C., Fox, K., Goldstein, L., & Grana, G. (2004). The interpersonal process model of intimacy: The role of self-disclosure, partner disclosure, and partner responsiveness in interactions between breast cancer patients and their partners. *Journal of Family Psychology, 18*, 589–599.

Manne, S.L., Ostroff, J.S., Winkel, G., Fox, K., Grana, G., Miller, E., et al. (2005). Couple-focused group intervention for women with early stage breast cancer. *Journal of Consulting and Clinical Psychology, 73*, 634–646.

Manne, S., Ostroff, J.S., Winkel, G., Goldstein, L., Fox, K., & Grana, G. (2004). Posttraumatic growth after breast cancer: Patient, partner, and couple perspectives. *Psychosomatic Medicine, 66*, 442–454.

Manne, S., Sherman, M., Ross, S., Ostroff, J., Heyman, R.E., & Fox, K. (2004). Couples' support-related communication, psychological distress, and relationship satisfaction among women with early stage breast cancer. *Journal of Consulting and Clinical Psychology, 72*, 660–670.

Mason, T. (2005). Information needs of wives of men following prostatectomy. *Oncology Nursing Forum, 32*, 557–563.

Monturo, C.A., Rogers, P.D., Coleman, M., Robinson, J.P., & Pickett, M. (2001). Beyond sexual assessment: Lessons learned from couples post radical prostatectomy. *Journal of the American Academy of Nurse Practitioners, 13*, 511–516.

Moore, K.N., & Estey, A. (1999). The early post-operative concerns of men after radical prostatectomy. *Journal of Advanced Nursing, 29*, 1121–1129.

Navon, L., & Morag, A. (2003). Advanced prostate cancer patients' ways of coping with the hormonal therapy's effect on body, sexuality, and spousal ties. *Qualitative Health Research, 13*, 1378–1392.

Neese, L.E., Schover, L.R., Klein, E.A., Zippe, C., & Kupelian, P.A. (2003). Finding help for sexual problems after prostate cancer treatment: A phone survey of men's and women's perspectives. *Psycho-Oncology, 12*, 463–473.

Phillips, C., Gray, R.E., Fitch, M.I., Labrecque, M., Fergus, K., & Klotz, L. (2000). Early postsurgery experience of prostate cancer patients and spouses. *Cancer Practice, 8*, 165–171.

Schultz, P.N., Klein, M.J., Beck, M.L., Stava, C., & Sellin, R.V. (2005). Breast cancer: Relationship between menopausal symptoms, physiologic health effects of cancer treatment and physical constraints on quality of life in long-term survivors. *Journal of Clinical Nursing, 14*, 204–211.

Scott, J.L., Halford, W.K., & Ward, B.G. (2004). United we stand? The effects of a couple-coping intervention on adjustment to early stage breast or gynecological cancer. *Journal of Consulting and Clinical Psychology, 72,* 1122–1135.

Shindel, A., Quayle, S., Yan, Y., Husain, A., & Naughton, C. (2005). Sexual dysfunction in female partners of men who have undergone radical prostatectomy correlates with sexual dysfunction of the male partner. *Journal of Sexual Medicine, 2,* 833–841.

Soloway, C.T., Soloway, M.S., Kim, S.S., & Kava, B.R. (2005). Sexual, psychological and dyadic qualities of the prostate cancer 'couple.' *BJU International, 95,* 780–785.

Steginga, S.K., Occhipinti, S., Dunn, J., Gardiner, R.A., Heathcote, P., & Yaxley, J. (2001). The supportive care needs of men with prostate cancer (2000). *Psycho-Oncology, 10,* 66–75.

Thornton, A., & Perez, M. (2006). Posttraumatic growth in prostate cancer survivors and their partners. *Psycho-Oncology, 15,* 285–296.

Tuinman, M.A., Fleer, J., Sleijfer, D.T., Hoekstra, H.J., & Hoekstra-Weebers, J.E. (2005). Marital and sexual satisfaction in testicular cancer survivors and their spouses. *Supportive Care in Cancer, 13,* 540–548.

Wagner, G., Fugl-Meyer, K., & Fugl-Meyer, A. (2000). Impact of erectile dysfunction on quality of life: Patient and partner perspectives. *International Journal of Impotence Research, 12,* S144–S146.

Wilson, K., Dowling, A., Abdolell, M., & Tannock, I. (2000). Perception of quality of life by patients, partners and treating physicians. *Quality of Life Research, 9,* 1041–1052.

Wimberly, S.R., Carver, C.S., Laurenceau, J.P., Harris, S.D., & Antoni, M.H. (2005). Perceived partner reactions to diagnosis and treatment of breast cancer: Impact on psychosocial and psychosexual adjustment. *Journal of Consulting and Clinical Psychology, 73,* 300–311.

CHAPTER 18

Gay and Lesbian Patients

Surprisingly, little is written in the literature about the experience of gays, lesbians, and bisexuals in the healthcare system, and in the cancer care system in particular. Conservative estimates suggest that 2%–3% of the U.S. population would self-identify as gay or lesbian (Blank, 2005), and, thus, most care providers would expect to encounter at least some gay or lesbian patients every year. This estimate includes some regional variation, with large metropolitan centers seeing more gay/lesbian/bisexual patients than smaller or rural ones. However, many gay/lesbian/bisexual patients choose to not disclose their sexual orientation, or they limit disclosure to care providers whom they trust or to very few care providers whom they deem as having to know about this.

Societal Attitudes

This reluctance to disclose or fear of the consequences of disclosure is related to two essential concepts: homophobia and heterosexism. Homophobia describes a fear, often irrational, of gay men and lesbian women on the part of heterosexuals. This fear usually is not based on experience or knowledge of gays and lesbians but rather on myths and assumptions. It often is manifested in derogatory language, jokes, and discriminatory treatment of individuals perceived or known to be gay or lesbian. At its very worst, it may involve extreme violence ("gay bashing") toward those perceived to be homosexual. Some gay/lesbian individuals may have subconsciously accepted this negative view that homosexuality is abnormal and even deviant and thus experience self-loathing and lack of self-acceptance; this is termed *internalized homophobia* and can result in risky behaviors, such as substance abuse and high-risk sexual activity.

Heterosexism, on the other hand, refers to viewing the world through the lens of heterosexuality and a lack of realization or acknowledgment that alternatives exist. This is evident in the assumption that everyone is heterosexual, and anything else is not "normal." Examples of heterosexism in healthcare systems abound. Asking a patient for his or her marital status is a heterosexist assumption because most gays or lesbians cannot be married. The choices under this classification include married, separated/divorced, widowed, or single. How does a lesbian woman who is in a long-term relationship answer this question? Heterosexism serves to alienate gays and lesbians, and although it is not as overtly threatening as homophobia, the social and psychological effects are far-reaching and are known to delay entry into the healthcare system.

Many healthcare providers describe themselves as being neutral in their practice regarding the sexual orientation of their patients. This is based on the belief that health care should be accessible to all and should not be based on the particular needs of any one group or population (Brotman, Ryan, Jalbert, & Rowe, 2002). This may result in healthcare providers not asking about sexual orientation when meeting new patients or ignoring disclosure in an attempt to appear accepting. Providers should acknowledge this disclosure and reflect acceptance and caring, which will further encourage patients to share sensitive information that may influence care (Williams-Barnard, Mendoza, & Shippee-Rice, 2001). In fact, patients may interpret neutral behavior as a negative response (Boehmer & Case, 2004).

Disclosure of Same-Sex Attraction or Relationship

Disclosure of sexual orientation is recognized as being difficult across the life span. The level of difficulty relates to the nature of the relationship (e.g., telling a parent), the age of the individual who is disclosing his or her sexuality (e.g., adolescent versus adult), and the value placed on the relationship. Concealment of sexual orientation is thought to lead to poor health outcomes (Cole, Kemeny, Taylor, & Visscher, 1996) and risk-taking behavior, including smoking and alcohol and substance abuse (Case et al., 2004).

Lesbians may find it more difficult to disclose their sexual orientation to healthcare providers (Klitzman & Greenberg, 2002), which may reflect the lack of power that many women feel in society in general and in the healthcare system in particular. Reasons for nondisclosure include fear of homophobia or a belief that sexual orientation is a private matter. However, those who have disclosed such information state that they did so when they felt that the environment was safe and that they had done some work in finding a healthcare provider whom others had described as sensitive and accepting to the needs of lesbians. Strategies for disclosure include altering forms to reflect relationship status (inserting the words "same-sex partner" when asked for marital status), bringing the partner to medical appointments and introducing her as "my partner," and telling healthcare providers early that one is homosexual so that if the patient needs to find another healthcare provider, this can be done before much time has passed (Boehmer & Case, 2004).

Healthcare Risks Related to Homosexuality

Healthcare providers are likely to make assumptions about both the healthcare status and the risks of disease of their gay/lesbian/bisexual patients. Examples of these include the notions that all gay men have anal intercourse and that self-identified lesbians never have penetrative sex with men. Both of these assumptions are false; many gay men do not include anal intercourse as part of their sexual repertoire, and some lesbians occasionally have penetrative sex with men for different reasons and yet continue to identify themselves as exclusively lesbian because this is where their emotional and intimate connections are best expressed.

Homosexuality and Cancer

Assumptions about risk for cancer abound. Lesbians are seen to be at low risk for cervical cancer and therefore may not be offered routine cervical screening (Carroll, 1999). These women might have been exposed to the human papillomavirus many years earlier, or, as previously discussed, may, in fact, be having penetrative intercourse. Lesbians also are less likely to participate in regular screening activities such as mammography and may have fewer interactions with the healthcare system if they do not become pregnant and do not have prenatal visits (Rankow, 1995). Lesbians may be at greater risk for breast and ovarian cancers because they might not benefit from the protective effects of pregnancy, breastfeeding, or use of oral contraceptives (Dibble, Roberts, & Nussey, 2004). Lesbians also tend to have higher body mass indexes than their heterosexual counterparts, which increases their risk of developing cardiovascular disease, diabetes, and ovarian cancer (Dibble, Roberts, Robertson, & Paul, 2002; Hughes & Evans, 2003).

The focus of health care for gay men in the past two decades has been on their risk of contracting HIV/AIDS. However, increasing evidence has shown that gay men who have receptive anal intercourse are at increased risk for anal cancer. Additionally, men who insert recreational drugs such as crystal meth or Ecstasy into their rectum are at increased risk for anal cancer (Ferri, 2004). Gay men with HIV/AIDS are at risk for acquiring cancers such as lymphoma as a result of the immune suppression caused by HIV infection. Gay men have the same risk for prostate cancer as men in the general population, but almost no patient education material on this topic exists that is specifically targeted to gay men (Blank, 2005).

Lesbians with breast cancer report varied experiences in the healthcare system. Although most do not describe being subjected to overt homophobia and discrimination because of their sexual orientation, some see themselves as being targeted or being denied standard care. For example, one woman recounted her experience of being told to remain stoic in the face of pain during a procedure because "lesbians are tough and should be able to tolerate pain" (Sinding, Barnoff, & Grassau, 2004).

Lesbians may experience less distress after a breast cancer diagnosis than heterosexual women. This is because lesbians often have a higher level of acceptance of their body image both before and after treatment. Furthermore, lesbians rate the support they receive from their partners as higher; female partners are seen to be more loving and caring, more willing to listen, and more helpful with daily tasks than the male partners of heterosexual women with breast cancer (Fobair et al., 2001). However, interactions with the healthcare system, particularly during a time of crisis such as a cancer diagnosis, remain fraught with anxiety for lesbians (Boehmer & Case, 2004). Some women report experiencing hostility from healthcare providers in response to their disclosure of sexual orientation (Matthews, 1998). Many others feel that they have to actively disclose because they are never asked outright if they are lesbian, and the common assumption is that all women are heterosexual. Lesbians who are in a partnered relationship more frequently disclose their sexual orientation to healthcare providers (Boehmer, Linde, & Freund, 2005). Many homosexual patients introduce their partner to the healthcare provider to promote the inclusion of the partner in their care and treatment and to ensure equality of care with their heterosexual counterparts (Matthews, Peterman, Delaney, Menard, & Brandenburg, 2002). Lesbians with cancer name their intimate partner as the most frequent source of support (Boehmer, Freund, & Linde, 2005); however, they also are well supported by friends rather than family of origin because of long-standing issues related to acceptance of their sexual orientation (Matthews, 1998). As time passes after diagnosis, the need for support and information may decline as coping improves and distress declines (Fobair et al., 2002). Women with breast cancer often find that support groups are helpful in adjusting to the diagnosis and treatment. Lesbians, however, may find that attending a support group of predominately heterosexual women is not very helpful. They may not feel comfortable enough in the situation to disclose their sexual orientation and may find that the heterosexist assumptions of the group are a barrier to receiving the support they need (Matthews et al., 2002).

The issues for gay men with prostate cancer have largely been ignored in the research literature. Traditionally, the consequences of treatment for prostate cancer are seen as the dominant quality-of-life issues that men with this cancer have to deal with (see Chapter 5). Almost all the patient education literature focuses on vaginal sex as the end point of sexual encounters for men, and the language used is heterosexist. This in itself presents a barrier to gay men's access to healthcare information. The literature on decision making for men with prostate cancer focuses on the role that the partner/spouse (almost always a woman) can play in helping patients to make a timely and appropriate decision. Gay men may feel that this language is exclusionary, particularly those patients who do not have a partner on whom they can rely for support, guidance, and assistance.

The nuances of gay sexual activity play a major role in the priority that gay men with prostate cancer place on erectile functioning. For example, men who are primarily anal receptive in their sexual activity may place less importance on their own ability to have an erection but will be more concerned about the potential for rectal pain and irritation following radiation therapy (Blank, 2005). Urologists are just as likely to be homophobic and heterosexist as any other healthcare providers. They may have very little knowledge about male homosexuality and thus might not provide the necessary information to enable gay patients to make treatment choices that address their health and sexual concerns and priorities.

Support groups for men with prostate cancer may not meet the needs of the homosexual population. Given that this is a disease of mainly older men, some of those attending these support groups may be conservative in their outlook and overtly homophobic. Larger metropolitan centers may offer support groups specifically for gay men; however, this does not mean that gay men or care providers know about these and can refer them. Support groups are available on the Internet that cater specifically to gay men. These can be particularly helpful to men in smaller centers or men who are not willing or able to attend a gay-specific support group.

Gay men with colorectal cancer experience the same sexual consequences as their heterosexual counterparts; however, for gay men who are anally receptive during sexual activity, the absence of a rectum may effectively shut down their usual form of sexual expression. Also, there is a perception, which may be seen as stereotypical, that gay men have a particular need for physical attractiveness, and for those who have spent many hours in the gym achieving this, the presence of a stoma and the need to wear an appliance may severely disrupt body image and integrity. For gay men who do not have a partner, this can be an overwhelming barrier to attracting a sexual partner and may lead to social isolation and depression.

Encouraging Inclusivity

How can healthcare providers be inclusive with gay, lesbian, and bisexual patients? The first step is for nurses to address their own assumptions, beliefs, and attitudes about homosexuality. As with the approach to sexuality in general, this most likely is reflective of the attitudes that have been absorbed growing up. Some healthcare professionals may reject a narrower heterosexist attitude, whereas others may not have explored their personal attitudes toward homosexuality. This is a good place to start. Nurses can think about their beliefs regarding homosexuality and where those beliefs came from. Have they changed over the years, or are they the same as they always were? Can you recall caring for a self-identified homosexual patient and the feelings that this experience invoked? What did you have to do to overcome assumptions or attitudes that got in the way of providing nonjudgmental care? Perhaps this has never presented a challenge to some, or perhaps others cannot recall ever taking care of a gay or lesbian patient. This most likely reflects the fact that the nurse has never asked the right questions or appeared to be nonaccepting, so a gay/lesbian patient never disclosed this information. Most professionals have encountered a gay or lesbian patient whether they know it or not.

Ask yourself if you regularly use inclusive language when taking a history from a new patient. Do you ask whether the patient has a partner and whether that partner is a man or woman? Most heterosexual patients will readily tell you that their partner is a man (or woman), and even if the gay/lesbian patient does not disclose to you at this point or states that he or she is not partnered at the present time, you have indicated by your choice of language that you are aware that there is something other than a heterosexual relationship. This may allow the gay/lesbian patient to be more open either at this time or at a future appointment. If the patient identifies as being gay/lesbian or bisexual, do not ignore the comment. Acknowledge this fact and inform the patient that his or her openness will allow for a better therapeutic relationship—and then make sure that this occurs. Another way of asking this question is to ask if the patient has sex with men, women, or both. This approach removes the notion that sex is something that happens only in the context of a relationship and may allow disclosure of bisexuality that occurs outside of an established relationship. Directly asking a patient if he or she is gay or lesbian can itself raise a barrier, as the patient may not self-identify as such but may, in fact, be having sexual relations with someone of the same or opposite sex.

Review the forms that patients are asked to complete. Is the language contained in these forms inclusionary or exclusionary? Consider advocating for a change in the section usually marked as "marital status." The section can be changed to "relationship or partner status" and can include the option of same-sex relationship (gay, lesbian, or bisexual) along with the usual choices of single, married, separated/divorced, or widowed.

Although considering one's personal attitudes, beliefs, and practices is important, it also is vital to confront these same attitudes and actions among coworkers and colleagues. Although the nurse may be gay positive, the receptionists, students, residents, and other healthcare professionals may not be. They have equal opportunities to interact with gay, lesbian, and bisexual patients and can cause harm through their words and actions. Include colleagues and coworkers in an exploration of attitudes, knowledge, and beliefs. This will provide a good idea of how easy or difficult it may be to change any homophobic or heterosexist attitudes and practices.

Review the educational materials that are provided to patients, and determine whether any images of same-sex couples are used as illustrations. These seemingly minor details can indicate to gay/lesbian patients who attend the clinic or hospital the safety in disclosing sexual orientation. Be familiar with gay- and lesbian-friendly resources in the community, and know the names and contact information for gay-positive or gay-identified counselors and other healthcare providers. Provide information to patients that includes Web sites and other resources that target gay, lesbian, and bisexual patients. Examples are provided in Figures 18-1 and 18-2 of ways of communicating using the PLISSIT (Annon, 1974) and BETTER models (Mick, Hughes, & Cohen, 2003) with gay, lesbian, and bisexual patients.

Figure 18-1. Example of the PLISSIT Model in Gay, Lesbian, and Bisexual Patients With Cancer

- **Permission:** An example of this level would be to include a general statement that normalizes the topic.

  "I ask all my patients about their sexual relationships, so I am now going to ask you a couple of questions. Do you have sex with men, women, or both?"

- **Limited information:** In the case of a couple where one person has had radiation therapy for prostate cancer, the nurse should be able to give general information about resuming intercourse.

  "If anal intercourse is part of your sexual repertoire, there are some general cautions that you need to be aware of. You should avoid intercourse during the weeks of treatment and for some weeks after. If you experience no pain, irritation, or bleeding, it is safe to resume anal intercourse as soon as you feel able."

- **Specific suggestion:** Information at this level includes anticipatory guidance related to possible sexual consequences of treatment.

  "If you are the receptive partner during anal intercourse, you are going to need to be careful both during and after the treatment. There is a risk of irritation to the rectum, and this may persist for a while. Be sure to use plenty of lubrication and go very gently."

- **Intensive therapy:** Nurses should know where to refer patients when problems or issues are disclosed that are beyond their scope of practice or expertise.

  "You have indicated to me that sex play with your partner tends to get rough, and it also sounds like this is something that you do not enjoy but are unable to deal with. Would you like to see a counselor who has experience dealing with relationships where communication is complex?"

Figure 18-2. Example of the BETTER Model With Gay, Lesbian, and Bisexual Patients With Cancer

- **Bringing up the topic:** Nurses are encouraged to raise the issue of sexuality with patients.

  "At some point during the diagnostic, treatment, or recovery process, most patients have questions or concerns about sexual functioning. We try to address these concerns when and if they arise, so please feel free to ask me anything."

- **Explaining that sex is a part of quality of life:** This helps to normalize the discussion and may help patients to feel less embarrassed or alone in having a problem.

  "Most women have concerns that touching the breast after surgery may feel different. Breast stimulation is an important part of sexual activity for many women, and I was wondering if this is something that you and your partner have talked about or have been concerned about."

- **Telling patients that resources will be found to address their concerns:** This step suggests to patients that even if the nurse does not have the immediate solution to the problem or question, others are available who can help.

  "I have never been asked that question before, but I know that one of my colleagues has worked with many lesbian patients and their partners. With your permission, I will ask her if she knows the answer, and then she can inform both of us at the same time."

- **Timing the intervention:** Patients may not be ready to deal with sexual issues at the time a problem is identified. However, patients can ask for information at any time in the future.

  "You will only be here with us for a brief period of time and may not feel like thinking about resuming sexual activity yet. Please be aware that you can always call to ask any questions that you or your partner have after your discharge. I also will include some reading material with your discharge instructions."

- **Educating patients about the sexual side effects of treatment:** Educating patients about potential side effects from treatments does not mean that they will occur. However, informing them about sexual side effects is as important as informing them about any other side effects.

  "It is important to keep the vagina open after radiation therapy, as you will need to have regular pelvic examinations for years to come. Is penetration with your own or your partner's fingers a usual part of your sexual activity? How comfortable are you with the idea of using a vaginal dilator to help to maintain patency of the vagina?"

- **Recording:** A brief notation that a discussion about sexuality or sexual side effects occurred is important.

  "The need for vaginal dilatation was discussed with the patient. Some strategies to accomplish this were discussed."

Case Study

R.J. is a 58-year-old man who is admitted to a surgical unit for radical prostatectomy. He appears tenser than would be expected. When the nurse asks him if he has any questions about the sexual or urinary side effects of the surgery, he states that this is of no concern to the nurse. He is evasive when the nurse asks if his spouse is going to wait while the surgery is being done. He is wearing a ring on the third finger of his left hand, and the nurse assumes based on this that he is married. A few minutes later there is a soft knock on the door, and a young man enters the room. The nurse greets him and asks him if he is R.J.'s son. This question is greeted with silence, and the nurse notices that the two of them exchange a long look.

Questions to consider:
• What assumptions has the nurse made in this case?
• What clues or cues did the nurse ignore or misinterpret?
• If she could go back to the beginning of this interaction, what, if anything, should the nurse do differently?
• How should nurses deal with a patient who appears reluctant to discuss a sensitive topic such as sexuality with them?

See Appendix B for answers to the case study questions.

Conclusion

Being diagnosed with cancer can be especially difficult for members of sexual minorities because of the fear of homophobia in healthcare settings and miscommunication. Although gays and lesbians may not be at greater risk for cancer than the general population, their experience might be significantly different. Homophobia and heterosexism are pervasive in our society and healthcare systems, and these affect the care that gay, lesbian, and bisexual patients with cancer receive.

References

Annon, J. (1974). *The behavioral treatment of sexual problems.* Honolulu, HI: Enabling Systems.

Blank, T.O. (2005). Gay men and prostate cancer: Invisible diversity. *Journal of Clinical Oncology, 23,* 2593–2596.

Boehmer, U., & Case, P. (2004). Physicians don't ask, sometimes patients tell: Disclosure of sexual orientation among women with breast carcinoma. *Cancer, 101,* 1882–1889.

Boehmer, U., Freund, K.M., & Linde, R. (2005). Support providers of sexual minority women with breast cancer: Who they are and how they impact the breast cancer experience. *Journal of Psychosomatic Research, 59,* 307–314.

Boehmer, U., Linde, R., & Freund, K.M. (2005). Sexual minority women's coping and psychological adjustment after a diagnosis of breast cancer. *Journal of Women's Health, 14,* 214–224.

Brotman, S., Ryan, B., Jalbert, Y., & Rowe, B. (2002). The impact of coming out on health and health care access: The experiences of gay, lesbian, bisexual and two-spirit people. *Journal of Health and Social Policy, 15,* 1–29.

Carroll, N.M. (1999). Optimal gynecologic and obstetric care for lesbians. *Obstetrics and Gynecology, 93,* 611–613.

Case, P., Austin, S.B., Hunter, D.J., Manson, J.E., Malspeis, S., Willett, W.C., et al. (2004). Sexual orientation, health risk factors, and physical functioning in the Nurses' Health Study II. *Journal of Women's Health, 13,* 1033–1047.

Cole, S.W., Kemeny, M.E., Taylor, S.E., & Visscher, B.R. (1996). Elevated physical health risk among gay men who conceal their homosexual identity. *Health Psychology, 15,* 243–251.

Dibble, S.L., Roberts, S.A., & Nussey, B. (2004). Comparing breast cancer risk between lesbians and their heterosexual sisters. *Women's Health Issues, 14,* 60–68.

Dibble, S.L., Roberts, S.A., Robertson, P.A., & Paul, S.M. (2002). Risk factors for ovarian cancer: Lesbian and heterosexual women. *Oncology Nursing Forum, 29,* E1–E7.

Ferri, R.S. (2004). Issues in gay men's health. *Nursing Clinics of North America, 39,* 403–410.

Fobair, P., Koopman, C., DiMiceli, S., O'Hanlan, K., Butler, L.D., Classen, C., et al. (2002). Psychosocial intervention for lesbians with primary breast cancer. *Psycho-Oncology, 11,* 427–438.

Fobair, P., O'Hanlan, K., Koopman, C., Classen, C., DiMiceli, S., Drooker, N., et al. (2001). Comparison of lesbian and heterosexual women's response to newly diagnosed breast cancer. *Psycho-Oncology, 10,* 40–51.

Hughes, C., & Evans, A. (2003). Health needs of women who have sex with women. *BMJ, 327,* 939–940.

Klitzman, R., & Greenberg, J. (2002). Patterns of communication between gay and lesbian patients and their health care providers. *Journal of Homosexuality, 42,* 65–75.

Matthews, A.K. (1998). Lesbians and cancer support: Clinical issues for cancer patients. *Health Care for Women International, 19,* 193–203.

Matthews, A.K., Peterman, A.H., Delaney, P., Menard, L., & Brandenburg, D. (2002). A qualitative exploration of the experiences of lesbian and heterosexual patients with breast cancer. *Oncology Nursing Forum, 29,* 1455–1462.

Mick, J., Hughes, M., & Cohen, M. (2003). Sexuality and cancer: How oncology nurses can address it BETTER. *Oncology Nursing Forum, 30*(Suppl. 2), 152–153.

Rankow, E.J. (1995). Breast and cervical cancer among lesbians. *Women's Health Issues, 5,* 123–129.

Sinding, C., Barnoff, L., & Grassau, P. (2004). Homophobia and heterosexism in cancer care: The experiences of lesbians. *Canadian Journal of Nursing Research, 36,* 170–188.

Williams-Barnard, C., Mendoza, D., & Shippee-Rice, R. (2001). The lived experience of college student lesbians' encounters with health care providers. *Journal of Holistic Nursing, 19,* 127–142.

Section IV

Treatment Modalities and Sexual Functioning

CHAPTER 19

Surgery

Surgery is the most common treatment for cancer and often is curative for individuals with localized disease confined to the primary site. Modern technologic advances such as laparoscopes, lasers, and robots have made surgery less invasive for many procedures and have lowered the risks for patients because of shorter operative time, less blood loss, faster recovery time, and less pain in the postoperative period (Frogge & Cunning, 2000). Surgery is performed to diagnose cancer through biopsies, to stage the disease, or to alleviate pain and suffering from advanced disease by debulking a tumor (Barclay, 2000). Surgery also is used as part of the rehabilitation process. Reconstructive surgery after treatment can significantly increase quality of life through improvements in function and self-esteem (Frogge & Cunning).

Surgery also can cause significant pain in both the long and short term and may leave patients with residual nerve and vascular damage that alters their daily functioning. Scarring also is permanent, and although scars fade with time, they serve as a constant and long-lasting reminder to patients of the cancer and its treatment. This can affect psychological well-being as individuals move from being a patient with cancer to a cancer survivor who is expected to return to normal life. Part of normal life for many adults is sexual functioning, and this is affected in many ways by surgery.

Breast Cancer

Surgery to the breast has the potential to cause significant sexual changes for women. For many women, the breasts are a source of sexual pleasure and an important contributor to sexual self-schema and body image. The diagnostic trajectory for women suspected of having breast cancer usually involves a surgical biopsy. When the diagnosis is confirmed, lumpectomy or, in some instances, mastectomy is performed.

Lumpectomy may leave one breast looking very different from the other because substantial amounts of breast tissue may be removed to ensure margins that are clear of disease. Alterations in sensation over the scar are common in the immediate postoperative period and beyond. Although these sensations may change over time, numbness and loss of sensation may persist. This may have significant sexual consequences for both patients and their partners. Some men may be reluctant to touch the affected breast for fear of causing pain, and women might interpret this reluctance as rejection. Many women report that they prefer not to be touched in the area of the scar, and this removes a source of pleasure that they had previously enjoyed as part of sex play.

Mastectomy does not have a direct effect on any aspect of the sexual response cycle; however, the resultant scarring and absence of the breast can have far-reaching emotional consequences for both women and their partners. Some women might avoid sexual contact because of fear of rejection of their new cancer-scarred body. Body image changes may be related to the scar on the breast from mastectomy. Some women experience lymphedema in the arm and/or shoulder of the affected side following lymph node removal (Morrell et al., 2005), which may result in persistent swelling, pain, and limitation in movement. Frustration with these limitations may lead to depression and social isolation if women restrict social activity because of embarrassment of the affected limb (McWayne & Heiney, 2005).

Women who have a mastectomy are more likely to report negative body image than those who have lumpectomy. However, reconstruction after mastectomy improves body image somewhat (Al-Ghazal, Fallowfield, & Blamey, 2000), and for many women, body image relates to sexual attractiveness. Immediate rather than delayed breast reconstruction results in less distress (Al-Ghazal, Sully, Fallowfield, & Blamey, 2000); however, fears of recurrence may be greater after breast-conserving treatment because women are not certain that all the cancer has been removed (Bredin, 1999). Women who have had breast reconstruction after mastectomy report that although the reconstructed breast is aesthetically pleasing, the area lacks sensation, which affects sexual pleasure (Wilmoth & Ross, 1997). Even with reconstruction, many women report that the breast looks and feels different (Nissen, Swenson, & Kind, 2002) and may be caressed less often during sexual activity (Schover et al., 1995). Women report experiencing altered sensation in the reconstructed breast (e.g., pins and needles, numbness), and the surgical scar remains a constant reminder of the cancer (Rowland et al., 2000).

Prostate Cancer

As described in Chapter 5, the most common treatment for prostate cancer is radical prostatectomy, in which the entire prostate gland and the seminal vesicles are surgically removed. Because of damage to the nerves responsible for erectile function, which lie on the outside of the prostate gland, erectile dysfunction is a common result of surgery. Depending on the amount of cancer spread throughout the prostate, it may not be possible to avoid excising one or both of the nerve bundles to remove all the malignant tissue (Vale, 2000). The nerve-sparing technique, in which one or both neurovascular bundles are preserved and not severed when the prostate gland is surgically removed, has somewhat improved preservation of erectile functioning (Walsh & Worthington, 2001).

Between 30% and 85% of men who have bilateral nerve-sparing surgery eventually will regain the ability to have an erection sufficient for penetration (Burnett, 2005; Gralnek, Wessells, Cui, & Dalkin, 2000; Stanford et al., 2000). However, most men will require some form of erectile aid (i.e., oral medication, vacuum pump, or intraurethral or intracorporal injection) to achieve this (Perez et al., 1997). Even with nerve-sparing surgical techniques, trauma to the nerve bundles from instrumentation, cautery, ischemia, or inflammation may occur, and erectile dysfunction can result (Meuleman & Mulders, 2003). Trauma to the blood vessels of the penis may lead to vascular insufficiency, and penile rigidity may not occur even with satisfactory nerve function (Nehra & Goldstein, 1999). Penile shortening also has been reported following surgery, with 71% of men experiencing some degree of shortening (Munding, Wessells, & Dalkin, 2001). This most likely is a result of early changes from nerve damage resulting in a hypotonic penis in the first three to six months after surgery (Mulhall, Land, Parker, Waters, & Flanigan, 2005). Structural changes to the corporal smooth muscle of the penis also occur, resulting in permanent damage to the nerves as well as hypoxia-induced collagen build-up.

Erectile dysfunction can persist for years following the surgery, although a trend toward improvement is seen up to five years later (Penson et al., 2005). Recovery of erectile function is dependent on age (younger men have greater success), erectile function before the surgery, size of prostate gland (smaller size has better outcomes), and surgical technique (Hollenbeck, Dunn, Wei, Montie, & Sanda, 2003). Men are distressed by this (Stanford et al., 2000), and their general quality of life, self-confidence, and self-esteem are all negatively affected (Clark et al., 2003). Masculine self-concept also is changed, which results in changes in social and intimate relationships (Bokhour, Clark, Inui, Silliman, & Talcott, 2001).

After surgery, orgasm still is possible in spite of lack of erections (Hollenbeck et al., 2003). However, ejaculation does not occur, because the source of fluid, the seminal vesicles, has been removed. This results in a qualitative change in the experience of orgasm, which will lack the propulsive sensation of ejaculation and may be accompanied by pelvic pain of variable duration.

Gynecologic Cancer

The potential for sexual consequences after surgery to the pelvis are fairly apparent. Most women with any form of gynecologic cancer will have a hysterectomy, which is known to cause disruption of sensory nerves in the pelvic area. Damage to autonomic nerves in the pelvis affects vasocongestion, lubrication, and enlargement of the vagina, all which are components of sexual arousal (Gruhmann, Robertson, Hacker, & Sommer, 2001). Although many women experience sexual dysfunction in the months following surgery, they also can experience consequences many years later. Cervical cancer survivors frequently are young women, and they report ongoing sexual problems 5–10 years after treatment, including vaginal dryness, which leads to pain with sexual activity (Wenzel et al., 2005). Some women report an awareness of the physical sensation of a shortened vagina after surgery (Juraskova et al., 2003).

Vulvectomy for cancer of the vulva involves a wide excision with removal of the distal urethra. Fatty tissue and pelvic lymph nodes also are removed, and the clitoris often is excised (Wallace, 1987; Willibrord et al., 1990). This extensive surgery results in a significant alteration in body image; the frequency of sexual activity decreases; and women tend to report lack of interest in sex and avoidance of sexual activity (Green et al., 2000). Scarring at the vaginal introitus causes pain with attempted penetration, and removal of the clitoris destroys orgasmic capacity. Loss of fatty tissue on the mons and absence of the labia also contribute to altered, absent, or painful sensations. Lymphadenectomy is implicated in edema of the lower limbs, and removal of the urethra can cause incontinence and dysuria.

Surgery for ovarian cancer usually involves not only removal of the ovaries, uterus, and uterine tubes but also debulking of tumor in the pelvis and sampling of pelvic lymph nodes and the omentum (Mannix, Jackson, & Raftos, 1999). Surgical menopause ensues in younger women, which affects energy levels and body image. Furthermore, psychological well-being is significantly affected by the real threat of death for women with this type of cancer, which has high rates of morbidity and mortality. Younger women tend to be more concerned about sexual issues after diagnosis (Stewart, Wong, Duff, Melancon, & Cheung, 2001). Scars from surgery serve as a visible reminder of the cancer, and weight loss or edema following surgery also can affect patients' sexual self-image.

Radical surgery for recurrent cervical, vulvar, or vaginal cancer involves removal of all the pelvic organs, including the uterus, ovaries, vagina, bladder, colon, and adjacent tissue. Newer surgical techniques allow for a urinary diversion and anal-sparing surgery, which avoids the need for ostomies and continence devices (Carter et al., 2004). The construction of a neovagina using a myocutaneous flap has greatly reduced the incidence of sexual dysfunction and has improved quality of life for these patients (Hawighorst-Knapstein, Schonefub, Hoffmann, & Knapstein, 1997; Mirhashemi et al., 2002; Ratliff et al., 1996). Radical surgery of this nature has enormous effects on body image, and many women are reluctant to talk to anyone about this or let family members see the changes to their bodies (Carter et al., 2004). Some women report that stimulation of the neovagina causes the sensation to be felt on the thigh, a result of the innervation of the flap used to create the neovagina. This tissue does not produce lubrication; thus, penetration is painful or impossible without the addition of a lubricant.

Colon Cancer

A major factor contributing to sexual difficulties for individuals with colon cancer is the change in body image related to creation of a stoma and the appliance worn to collect feces. Ostomates often will react with shock when they see the stoma soon after surgery, and they report feeling sexually unattractive. Fear of the reaction of the sexual partner to the stoma and appliance further complicates this reaction. Some partners respond negatively to the stoma, others are cautious in their response, and some will be positive (Gloeckner, 1991). Patients are concerned about the appearance of the stoma and anxious about harming the stoma or causing pain if it is touched during sexual activity. Ostomates also may be concerned about odor, leakage, gas, or noises emitted by the appliance (Golis, 1996).

Alterations in body image and sexual self-schema occur in both men and women. The speed with which cancer surgery is carried out may have something to do with this, as there often is little time for preparation and education. Patients may be more concerned with threat to life than anticipating what the stoma may look like and how it will affect body image (Golis, 1996; Shell, 1992).

Testicular Cancer

Surgery for testicular cancer usually involves an orchiectomy, which generally does not interfere with physiologic functioning. However, although testosterone levels remain within the normal range (Lackner et al., 2005), some men will experience loss of libido following this surgery (Jonker-Pool et al., 2001). This may be psychological in nature and related to the stress of the cancer diagnosis, anxiety, and fear of the unknown. Men also report orgasmic dysfunction following the surgery. The cause of this is not known, as the surgical removal of one testicle should not interfere with either the physical sensation of orgasm or the reflex arc involved. Once again, this may be psychological in nature (Fegg et al., 2003).

Ejaculatory problems are common because both lymph node dissection and secondary resection of a retroperitoneal tumor mass interfere with normal ejaculation (Jonker-Pool et al., 2001). Many men experience "dry ejaculation," especially if bilateral lymph node dissection was performed (Aass, Grunfeld, Kaalhus, & Fossa, 1993). More modern surgical techniques that spare the nerves may reduce the incidence and severity of this side effect (Jonker-Pool et al.).

Counseling of the Postsurgical Patient

In the immediate postoperative period, most patients have little or no desire for sexual activity. However, the need for touch is a relative constant in the lives of human beings, and many people experience pleasure from the touch of an intimate partner during recovery. Partners may be fearful of hurting or harming the patient and may avoid any kind of touch. The nurse can reassure both the patient and his or her partner that gentle massage or stroking of unaffected body parts can be therapeutic and can help the patient to relax. This is important information for the couple, as they may be hesitant to resume any form of touching after discharge and may grow distant over time.

Some patients will ask about the resumption of sexual activity after surgery, but for patients with cancer, the distress of the diagnosis and anticipation of further treatment may preclude asking these questions. The nurse should discuss resuming sexual activity with the patient, either alone or when the partner is visiting. This will give permission for other questions to be asked and will allow the nurse to introduce the topic and to indicate that if further information is necessary, healthcare providers are willing to talk about this topic and give additional advice.

Pain

When patients have recovered from surgery, they are able to resume sexual activity. Postsurgical pain is a significant barrier to the resumption of sexual activity, but a number of strategies can alleviate or prevent this. For the patient who continues to experience pain, taking an analgesic one-half to one hour before sexual activity can be helpful. A warm bath or shower also can help the person to relax, and including the partner in this can begin the sexual experience for the couple through touching and sex play (often described as foreplay). For some couples, this may be as much as they want to participate in, and it can draw them closer and allow for pleasurable sensations without the pressure to have penetrative intercourse.

The patient may need to be given permission to try different sexual activities if penetrative intercourse is too painful or not desirable. Mutual masturbation, oral sex, the use of vibrators for sexual stimulation, or sensual massage all can be substituted; however, the patient and partner may not normally use these forms of sexual expression and may be more or less interested in trying alternatives to penetrative intercourse. Using a different position for intercourse also can help to prevent or alleviate pain, especially when the patient has an abdominal wound and the traditional missionary position causes pain (or the fear of pain) for the woman. The side-lying, rear-entry, or woman-on-top positions can be helpful for this. Couples may need to be referred to a book (see Chapter 24 for resources) for detailed descriptions or diagrams that illustrate these positions. Placing a small pillow or folded towel over an abdominal wound also can help to prevent or alleviate pressure on the wound.

Fatigue

Fatigue is a common symptom of both cancer and recovery from surgery. Couples may want to try alternative activities to penetrative intercourse, as these often require less energy. Identifying the time of day when energy levels are higher is one strategy that facilitates engaging in sexual activity when it is desired. Using a vibrator to stimulate the clitoris requires very little energy from either partner and is highly effective in facilitating orgasm. Many couples may not know where to buy a vibrator or how to use it, and the nurse can direct the couple to any number of resources to obtain this information. The couple does not need to buy a special vibrator; the wand massagers commonly found in drugstores or department stores are as effective and may be less expensive and more acceptable to the couple.

Specific intervention strategies for various cancers are given in the appropriate chapters in Section II of this text.

Conclusion

Surgery affects sexual functioning in the immediate postoperative period. In addition, scarring, pain, alterations in mobility, and recovery all have a significant and, for some, prolonged impact on sexual activity. Although most patients recover in about six weeks, some may find that the sexual consequences last for much longer and may require the assistance of a specialist to recover sexual function or find alternative routes to sexual satisfaction.

References

Aass, N., Grunfeld, B., Kaalhus, O., & Fossa, S.D. (1993). Pre- and post-treatment sexual life in testicular cancer patients: A descriptive investigation. *British Journal of Cancer, 67,* 1113–1117.

Al-Ghazal, S.K., Fallowfield, L., & Blamey, R.W. (2000). Comparison of psychological aspects and patient satisfaction following breast conserving surgery, simple mastectomy and breast reconstruction. *European Journal of Cancer, 36,* 1938–1943.

Al-Ghazal, S.K., Sully, L., Fallowfield, L., & Blamey, R.W. (2000). The psychological impact of immediate rather than delayed breast reconstruction. *European Journal of Surgical Oncology, 26,* 17–19.

Barclay, M. (2000). Cancer surgery. In B. Nevidjon & K. Sowers (Eds.), *A nurse's guide to cancer care* (pp. 192–198). Philadelphia: Lippincott Williams & Wilkins.

Bokhour, B.G., Clark, J.A., Inui, T.S., Silliman, R.A., & Talcott, J.A. (2001). Sexuality after treatment for early prostate cancer: Exploring the meanings of "erectile dysfunction." *Journal of General Internal Medicine, 16,* 649–655.

Bredin, M. (1999). Mastectomy, body image and therapeutic massage: A qualitative study of women's experiences. *Journal of Advanced Nursing, 29,* 1113–1120.

Burnett, A.L. (2005). Erectile dysfunction following radical prostatectomy. *JAMA, 293,* 2648–2653.

Carter, J., Chi, D., Abu-Rustum, N., Brown, C., McCreath, W., & Barakat, R. (2004). Brief report: Total pelvic exenteration—a retrospective clinical needs assessment. *Psycho-Oncology, 13,* 125–131.

Clark, J.A., Inui, T.S., Silliman, R.A., Bokhour, B.G., Krasnow, S.H., Robinson, R.A., et al. (2003). Patients' perceptions of quality of life after treatment for early prostate cancer. *Journal of Clinical Oncology, 21,* 3777–3784.

Fegg, M.J., Gerl, A., Vollmer, T.C., Gruber, U., Jost, C., Meiler, S., et al. (2003). Subjective quality of life and sexual functioning after germ-cell tumour therapy. *British Journal of Cancer, 89,* 2202–2206.

Frogge, M., & Cunning, S. (2000). Surgical therapy. In C.H. Yarbro, M.H. Frogge, M. Goodman, & S.L. Groenwald (Eds.), *Cancer nursing: Principles and practice* (5th ed., pp. 272–285). Sudbury, MA: Jones and Bartlett.

Gloeckner, M. (1991). Perceptions of sexuality after ostomy surgery. *Journal of Enterostomal Therapy, 18,* 36–38.

Golis, A. (1996). Sexual issues for the person with an ostomy. *Journal of Wound, Ostomy, and Continence Nursing, 23,* 33–37.

Gralnek, D., Wessells, H., Cui, H., & Dalkin, B.L. (2000). Differences in sexual function and quality of life after nerve sparing and nonnerve sparing radical retropubic prostatectomy. *Journal of Urology, 163,* 1166–1169.

Green, M.S., Naumann, R.W., Elliot, M., Hall, J.B., Higgins, R.V., & Grigsby, J.H. (2000). Sexual dysfunction following vulvectomy. *Gynecologic Oncology, 77,* 73–77.

Gruhmann, M., Robertson, R., Hacker, N., & Sommer, G. (2001). Sexual functioning in patients following radical hysterectomy for stage IB cancer of the cervix. *International Journal of Gynecological Cancer, 11,* 372–380.

Hawighorst-Knapstein, S., Schonefub, G., Hoffmann, S., & Knapstein, P. (1997). Pelvic exenteration: Effects of surgery on quality of life and body image—a prospective longitudinal study. *Gynecologic Oncology, 66,* 495–500.

Hollenbeck, B.K., Dunn, R.L., Wei, J.T., Montie, J.E., & Sanda, M.G. (2003). Determinants of long-term sexual health outcome after radical prostatectomy measured by a validated instrument. *Journal of Urology, 169,* 1453–1457.

Jonker-Pool, G., van de Wiel, H.B., Hoekstra, H.J., Sleijfer, D.T., Van Driel, M.F., Van Basten, J.P., et al. (2001). Sexual functioning after treatment for testicular cancer—review and meta-analysis of 36 empirical studies between 1975–2000. *Archives of Sexual Behavior, 30,* 55–74.

Juraskova, I., Butow, P., Robertson, R., Sharpe, L., McLeod, C., & Hacker, N. (2003). Post-treatment sexual adjustment following cervical and endometrial cancer: A qualitative insight. *Psycho-Oncology, 12,* 267–279.

Lackner, J., Schatzl, G., Koller, A., Mazal, P., Waldhoer, T., Marberger, M., et al. (2005). Treatment of testicular cancer: Influence on pituitary-gonadal axis and sexual function. *Urology, 66,* 402–406.

Mannix, J., Jackson, D., & Raftos, M. (1999). Ovarian cancer: An update for nursing practice. *International Journal of Nursing Practice, 5,* 47–50.

McWayne, J., & Heiney, S.P. (2005). Psychologic and social sequelae of secondary lymphedema: A review. *Cancer, 104,* 457–466.

Meuleman, E.J., & Mulders, P.F. (2003). Erectile function after radical prostatectomy: A review. *European Urology, 43,* 95–101.

Mirhashemi, R., Averette, H., Lambrou, N., Penalver, M., Mendez, L., Ghurani, G., et al. (2002). Vaginal reconstruction at the time of pelvic exenteration: A surgical and psychosexual analysis of techniques. *Gynecologic Oncology, 87,* 39–45.

Morrell, R.M., Halyard, M.Y., Schild, S.E., Ali, M.S., Gunderson, L.L., & Pockaj, B.A. (2005). Breast cancer-related lymphedema. *Mayo Clinic Proceedings, 80,* 1480–1484.

Mulhall, J., Land, S., Parker, M., Waters, W.B., & Flanigan, R.C. (2005). The use of an erectogenic pharmacotherapy regimen following radical prostatectomy improves recovery of spontaneous erectile function. *Journal of Sexual Medicine, 2,* 532–540.

Munding, M., Wessells, H., & Dalkin, B. (2001). Pilot study of changes in stretched penile lengths 3 months after radical retropubic prostatectomy. *Urology, 58,* 567–569.

Nehra, A., & Goldstein, I. (1999). Sildenafil citrate (Viagra) after radical retropubic prostatectomy: Con. *Urology, 54,* 587–589.

Nissen, M.J., Swenson, K.K., & Kind, E.A. (2002). Quality of life after postmastectomy breast reconstruction. *Oncology Nursing Forum, 29,* 547–553.

Penson, D.F., McLerran, D., Feng, Z., Li, L., Albertsen, P.C., Gilliland, F.D., et al. (2005). 5-year urinary and sexual outcomes after radical prostatectomy: Results from the prostate cancer outcomes study. *Journal of Urology, 173,* 1701–1705.

Perez, M.A., Meyerowitz, B.E., Lieskovsky, G., Skinner, D.G., Reynolds, B., & Skinner, E.C. (1997). Quality of life and sexuality following radical prostatectomy in patients with prostate cancer who use or do not use erectile aids. *Urology, 50,* 740–746.

Ratliff, C., Gershenson, D., Morris, M., Burke, T., Levenback, C., Schover, L., et al. (1996). Sexual adjustment of patients undergoing gracilis myocutaneous flap vaginal reconstruction in conjunction with pelvic exenteration. *Cancer, 78,* 2229–2235.

Rowland, J.H., Desmond, K.A., Meyerowitz, B.E., Belin, T.R., Wyatt, G.E., & Ganz, P.A. (2000). Role of breast reconstructive surgery in physical and emotional outcomes among breast cancer survivors. *Journal of the National Cancer Institute, 92,* 1422–1429.

Schover, L.R., Yetman, R., Tuason, L., Meisler, E., Esselstyn, C., Hermann, R., et al. (1995). Partial mastectomy and breast reconstruction: A comparison of their effects on psychosocial adjustment, body image, and sexuality. *Cancer, 75,* 54–64.

Shell, J.A. (1992). The psychosexual impact of ostomy surgery. *Progressions: Developments in Ostomy and Wound Care, 4*(1), 3–15.

Stanford, J.L., Feng, Z., Hamilton, A.S., Gilliland, F.D., Stephenson, R.A., Eley, J.W., et al. (2000). Urinary and sexual function after radical prostatectomy for clinically localized prostate cancer: The Prostate Cancer Outcomes Study. *JAMA, 283,* 354–360.

Stewart, D., Wong, F.W., Duff, S., Melancon, C., & Cheung, A. (2001). "What doesn't kill you makes you stronger": An ovarian cancer survivor survey. *Gynecologic Oncology, 83,* 537–542.

Vale, J. (2000). Erectile dysfunction following radical therapy for prostate cancer. *Radiotherapy and Oncology, 57,* 301–305.

Wallace, L. (1987). Psychological aspects of physical illness: Sexual adjustment after radical genital surgery. *Nursing Times, 83*(51), 41–43.

Walsh, P.C., & Worthington, J. (2001). *Dr. Patrick Walsh's guide to surviving prostate cancer.* New York: Warner Books.

Wenzel, L., DeAlba, I., Habbal, R., Kluhsman, B., Fairclough, D., Krebs, L., et al. (2005). Quality of life in long-term cervical cancer survivors. *Gynecologic Oncology, 97,* 310–317.

Willibrord, C., Weijmar Schultz, W., van de Wiel, H., Bouma, J., Hanssens, J., & Littlewood, J. (1990). Psychosexual functioning after the treatment of cancer of the vulva. *Cancer, 66,* 402–407.

Wilmoth, M.C., & Ross, J.A. (1997). Women's perception: Breast cancer treatment and sexuality. *Cancer Practice, 5,* 353–359.

CHAPTER 20

Chemotherapy

Chemotherapy is used to treat many different kinds of cancer. Because it is a systemic treatment, it has the ability to target cancer cells that may have spread to other parts of the body. Chemotherapy often is given as an adjunct to surgery and/or radiation either before these forms of treatment (neoadjuvant), at the same time, or after (Painter, 2000). Chemotherapy predominately affects rapidly dividing cells, and the effects are dose dependent. Cells that are rapidly dividing are commonly found in the gastrointestinal tract, hair follicles, gonads, and bone marrow. The common side effects of chemotherapy are related to the effects on these cells and include nausea and vomiting, alopecia, fertility, sexual problems, and risk of infection (Camp-Sorrell, 2000).

Chemotherapy and Sexual Side Effects

Very little information exists in the literature that is directly related to the effects of chemotherapy on sexual functioning beyond agents that are known to target the gonads. Much of what is known comes from anecdotal evidence from qualitative studies in which participants mention alterations in sexual functioning while on chemotherapy. This may be because when phase 1 and phase 2 clinical trials are conducted, targeted questions are not asked of trial participants because the assumption is that people dealing with acute cancer either are not interested in sex or are not able to have sex. Participants in these trials are commonly asked a long list of questions related to symptoms, and if sexual functioning is not mentioned or is merely mentioned in a global statement, the individual may not volunteer information about something that not only is intensely private but also appears to be of little interest to the research nurse or clinical investigator. However, many patients on

213

chemotherapy report a significant impact on sexual functioning through all stages of the sexual response cycle. This impact is well known to negatively affect patients' quality of life, self-image, and partner relationships.

Breast Cancer

Chemotherapy causes a profound impact on sexual activity for patients with breast cancer because of hormonal changes from cessation of ovarian activity. The effect is most profound for premenopausal women and mainly is seen if an alkylating agent such as cyclophosphamide is used (Stead, 2003). The incidence of sexual dysfunction in women receiving adjuvant chemotherapy is significant. Most report no sexual desire at all, whereas some report low desire (Barni & Mondin, 1997). Dyspareunia is another common complaint caused by vaginal dryness as a result of reduced estrogen levels (Knobf, 2001). Patients have reported sexual changes up to five years after treatment (Meyerowitz, Desmond, Rowland, Wyatt, & Ganz, 1999). Not only does ovarian failure result in loss of circulating estrogen, but levels of testosterone also may fall (Speer et al., 2005), which is, in part, theorized to create problems with decreased libido and lack of sexual thoughts and fantasies.

Chemotherapy-induced ovarian failure, which is experienced as the sudden onset of severe menopausal symptoms, is extremely distressing. Symptoms of chemically induced menopause are dramatic, and women report menstrual cycle changes, hot flashes, insomnia, vaginal dryness, dyspareunia, and weight gain (Knobf, 2001). Although many studies suggest that menopausal symptoms are worse for women who were premenopausal when diagnosed (Rogers & Kristjanson, 2002), others suggest that postmenopausal women are five to seven times more likely to suffer severe menopausal symptoms than younger women (Crandall, Petersen, Ganz, & Greendale, 2004). Changes in arousal and orgasm also are common for women treated with chemotherapy, particularly for women younger than 50. However, women continue to report satisfaction in their relationships in spite of ongoing sexual challenges (Ganz, Rowland, Desmond, Meyerowitz, & Wyatt, 1998). Long-term breast cancer survivors have reported significant global decreases in sexual functioning, including decreased libido, reduced ability to relax and enjoy sex, decreased ability to become aroused, and difficulty achieving orgasm. These are all strongly associated with vaginal dryness (Broeckel, Thors, Jacobsen, Small, & Cox, 2002).

As a result of decreased levels of circulating estrogen, the vaginal mucosa thins, and less lubrication is produced, thus resulting in vaginal dryness. As a result, women experience pain when penetration is attempted (dyspareunia). This may lead to a chronic condition known as vaginismus (Barni & Mondin, 1997), which is when the muscles of the vaginal introitus contract with any attempt at penetration. There also is a psychogenic component to this—intercourse becomes something to fear because of the pain, and so a vicious circle of pain and fear begins. Some women also experience urinary tract infections (UTIs) after attempts at sexual intercourse. The alteration in the vaginal pH caused by estrogen deficiency also predisposes women to UTIs (Ponzone et al., 2005). This too can contribute to decreased interest in sex if the result is a painful infection.

Undergoing chemotherapy also affects body image. For many women, weight is an important body image issue that is closely connected to sexual self-schema and perception of sexual attractiveness (Wilmoth, Coleman, Smith, & Davis, 2004). The weight gain experienced in the months and years after chemotherapy, usually in the range of 10 pounds or more (McInnes & Knobf, 2001), can affect how women perceive themselves in the context of their sexual lives and relationships. The hair loss commonly experienced as a side effect of chemotherapy also can have a major impact on body image. The loss of pubic hair can have an impact on women's perceptions of themselves as sexual beings. Many women find that they are embarrassed by the loss of pubic hair, and this is a barrier to feeling and acting like an adult sexual partner.

Another factor associated with menopausal symptoms and sexual dysfunction in postmenopausal women is the incidence of urinary incontinence. In the postmenopausal years, many women experience stress or urgency incontinence, which can be a significant predictor of problems in sexual functioning (Greendale, Petersen, Zibecchi, & Ganz, 2001). Urinary incontinence may occur with deep vaginal penetration, abdominal pressure, and clitoral stimulation and is a source of great embarrassment to most women.

Tamoxifen, a selective estrogen receptor modulator (SERM), lowers serum estrogen and progesterone levels (Angelopoulos, Barbounis, Livadas, Kaltsas, & Tolis, 2004). It is used as adjuvant treatment for women with estrogen receptor–positive breast cancer and is now the standard of care. Tamoxifen is known to affect menopausal symptoms and sexuality. Women taking tamoxifen commonly experience hot flashes (Young-McCaughan, 1996). Although women report a decrease in libido (Hunter et al., 2004), this complex construct is multifactorial and not related to the use of a SERM alone (Angelopoulos et al.). Tamoxifen has mildly estrogenic effects on the vaginal mucosa, which provides some women with relief from the vaginal dryness experienced as a result of chemotherapy-induced vaginal atrophy (Rogers & Kristjanson, 2002). The side effects of tamoxifen appear to be most severe in premenopausal women with breast cancer; postmenopausal women seem to experience fewer or less-distressing negative side effects (Ganz et al., 1998). Aromatase inhibitors now are being used in place of tamoxifen. These drugs appear to have similar estrogen-suppressive side effects, including hot flashes and vaginal dryness (Bentrem & Jordan, 2002). Anecdotal reports of severe vaginal atrophy with aromatase inhibitors also exist, with the subsequent development of vaginal stenosis.

Prostate Cancer

Prostate cancer is an androgen-dependent cancer, and androgen ablation therapy (also known as androgen deprivation or hormone therapy) is used to treat men who are diagnosed with advanced prostate cancer. Androgen ablation today is most commonly achieved through the use of injectable luteinizing hormone-releasing hormone (LHRH) agonists and nonsteroidal antiandrogens. Androgen deprivation therapy has a global effect on all aspects of sexual functioning. The most profound of these is the impact of androgen deprivation on sexual desire. Men taking these medications report that sexual dreams and fantasies stop completely, and they experience a lack of interest in anything sexual along with a complete end to any sexual pleasure (Navon & Morag, 2003). They also report changes in body image, perception of their masculinity, and, as a result, alterations in their spousal relationships (Clark et al., 1997). Testosterone levels will, however, rise to normal levels 18–24 weeks after treatment is stopped (Murthy et al., 2006), but some men may have to remain on this treatment indefinitely. Androgen ablation also affects the ability to have an erection, and men with low or no interest in sex appear to experience less distress when they cannot achieve an erection than men who still desire sex but cannot have an erection (Dahn et al., 2004). Other side effects of these drugs include feminization, hot flashes, and gynecomastia (increase in volume of breast tissue) (Anderson, 2001). These side effects are regarded as extremely bothersome by many men (Lubeck, Grossfeld, & Carroll, 2001) and contribute to lower quality of life. Orchiectomy, or surgical castration, is an alternative to medical treatment. However, the thought of being castrated is a source of extreme distress for many men (Cleary, Morrissey, & Oster, 1995), who may choose to refuse treatment rather than undergo this surgical procedure. Since the advent of injectable LHRH agonists and nonsteroidal antiandrogens, older treatments such as surgical castration are no longer favored (Potosky et al., 2002).

Gynecologic Cancer

Women with gynecologic cancer are treated with chemotherapy as an adjunct to surgery and radiation. Most women with ovarian cancer begin chemotherapy shortly after surgery, and the global effects of these drugs further influence patients' well-being and sexual functioning, particularly sexual desire (Carmack Taylor, Basen-Engquist, Shinn, & Bodurka, 2004). The fatigue that women with ovarian cancer frequently experience may persist months after completion of treatment. Fatigue is associated with changes in quality of life and depression, which have an impact on sexuality (Holzner et al., 2003). As with women with breast cancer, loss of hair during chemotherapy has a major impact on body image (Fitch, 2003). Women may not expect that they will lose all their body hair, including pubic hair. This can have a devastating effect on how the woman and her partner view her sexuality. Women report that without pubic hair, they do not feel like adults, so sexual touching is difficult. Ovarian cancer can leave a woman feeling inadequate in her role as partner (Lammers, Schaefer, Ladd, & Echenberg, 2000). This causes distress for women who may be fearful that lack of sexual activity may cause problems in the relationship (Sun et al., 2005).

Testicular Cancer

Chemotherapy for testicular cancer has a significant global impact on sexual functioning, with up to one-third of men experiencing loss of libido, orgasmic and ejaculatory problems, and a subsequent decrease in level of sexual activity (Jonker-Pool et al., 2001). In the period during and immediately after chemotherapy, when nausea and fatigue are at their worst (Brown, 2003), this is to be expected. However, these problems appear to persist for at least the first six months after completion of treatment (Heidenreich & Hofmann, 1999). This inability to perform sexually can lower the man's confidence in himself as a sexual partner and can have psychological consequences that may last for a significant period of time.

Hematologic Cancer

Chemotherapy for leukemia is given based on the type of disease (acute or chronic, myeloid or lymphocytic), and all chemotherapy has the potential to affect sexual functioning. The alkylating agents (busulfan, cyclophosphamide, ifosfamide, nitrogen mustard) cause significant nausea and vomiting, which decreases patients' desire and ability to engage in sexual activity. Antimetabolites (cladribine, cytarabine, hydroxyurea, methotrexate) cause general malaise, mucositis, and nausea and vomiting, all of which affect sexual functioning. Antitumor antibiotics (daunorubicin, doxorubicin, mitoxantrone) also cause nausea and vomiting and mucositis. Plant alkaloids (vincristine) cause peripheral neuropathy, which may affect sensation in the hands and fingers (Schwartz & Plawecki, 2002). All these agents are used in various combinations, and the side effects may be cumulative (Lubejko & Ashley, 1998).

The chemotherapeutic agents used in the treatment of Hodgkin lymphoma include alkylating agents (carmustine, cyclophosphamide, dacarbazine, nitrogen mustard, thiotepa), antitumor agents (bleomycin, doxorubicin), and plant alkaloids (etoposide, vincristine). Non-Hodgkin lymphoma is treated with alkylating agents (carmustine, ifosfamide, thiotepa), antimetabolites (cytarabine, methotrexate), antitumor agents (bleomycin, doxorubicin), and plant alkaloids (vinblastine, vincristine) (Lubejko & Ashley, 1998). Nausea and vomiting are common with all forms of chemotherapy, as are general malaise and feelings of being unwell. Hair loss also is a common side effect of chemotherapy, and the loss of hair makes both men and women feel less attractive and has the effect of infantilizing the patient as previously discussed.

Counseling of Patients Receiving Chemotherapy

Nurses can provide some key pieces of information related to chemotherapy and sexual activity to patients and their partners. Individuals who are feeling nauseated are unlikely to be interested in sexual activity; however, sexual activity itself may cause some nausea, particularly when abdominal pressure occurs because of sexual positioning. Patients may be counseled to take an antiemetic before sexual activity or to choose a sexual position that avoids abdominal pressure. Moreover, sexual intercourse is not always the end goal of sexual touch, and patients and their partners should be encouraged to find other ways of sexual pleasuring that do not provoke fatigue or nausea in patients but that satisfy both the patients' and their partners' need and desire for intimate touch.

Important to note is that when alopecia is discussed, both in the literature and in the clinical arena, the loss of hair on the head most often is described, and very rarely, if ever, is the loss of pubic hair discussed (Batchelor, 2001). Although head hair is something that is visible to others and alopecia is a significant factor in social and intimate interactions, avoiding the topic of loss of pubic hair sets patients up for a shock when this occurs, as they most often are not prepared. As previously discussed, many individuals find the loss of pubic hair to be disturbing; however, some individuals find this sexually stimulating and may enjoy the altered sensations that flow from a hairless scrotum, mons pubis, and labia. What is important is that patients and partners are prepared for this.

One of the common manifestations of mucositis in women is vaginal irritation or vaginitis. Women commonly will experience both irritation to the vagina (which is internal) and vulvar irritation. Symptoms include itching, discharge, soreness, bleeding, and odor. This usually occurs three to five days after infusion of chemotherapy and lasts for up to 10 days. Interventions for these symptoms focus on prevention, such as avoiding tight-fitting pants and pantyhose, wearing cotton underwear, and maintaining fastidious personal hygiene. Women should be encouraged to use mild soap and water for cleansing and to avoid bubble baths, douche, and chemical irritants such as genital deodorant sprays. Cool sitz baths and warm compresses can provide some local relief. Concomitant bacterial infections such as *Candida albicans* or *Trichomonas vaginitis* also should be ruled out and treated appropriately if they are present. The use of additional lubrication for sexual touching and penetrative intercourse will help to make the activity more comfortable and may prevent vaginal irritation.

For individuals who wish to participate in penetrative intercourse while undergoing chemotherapy, some special caveats apply. Intercourse should be avoided when neutrophil and platelet counts are low (Camp-Sorrell, 2000). This will prevent infection and bleeding. Condoms should be used both to prevent transmission of infection and to prevent exposure of the partner to chemotherapeutic agents in the patient's body fluids. Patients should exercise caution in choosing which condoms to use, as those that are lubricated usually contain nonoxynol-9, which can be irritating to vaginal tissue.

Conclusion

Chemotherapy and the attendant systemic effects of the drugs can alter a patient's sense of self as a sexual being. Anorexia, nausea, alopecia, and other common side effects of treatment all can have a negative impact on sexuality. Chemotherapy is used to treat many different types of cancer and also is used in the adjuvant setting. The cumulative effects of chemotherapy in addition to surgery and/or radiation increase the potential for side effects that significantly alter the patient's interest in and capacity for sexual activity.

References

Anderson, J. (2001). Quality of life aspects of treatment options for localized and locally advanced prostate cancer. *European Urology, 40*(Suppl. 2), 24–30.

Angelopoulos, N., Barbounis, V., Livadas, S., Kaltsas, D., & Tolis, G. (2004). Effects of estrogen deprivation due to breast cancer treatment. *Endocrine-Related Cancer, 11*, 523–535.

Barni, S., & Mondin, R. (1997). Sexual dysfunction in treated breast cancer patients. *Annals of Oncology, 8*, 149–153.

Batchelor, D. (2001). Hair and cancer chemotherapy: Consequences and nursing care—a literature study. *European Journal of Cancer Care, 10*, 147–163.

Bentrem, D., & Jordan, C. (2002). Role of antiestrogens and aromatase inhibitors in breast cancer treatment. *Current Opinion in Obstetrics and Gynecology, 14*, 5–12.

Broeckel, J.A., Thors, C.L., Jacobsen, P.B., Small, M., & Cox, C.E. (2002). Sexual functioning in long-term breast cancer survivors treated with adjuvant chemotherapy. *Breast Cancer Research and Treatment, 75*, 241–248.

Brown, C.G. (2003). Testicular cancer: An overview. *Medsurg Nursing, 12*, 37–43.

Camp-Sorrell, D. (2000). Chemotherapy: Toxicity management. In C.H. Yarbro, M.H. Frogge, M. Goodman, & S.L. Groenwald (Eds.), *Cancer nursing: Principles and practice* (5th ed., pp. 445–486). Sudbury, MA: Jones and Bartlett.

Carmack Taylor, C.L., Basen-Engquist, K., Shinn, E.H., & Bodurka, D.C. (2004). Predictors of sexual functioning in ovarian cancer patients. *Journal of Clinical Oncology, 22,* 881–889.

Clark, J., Wray, N., Brody, B., Ashton, C., Giesler, B., & Watkins, H. (1997). Dimensions of quality of life expressed by men treated for metastatic prostate cancer. *Social Science and Medicine, 45,* 1299–1309.

Cleary, P., Morrissey, G., & Oster, G. (1995). Health-related quality of life in patients with advanced prostate cancer: A multinational perspective. *Quality of Life Research, 4,* 207–220.

Crandall, C., Petersen, L., Ganz, P.A., & Greendale, G.A. (2004). Association of breast cancer and its therapy with menopause-related symptoms. *Menopause, 11,* 519–530.

Dahn, J.R., Penedo, F.J., Gonzalez, J.S., Esquiabro, M., Antoni, M.H., Roos, B.A., et al. (2004). Sexual functioning and quality of life after prostate cancer treatment: Considering sexual desire. *Urology, 63,* 273–277.

Fitch, M.I. (2003). Psychosocial management of patients with recurrent ovarian cancer: Treating the whole patient to improve quality of life. *Seminars in Oncology Nursing, 19,* 40–53.

Ganz, P.A., Rowland, J.H., Desmond, K., Meyerowitz, B.E., & Wyatt, G.E. (1998). Life after breast cancer: Understanding women's health-related quality of life and sexual functioning. *Journal of Clinical Oncology, 16,* 501–514.

Greendale, G.A., Petersen, L., Zibecchi, L., & Ganz, P.A. (2001). Factors related to sexual function in postmenopausal women with a history of breast cancer. *Menopause, 8,* 111–119.

Heidenreich, A., & Hofmann, R. (1999). Quality-of-life issues in the treatment of testicular cancer. *World Journal of Urology, 17,* 230–238.

Holzner, B., Kemmler, G., Meraner, V., Maislinger, A., Kopp, M., Bodner, T., et al. (2003). Fatigue in ovarian carcinoma patients: A neglected issue? *Cancer, 97,* 1564–1572.

Hunter, M., Grunfeld, E., Mittal, S., Sikka, P., Ramirez, A., Fentiman, I., et al. (2004). Menopausal symptoms in women with breast cancer: Prevalence and treatment preferences. *Psycho-Oncology, 13,* 769–778.

Jonker-Pool, G., van de Wiel, H.B., Hoekstra, H.J., Sleijfer, D.T., Van Driel, M.F., Van Basten, J.P., et al. (2001). Sexual functioning after treatment for testicular cancer—review and meta-analysis of 36 empirical studies between 1975–2000. *Archives of Sexual Behavior, 30,* 55–74.

Knobf, M.T. (2001). The menopausal symptom experience in young mid-life women with breast cancer. *Cancer Nursing, 24,* 201–210.

Lammers, S.E., Schaefer, K.M., Ladd, E.C., & Echenberg, R. (2000). Caring for women living with ovarian cancer: Recommendations for advanced practice nurses. *Journal of Obstetric, Gynecologic, and Neonatal Nursing, 29,* 567–573.

Lubeck, D., Grossfeld, G., & Carroll, P. (2001). The effect of androgen deprivation therapy on health-related quality of life in men with prostate cancer. *Urology, 58,* 94–100.

Lubejko, B.G., & Ashley, B.W. (1998). Chemotherapy. In C. Ziegfeld, B. Lubejko, & B. Shelton (Eds.), *Oncology fact finder: Manual of cancer nursing* (pp. 30–47). Philadelphia: Lippincott Williams & Wilkins.

McInnes, J.A., & Knobf, M.T. (2001). Weight gain and quality of life in women treated with adjuvant chemotherapy for early-stage breast cancer. *Oncology Nursing Forum, 28,* 675–684.

Meyerowitz, B.E., Desmond, K.A., Rowland, J.H., Wyatt, G.E., & Ganz, P.A. (1999). Sexuality following breast cancer. *Journal of Sex and Marital Therapy, 25,* 237–250.

Murthy, V., Norman, A., Shahidi, M., Parker, C., Horwich, A., Huddart, R., et al. (2006). Recovery of serum testosterone after neoadjuvant androgen deprivation therapy and radical radiotherapy in localized prostate cancer. *BJU International, 97,* 476–479.

Navon, L., & Morag, A. (2003). Advanced prostate cancer patients' relationships with their spouses following hormonal therapy. *European Journal of Oncology Nursing, 7,* 73–80.

Painter, J. (2000). Chemotherapy administration. In B. Nevidjon & K. Sowers (Eds.), *A nurse's guide to cancer care* (pp. 199–214). Philadelphia: Lippincott Williams & Wilkins.

Ponzone, R., Biglia, N., Jacomuzzi, M.E., Maggiorotto, F., Mariani, L., & Sismondi, P. (2005). Vaginal oestrogen therapy after breast cancer: Is it safe? *European Journal of Cancer, 41,* 2673–2681.

Potosky, A.L., Reeve, B.B., Clegg, L.X., Hoffman, R.M., Stephenson, R.A., Albertsen, P.C., et al. (2002). Quality of life following localized prostate cancer treated initially with androgen deprivation therapy or no therapy. *Journal of the National Cancer Institute, 94,* 430–437.

Rogers, M., & Kristjanson, L.J. (2002). The impact on sexual functioning of chemotherapy-induced menopause in women with breast cancer. *Cancer Nursing, 25,* 57–65.

Schwartz, S., & Plawecki, H.M. (2002). Consequences of chemotherapy on the sexuality of patients with lung cancer. *Clinical Journal of Oncology Nursing, 6,* 212–216.

Speer, J.J., Hillenberg, B., Sugrue, D.P., Blacker, C., Kresge, C.L., Decker, V.B., et al. (2005). Study of sexual functioning determinants in breast cancer survivors. *Breast Journal, 11,* 440–447.

Stead, M.L. (2003). Sexual dysfunction after treatment for gynecologic and breast malignancies. *Current Opinion in Obstetrics and Gynecology, 15,* 57–61.

Sun, C.C., Bodurka, D.C., Weaver, C.B., Rasu, R., Wolf, J.K., Bevers, M.W., et al. (2005). Rankings and symptom assessments of side effects from chemotherapy: Insights from experienced patients with ovarian cancer. *Supportive Care in Cancer, 13,* 219–227.

Wilmoth, M.C., Coleman, E.A., Smith, S.C., & Davis, C. (2004). Fatigue, weight gain, and altered sexuality in patients with breast cancer: Exploration of a symptom cluster. *Oncology Nursing Forum, 31,* 1069–1075.

Young-McCaughan, S. (1996). Sexual functioning in women with breast cancer after treatment with adjuvant therapy. *Cancer Nursing, 19,* 308–319.

CHAPTER 21

Radiation Therapy

Radiation therapy is used to treat patients throughout the disease spectrum with the intent to cure, to control the growth or spread of a malignant lesion, to downstage large and bulky tumors, and as adjuvant therapy to reduce the risk of local recurrence at the site of the tumor. It also can be used as palliation to control pain or other symptoms. Radiation can be given externally or internally through the placement of radioactive seeds or a temporary intracavity implant. When radiation is used in combination with surgery and/or chemotherapy, the intent is to reduce the chance of failure of all modalities; however, this will increase the incidence and severity of side effects. Both acute and long-term toxicities are associated with the use of radiation therapy, and these all can affect sexuality.

Breast Cancer

Radiation therapy for breast cancer affects sexuality by virtue of its impact on energy and local changes to the skin of the treated breast. Fatigue is a common side effect of radiation therapy, and this can significantly affect libido. Many women continue to work and maintain their normal family and household duties while undergoing radiation therapy; this can have a measurable effect on fatigue, which may influence patients' libido and ability to engage in sexual activity. Radiation damage to the skin may affect sexual response to caressing, and some women experience shooting pains in the breast as well as nipple discomfort (Wilmoth & Botchway, 1999). Skin discoloration caused by burning from the radiation might be both painful and disfiguring (Wilmoth & Botchway). The tattoo marks left on the skin of the chest can be a constant reminder of the cancer, which can have long-lasting emotional and sexual side effects.

Prostate Cancer

In men with prostate cancer treated with radiation, erectile dysfunction is common, with up to 84% of patients reporting some erectile dysfunction depending on the kind of radiation given (Incrocci, 2004). The cause of erectile dysfunction after radiation therapy is not clear, and there appears to be venous, arterial (Incrocci, 2004), and neural etiology (Incrocci, 2006; Mulhall & Yonover, 2001). Radiation to the bulb of the penis is thought to be a contributing cause of tissue damage (Merrick et al., 2005). Patients who receive less than 40 Gy to 70% of the bulb of the penis appear to have an increased chance of maintaining erectile function (Fisch, Pickett, Weinberg, & Roach, 2001). Tissue fibrosis is an important contributor to erectile dysfunction, as it usually is caused by reduced blood flow to the corpora cavernosa with resultant oxygen deprivation (Fitzpatrick et al., 1998). In men who have had brachytherapy, the theory is that trauma to the tissues during insertion of the needles used to place the radioactive seeds is associated with erectile dysfunction (Macdonald et al., 2005).

Erectile function tends to decline in the years following external beam radiation therapy (EBRT) beginning 12 months after treatment, with a nadir being reached at 22–24 months (Turner, Adams, Bull, & Berry, 1999; Zelefsky et al., 1999). Fifty percent of men will experience erectile dysfunction three years after treatment (Merrick et al., 2005), and further decline will be seen up to five years after treatment (Potosky et al., 2004). Men receiving brachytherapy tend to preserve erectile functioning, as compared to other forms of radiation therapy (Stock, Stone, & Iannuzzi, 1996), and generally are satisfied with their level of functioning three years after treatment (Mabjeesh, Chen, Beri, Stenger, & Matzkin, 2005). Men with more advanced prostate cancer who receive a combination of brachytherapy and EBRT are at increased risk for sexual dysfunction, and the addition of hormone ablation therapy further negatively affects the ability to have an erection (Speight et al., 2004).

The ability to achieve an erection is just one part of sexual functioning for men. After radiation treatment for prostate cancer, ejaculatory disturbances are common, with reduction in volume of ejaculate, absence of ejaculation, and pain with orgasm being noted (Incrocci, Slob, & Levendag, 2002). Men often will choose radiation therapy because of the lower side-effect profile (Hall, Boyd, Lippert, & Theodorescu, 2003). They need to be informed not only about the risk for erectile dysfunction but also about the temporal nature of sexual decline and that ejaculation will change.

Gynecologic Cancer

Radiation therapy has been used for many years to treat cervical cancer. Radiation may be given either externally or internally (brachytherapy) and sometimes in combination. When brachytherapy is given, applicators are inserted into the vagina, and the radiation source (either high or low dose) is loaded into the applicator. This remains in place for a predetermined period of time and then is removed. The treatment may be repeated a number of times depending on the radiation source (Lancaster, 2004). The tissues of the vagina react to this treatment with changes in the vasculature in the walls, leading to fibrosis of tissues (Katz et al., 2001), and the vaginal epithelium may be destroyed (Pras et al., 2003). This may reduce the length of the vagina, which causes pain during intercourse. Furthermore, the vagina will lack lubrication, which also causes pain with penetration. Radiation also affects the ovaries, resulting in estrogen deficiency and further thinning of the vaginal walls (Lamb, 1998). Anecdotal reports of the consequences of radiation therapy include extreme sensitivity at the vaginal introitus, friable mucous membranes, and burning with exposure to semen when intercourse is attempted (Jenkins, 1986).

Radiation exposure of adjacent tissues has the potential to affect both the bladder and the bowel, which also may have an impact on sexual functioning (Burke, 1996). Women with cervical cancer are known to experience significant dysfunction in all phases of the sexual response cycle after treatment (Andersen, Anderson, & deProsse, 1989). Over time, these negative changes may decline, but sexual functioning does not return to pretreatment levels. Women with cervical cancer treated by both hysterectomy and radiotherapy carry a double burden and describe feeling sexually unattractive. They also report feeling pain with intercourse and are concerned that sexual activity might provoke a recurrence or spread of their disease (Cull et al., 1993; Kritcharoen, Suwan, & Jirojwong, 2005).

Women who have undergone radiation therapy are required to perform regular vaginal dilatation to maintain patency for both sexual activity and pelvic examinations. Details of what this entails are provided in Chapter 6. An alternative to this is regular sexual intercourse (Gosselin & Waring, 2001); however, this may not be possible because of pain. Social considerations also are important, as the patient may not be in a partnered relationship, her partner may not be able to perform sexually, or the couple may not wish to have intercourse. Despite the considerable discomfort and difficulties following radiation therapy, many women continue to be sexually active following treatment (Jensen et al., 2003).

Testicular Cancer

The addition of radiation therapy to the treatment regimen for men with testicular cancer has significant effects on patients' ability to have erections and to experience ejaculation (Jonker-Pool et al., 2001). Treated men tend to have fewer morning erections, and these often are insufficient or do not last long enough for penetration

(Tinkler, Howard, & Kerr, 1992). These men also may experience reduced volume of ejaculate (Arai, Kawakita, Okada, & Yoshida, 1997).

Hematologic Cancer

When radiation therapy is given for lymphoma, the side effects are dictated by site (e.g., chest, abdomen, brain, spine) and amount of radiation given (low or high dose). Generally, the ovaries and testicles are shielded if radiation is given to the abdomen, with the intent of preserving fertility whenever possible. Cranial-spinal radiation is used as prophylaxis for patients with leukemia and non-Hodgkin lymphoma. This has a direct effect on the hypothalamus, influencing the production of gonadotropin-releasing hormone (Byrne et al., 2004) and leading to ovarian failure. This will affect long-term fertility as well as predispose women to early menopause and its attendant symptoms, which may affect sexuality.

Counseling for Patients Undergoing Radiation Therapy

Nurses caring for patients undergoing radiation therapy can offer assistance and information specifically related to the sexual side effects of this form of treatment. Fatigue is an almost ubiquitous experience of patients undergoing radiation therapy of any kind, and this will affect their general quality of life and, specifically, their sexuality. As described in this chapter and in all the chapters of Section II, the fatigue that results from radiation therapy primarily affects patients' libido or interest in being sexual. The experience of fatigue is unique to each individual but generally involves feeling tired, weak, exhausted, and unwell, along with an impaired ability to concentrate or participate in activities of daily living (Maher, 2000a). Fatigue also can be part of clinical depression. It often is very difficult and frustrating for both patients and families to deal with this symptom, and preparatory counseling should be provided so that this is not an unexpected surprise when it occurs. Fatigue tends to be cumulative, usually appears a few weeks into treatment, and may persist for weeks or months after treatment is completed (Maher, 2000b).

Skin damage from radiation may last for an extended period of time, and ongoing symptoms of neuropathy and contractions may interfere with sexual touch (Maher, 2000b). The skin is an important organ in sexual activity because it is extremely sensitive to touch and pressure, and sensual touch often is part of the sexual encounter. Prevention of skin changes and prompt treatment of skin damage form the cornerstones of nursing care for patients undergoing radiation therapy.

Inevitably, patients' body image will be affected, and, as discussed in previous chapters, body image is an important component of sexual self-schema. Patients may need advice on how best to conceal parts of the body that have been affected by radiation or how to find alternative clothing or underwear that will allow sexual expression without exposing too much. Extreme sensitivity to touch is difficult to manage, and the couple may need help in exploring other ways of touching that do not result in discomfort for patients or avoidance by partners.

Specific issues apply according to the site of the cancer and the area exposed to radiation. These are discussed in the appropriate chapters in Section II of this text.

Conclusion

Similar to chemotherapy, radiation has systemic effects on patients with cancer, but it also produces significant local complications such as tissue damage that alter sexual functioning for individuals with cancer. Nurses can provide both anticipatory and targeted advice for patients undergoing radiation therapy that will help to prepare them for sexual changes and also can help to find solutions to specific problems related to this form of therapy.

References

Andersen, B., Anderson, B., & deProsse, C. (1989). Controlled prospective longitudinal study of women with cancer: I. Sexual functioning outcomes. *Journal of Consulting and Clinical Psychology, 6,* 683–691.

Arai, Y., Kawakita, M., Okada, Y., & Yoshida, O. (1997). Sexuality and fertility in long-term survivors of testicular cancer. *Journal of Clinical Oncology, 15,* 1444–1448.

Burke, L. (1996). Sexual dysfunction following radiotherapy for cervical cancer. *British Journal of Nursing, 5,* 239–244.

Byrne, J., Fears, T., Mills, J., Zeltzer, L., Sklar, C., & Nicholson, H. (2004). Fertility in women treated with cranial radiotherapy for childhood acute lymphoblastic leukemia. *Pediatric Blood and Cancer, 4,* 589–597.

Cull, A., Cowie, V., Farquharson, D., Livingstone, J., Smart, G., & Elton, R. (1993). Early stage cervical cancer: Psychosocial and sexual outcomes of treatment. *British Journal of Cancer, 68,* 1216–1220.

Fisch, B.M., Pickett, B., Weinberg, V., & Roach, M. (2001). Dose of radiation received by the bulb of the penis correlates with risk of impotence after three-dimensional conformal radiotherapy for prostate cancer. *Urology, 57,* 955–959.

Fitzpatrick, J.M., Kirby, R.S., Krane, R.J., Adolfsson, J., Newling, D.W., & Goldstein, I. (1998). Sexual dysfunction associated with the management of prostate cancer. *European Urology, 33,* 513–522.

Gosselin, T.K., & Waring, J.S. (2001). Nursing management of patients receiving brachytherapy for gynecologic malignancies. *Clinical Journal of Oncology Nursing, 5,* 59–63.

Hall, J.D., Boyd, J.C., Lippert, M.C., & Theodorescu, D. (2003). Why patients choose prostatectomy or brachytherapy for localized prostate cancer: Results of a descriptive survey. *Urology, 61,* 402–407.

Incrocci, L. (2004). Radiotherapy for prostate cancer and sexual functioning. *Hospital Medicine, 65,* 605–608.

Incrocci, L. (2006). Sexual function after external-beam radiotherapy for prostate cancer: What do we know? *Critical Reviews in Oncology/Hematology, 57,* 165–173.

Incrocci, L., Slob, A.K., & Levendag, P.C. (2002). Sexual (dys)function after radiotherapy for prostate cancer: A review. *International Journal of Radiation Oncology, Biology, Physics, 52,* 681–693.

Jenkins, B.Y. (1986). Sexual healing after pelvic irradiation. *American Journal of Nursing, 86,* 920–922.

Jensen, P.T., Groenvold, M., Klee, M.C., Thranov, I., Petersen, M.A., & Machin, D. (2003). Longitudinal study of sexual function and vaginal changes after radiotherapy for cervical cancer. *International Journal of Radiation Oncology, Biology, Physics, 56,* 937–949.

Jonker-Pool, G., van de Wiel, H.B., Hoekstra, H.J., Sleijfer, D.T., Van Driel, M.F., Van Basten, J.P., et al. (2001). Sexual functioning after treatment for testicular cancer—review and meta-analysis of 36 empirical studies between 1975–2000. *Archives of Sexual Behavior, 30,* 55–74.

Katz, A., Njuguna, E., Rakowsky, E., Sulkes, A., Sulkes, J., & Fenig, E. (2001). Early development of vaginal shortening during radiation therapy for endometrial or cervical cancer. *International Journal of Gynecological Cancer, 11,* 234–235.

Kritcharoen, S., Suwan, K., & Jirojwong, S. (2005). Perceptions of gender roles, gender power relationships, and sexuality in Thai women following diagnosis and treatment for cervical cancer. *Oncology Nursing Forum, 32,* 682–688.

Lamb, M. (1998). Questions women ask about gynecologic cancer and sexual functioning. *Developments in Supportive Cancer Care, 1,* 11–13.

Lancaster, L. (2004). Preventing vaginal stenosis after brachytherapy for gynaecological cancer: An overview of Australian practices. *European Journal of Oncology Nursing, 8,* 30–39.

Mabjeesh, N., Chen, J., Beri, A., Stenger, A., & Matzkin, H. (2005). Sexual function after permanent 125I-brachytherapy for prostate cancer. *International Journal of Impotence Research, 17,* 96–101.

Macdonald, A.G., Keyes, M., Kruk, A., Duncan, G., Moravan, V., & Morris, W.J. (2005). Predictive factors for erectile dysfunction in men with prostate cancer after brachytherapy: Is dose to the penile bulb important? *International Journal of Radiation Oncology, Biology, Physics, 63,* 155–163.

Maher, K.E. (2000a). Principles of radiation therapy. In B. Nevidjon & K. Sowers (Eds.), *A nurse's guide to cancer care* (pp. 215–240). Philadelphia: Lippincott Williams & Wilkins.

Maher, K.E. (2000b). Radiation therapy: Toxicities and management. In C.H. Yarbro, M.H. Frogge, M. Goodman, & S.L. Groenwald (Eds.), *Cancer nursing: Principles and practice* (5th ed., pp. 323–351). Sudbury, MA: Jones and Bartlett.

Merrick, G.S., Butler, W.M., Wallner, K.E., Galbreath, R.W., Anderson, R.L., Kurko, B.S., et al. (2005). Erectile function after prostate brachytherapy. *International Journal of Radiation Oncology, Biology, Physics, 62,* 437–447.

Mulhall, J.P., & Yonover, P.M. (2001). Correlation of radiation dose and impotence risk after three-dimensional conformal radiotherapy for prostate cancer. *Urology, 58,* 828.

Potosky, A.L., Davis, W.W., Hoffman, R.M., Stanford, J.L., Stephenson, R.A., Penson, D.F., et al. (2004). Five-year outcomes after prostatectomy or radiotherapy for prostate cancer: The Prostate Cancer Outcomes Study. *Journal of the National Cancer Institute, 96,* 1358–1367.

Pras, E., Wouda, J., Willemse, P., Midden, M., Zwart, M., de Vries, E., et al. (2003). Pilot study of vaginal plethysmography in women treated with radiotherapy for gynecological cancer. *Gynecologic Oncology, 91,* 540–546.

Speight, J.L., Elkin, E.P., Pasta, D.J., Silva, S., Lubeck, D.P., Carroll, P.R., et al. (2004). Longitudinal assessment of changes in sexual function and bother in patients treated with external beam radiotherapy or brachytherapy, with and without neoadjuvant androgen ablation: Data from CaPSURE. *International Journal of Radiation Oncology, Biology, Physics, 60,* 1066–1075.

Stock, R.G., Stone, N.N., & Iannuzzi, C. (1996). Sexual potency following interactive ultrasound-guided brachytherapy for prostate cancer. *International Journal of Radiation Oncology, Biology, Physics, 35,* 267–272.

Tinkler, S.D., Howard, G.C., & Kerr, G.R. (1992). Sexual morbidity following radiotherapy for germ cell tumours of the testis. *Radiotherapy and Oncology, 25,* 207–212.

Turner, S.L., Adams, K., Bull, C.A., & Berry, M.P. (1999). Sexual dysfunction after radical radiation therapy for prostate cancer: A prospective evaluation. *Urology, 54,* 124–129.

Wilmoth, M.C., & Botchway, P. (1999). Psychosexual implications of breast and gynecologic cancer. *Cancer Investigation, 17,* 631–636.

Zelefsky, M.J., Wallner, K.E., Ling, C.C., Raben, A., Hollister, T., Wolfe, T., et al. (1999). Comparison of the 5-year outcome and morbidity of three-dimensional conformal radiotherapy versus transperineal permanent iodine-125 implantation for early-stage prostatic cancer. *Journal of Clinical Oncology, 17,* 517–522.

Section V

Tools for Healthcare Providers

CHAPTER 22

Sexuality Counseling

Sexuality counseling should not be confused with sex therapy, which treats the symptoms of sexual dysfunctions such as erectile dysfunction, arousal disorders, difficulty achieving orgasm, rapid ejaculation, and pain disorders associated with penetrative intercourse (Kleinplatz, 2001). Sexuality counseling also deals with relationship and communication issues that are manifested as sexual problems or sexual problems that stem from relationship and communication issues. Many different models or methods of using sex therapy exist, beginning with the landmark work of Masters and Johnson in the 1960s and continuing with the work of Helen Singer Kaplan in the 1970s and 1980s. Today there are feminist sex therapists, intimacy-based sex therapists, narrative sex therapists, sex therapists who provide group therapy, and sex therapists who specialize in working with survivors of sexual abuse, same-sex couples, and other populations.

Identification of Sexual Problems

For nurses or other healthcare providers who work with patients with cancer, the first step in providing assistance to individuals and couples affected by this disease is to address the topic with them. As detailed in Chapter 3, this begins with taking a sexual history from the patient as part of the routine health history. The purposes of taking a sexual health history are to find out if there is a problem associated with the disease or treatment or if the problem is of a long-standing nature, to learn about the patient's sexual history, to make the patient feel comfortable with the conversation, and to take the necessary steps to manage the problem or find the patient additional help (Bartlik, Rosenfeld, & Beaton, 2005). If a problem is identified—for example, a male patient with prostate cancer is having difficulty with erections—the oncology care provider needs to decide what to do with this information. One possibility is to refer the patient to a sex therapist. This may not be necessary, though, because the solution or resolution of the problem might not necessitate in-depth counseling and may, in fact, be addressed through sharing information or by providing a prescription for medication that can improve erections. In the case of the man described previously, a few carefully selected questions and a review of the man's medical and surgical history may provide the answers. For example, if the man had non-nerve-sparing surgery, the possibility of him having an erection is minimal. This information can be obtained from the patient himself ("Do you know whether the surgeon performed nerve-sparing surgery?"), from the surgeon, or from the patient's chart, where the operative report would state the extent of the surgery and whether the nerves were spared. In this instance, medication would be of limited benefit, and the man may instead be referred to a sexuality counselor who could explore with him and his partner how to find alternatives to penetrative intercourse.

The sexual health assessment models suggested in Chapter 3 are part of the sexuality counseling that many oncology care providers can offer to their patients. The PLISSIT and BETTER models allow for information related to sexuality to be incorporated in the care of patients with cancer. The most frequently used model is the PLISSIT model (Annon, 1974). The first level of this model involves giving the patient or client *permission* to talk about sexual issues. The second level, *limited information,* refers to factual information given to the patient in response to a question or observation. The third level involves making a *specific suggestion* to the client or patient. Finally, the fourth level refers to *intensive therapy* needed for severe or more long-standing sexual problems.

The first three levels (permission, limited information, and specific suggestion) of the PLISSIT model comprise a limited form of sexuality counseling and are within the scope of practice of most oncology care providers. They essentially include patient education and information sharing, which should be provided by all healthcare providers as part of routine care. The final level, intensive therapy, should be offered when the problem identified is out of the care provider's scope of practice. For example, if the patient identifies that he or she has been subjected to sexual abuse in the near or distant past, this would be a topic that is best handled by a specialist in the area. Care providers can acknowledge that this is an issue they are not qualified to deal with, but if the patient is willing, they will provide a referral to a specialist.

Another model described in Chapter 3 is the BETTER model (Mick, Hughes, & Cohen, 2003), which was developed to assist healthcare providers in including sexuality assessment in the care of patients with cancer. It is similar to the PLISSIT model in that the first level of intervention involves *bringing up* the topic. The second step involves *explaining* that sexuality is part of quality of life, and patients should be aware that they can talk about this with the nurse. Care providers then should *tell* patients that appropriate resources will be found to address their concerns, and that although the *timing* may not be appropriate now, they can ask for information at any time. Patients should be *educated* about the sexual side effects of their treatment, and finally, nurses should *record* in the patients' charts that this topic has been discussed.

As with the PLISSIT model, the first five stages of this model include information sharing between nurses and patients and their partners. This certainly is within the scope of practice of most healthcare professionals.

The third model described in Chapter 3 is the ALARM model (Andersen, 1990), which was developed as a brief assessment of sexual activity and the sexual response cycle. It is based on Masters and Johnson's four-stage sexual response cycle and is more biomedical in approach than the preceding two models. This model asks questions about sexual activity, libido, arousal and orgasm, resolution, and pertinent medical history. The biomedical perspective of this model requires healthcare providers to ask very specific questions about aspects of the sexual response cycle, which many nurses would not be comfortable doing. However, this should not preclude nurses from using this model. Nurses with more extensive experience caring for specific populations who commonly experience sexual problems as part of the disease process or treatment (for example, nurses working in gynecology oncology clinics) may find that they are comfortable asking specific questions about desire, arousal, and orgasm. However, they also must be aware of the limitations of their practice and skill and need to refer patients and partners for more in-depth counseling when information sharing is insufficient.

The New View of Women's and Men's Sexual Problems

All the models discussed previously take a fairly biologic approach to sexual problems, although psychological and social issues can be included. Another way of looking at sexual problems is from a sociopolitical perspective. The framework presented by the New View Working Group provides some interesting alternatives to the traditional biomedical approach (Working Group for a New View of Women's Sexual Problems, 2001). According to this model, sexual problems are defined as discontent or dissatisfaction with any emotional, physical, or relational aspect of sexual experience and may arise in one or more of the following interrelated aspects of women's and men's sexual lives. Sexual problems are seen to occur in four major domains as presented. This model has been modified to address the sexual problems of both women and men (Tiefer, Snyder, & McNeel, 2006).

I. Sexual Problems Due to Sociocultural, Political, or Economic Factors
   A. Ignorance or anxiety because of inadequate sex education, lack of access to health services, or other social constraints, including
      1. Lack of vocabulary to describe subjective or physical experience
      2. Lack of information about human sexual biology and life-stage changes
      3. Lack of information about how gender roles and cultural norms influence men's and women's sexual expectations, beliefs, and behaviors
      4. Inadequate access to information and services regarding contraception and abortion, sexually transmitted disease (STD) prevention and treatment, sexual trauma, and domestic violence
   B. Sexual avoidance, distress, or lack of pleasure caused by a perceived inability to meet cultural norms regarding correct or ideal sexuality, including
      1. Anxiety or shame about one's body, sexual attractiveness, or sexual responses
      2. Confusion or shame about one's sexual orientation or identity or about sexual fantasies, desires, and preferences
      3. Fear of judgment or punishment by cultural, community, or religious institutions
   C. Inhibitions resulting from conflict between the sexual norms of one's subculture or culture of origin and those of the dominant culture
   D. Lack of interest, fatigue, or lack of time because of family, work, or other obligations
II. Sexual Problems Due to Partner and Relationship
   A. Inhibition, avoidance, or distress arising from
      1. Betrayal, dislike, fear, or resentment of partner, abuse or exploitation by partner, or unequal power status between partners
      2. Discrepancies in desire for frequency or nature of sexual activity.
      3. Inability to communicate effectively about preferences for initiation, pacing, or shaping of sexual activities
      4. Disagreements, spoken or assumed, about the terms of the relationship, the degree or meaning of commitment, or the desire for monogamy or non-monogamy
   B. Loss of sexual interest and reciprocity as a result of ongoing conflicts over commonplace issues such as money, schedules, or relatives, or resulting from traumatic experiences, such as infertility or the death of a child
   C. Inhibitions in arousal or spontaneity in response to partner's health status or sexual problems

III. Sexual Problems Due to Psychological Factors
    A. Actual or perceived lack of choice in sexual behaviors or attitudes, ranging from aversion or ambivalence about sexual pleasure to sexual obsessions or compulsive behaviors
    B. Consequences of past negative sexual, physical, or emotional experiences
    C. Guilt or shame about sexual desires or fantasies
    D. Effects of depression or anxiety
    E. General personality problems with attachment, rejection, cooperation, or entitlement
    F. Sexual inhibition because of possible negative consequences (e.g., pain during sex, pregnancy, STD, loss of reputation, rejection, abandonment by partner)
    G. Deeply held negative beliefs about one's self-worth or desirability
    H. Not accepting age-related life changes
IV. Sexual Problems Due to Physiologic or Medical Factors
Pain or lack of physical sensation or response during sexual activity despite a supportive and safe interpersonal situation, adequate sexual knowledge, and positive sexual attitudes. Such problems may arise from
    A. Local or systemic medical conditions affecting neurologic, vascular, circulatory, endocrine, musculoskeletal, or other systems of the body
    B. Pregnancy, fertility treatments, STD, or other sex or reproductive conditions
    C. Side effects of drugs, medications, or medical treatments
    D. Overuse of or dependence on alcohol, other recreational or prescribed drugs, or other substances.

Information Sharing

Many individuals with cancer will face challenges to their knowledge base about their own bodies and the effect that cancer has on the body and its functioning, including sexual functioning. The functions of the human body are a mystery to many or are simply taken for granted; not until the body is challenged by illness do people realize that they do not know how or why things work as they do and the reasons for alterations in that functioning. Providing patients with this knowledge at a time of heightened need and anxiety is one of the hallmarks of nursing care, and of exemplary nursing care in particular. Knowing when and how to give the information are some of the attributes of the expert nurse, and the provision of information related to sexual functioning requires a specific skill set and good communication skills.

Many reasons exist for why individuals display a knowledge deficit related to their condition or to themselves as sexual beings. Most people have not had specific education about how the body works and responds to illness. They may be old enough that they have forgotten what they were taught at school in the basic biology course they took. They may have led healthy lives until the cancer diagnosis and did not have reason to explore how the body works. Sexuality education may have been something that was entirely missing from their lives because of their age, the political climate when they were in school, the religious or social views of their parents, or other factors.

Some people have great difficulty expressing themselves clearly. They may think that they do not know the "correct" or professional terms to describe their anatomy or sexual practices. They may thus be reluctant to say anything or ask questions for fear of embarrassing themselves, their partner, or the healthcare provider. By using simple language and checking that the patients and partners understand, healthcare professionals can quickly assess the level of their comfort and understanding and can modify their language accordingly.

Information sharing with patients often begins with an explanation of how their sexual and reproductive organs work (see Chapter 2) and how these are affected by a specific disease process or treatment regimen. Healthcare professionals should ask patients what they understand about the nature of the disease and how it may affect their life. Patients often have a great deal of misunderstanding regarding what the diagnosis means and how the disease or treatment may affect them. Clearing up misconceptions and misunderstandings often solves the problem, which was based on inaccurate recall of conversations with other care providers or on the patient receiving information at a time when he or she could not comprehend the information because of heightened anxiety, shock, or fear.

When dealing with a couple who are experiencing difficulties in their sexual life as a result of treatment, nurses should be careful to avoid assuming that problems are new and related to the disease and/or treatment. Stress of the diagnosis and treatment may be causing old issues to surface, and the couple may see the cancer as an opportunity to ask for help. Encouraging the couple to describe what is happening in their life together and as individuals will allow nurses to gain a better understanding of the depth and breadth of the issue. As much attention should be given to *how* the couple communicates as to *what* they are saying. Do they use "I" statements when describing feelings (as in "I feel hurt when you turn away from me"), or do they use "you" statements that tend to assign blame ("You really hurt me when you turn away from me")? Observing how the couple listens to one another also is valuable. What appears to be active listening by a partner may, in fact, be tuning out or merely nodding and appearing to listen when the listener is more involved with his or her own thoughts rather than focusing on what the other person is saying. Asking the listener to repeat what he or she has heard is a useful method to check attentiveness and to illustrate how easy and common it is to interpret what another person is saying in the context of one's own feelings and state of mind.

Nurses may find it useful to ask the couple what they understand from the information that they have shared with them about the specifics of the disease and treatment and their effects on sexuality. One or both members of the couple may not have heard the nurse because they are not ready for the level of information that was provided, are not familiar with the terminology used, or are just too stressed by other factors to be able to listen, absorb, and integrate new knowledge.

Knowing when to share information and how much to share is a skill and an art that grows with experience and expertise. The timing of information is especially important, as many patients do not hear much after they have heard the words "you have cancer." Although imparting information about sexuality is important, it is not the most important piece of information that patients need in the early stages of the disease. Information about this topic generally can be discussed at a later time; however, if it is a high priority with patients and/or their partners, they will ask questions about it, especially if they have been given permission to do so by the nurse.

Referral for Specialized Counseling

Some patients will require the specialized skills of a sex therapist or specialty sexuality counselor who has expertise in the area of sex therapy and cancer care. Some social workers, psychologists, psychiatrists, or advanced practice nurses may possess these skills. Nurses should know the names and contact information of these healthcare professionals so that they can refer patients in a timely manner. It is beneficial for them to have personal contact with these individuals before they start referring patients. This allows them to have an idea of their style and model of treatment, any charges that patients may incur, the anticipated length of time they may wait for an appointment, and the preferred method of sending referrals. Nurses also should have an understanding of what information will be sent back to the referring care provider or organization. A list of certified sex therapists or counselors in one's area is available on the Web site of the American Association of Sex Educators, Counselors, and Therapists at www.aasect.org.

If an organization has one or more professionals on staff who provide this kind of counseling, it always is helpful to involve them in team conferences where a shared patient is being discussed. They may be able to provide valuable information about the specific patient to the rest of the team along with more general information about sexual issues and concerns that occur with different types of cancer.

Conclusion

Counseling patients with cancer who are experiencing sexual changes varies in the amount and depth of information provided. This information is always based on an assessment of what the patient knows and understands about his or her condition in the context of normal sexual functioning. A number of models exist that facilitate the sharing of information with patients and their partners. Nurses can achieve solutions for problems presented by providing accurate and timely information or by referring patients to a specialist in this area.

References

Andersen, B.L. (1990). How cancer affects sexual functioning. *Oncology, 4*, 81–94.

Annon, J. (1974). *The behavioral treatment of sexual problems*. Honolulu, HI: Enabling Systems.

Bartlik, B., Rosenfeld, S., & Beaton, C. (2005). Assessment of sexual functioning: Sexual history taking for practitioners. *Epilepsy and Behavior, 7*(Suppl. 2), S15–S21.

Kleinplatz, P.J. (2001). *New directions in sex therapy: Innovations and alternatives*. Philadelphia: Brunner-Routledge.

Mick, J., Hughes, M., & Cohen, M. (2003). Sexuality and cancer: How oncology nurses can address it BETTER. *Oncology Nursing Forum, 30*(Suppl. 2), 152–153.

Tiefer, L., Snyder, U., & McNeel, D. (2006, July 26). *The "New View" approach to men's sexual problems*. Retrieved January 17, 2007, from http://www.medscape.com/viewprogram/5737

Working Group for a New View of Women's Sexual Problems. (2001). A new view of women's sexual problems. *Women and Therapy, 24*(1/2), 1–8.

CHAPTER 23

Research in Sexuality

This chapter will discuss some ethical issues in the area of sexual history taking and counseling. Frequently used instruments will be presented and evaluated so that readers interested in conducting research in this area will have some of the tools needed.

Most of the information presented in the previous sections and chapters of this book is based on research findings from both qualitative and quantitative studies in medical, nursing, and social science journals. Recent decades have seen an increase in the number of studies of sexuality and sexual functioning, including those focusing on participants with cancer. However, most of the research has focused on cancers (e.g., breast, ovarian, uterine, prostate) that specifically affect sexual or reproductive organs, and the research in this area on other kinds of cancer lags far behind.

Many of the studies do not use instruments or measures that are specifically designed to measure sexual functioning but rather ask a few questions related to sexuality. The questions asked relate to frequency of sexual intercourse, ability to have an erection, or orgasm. These kinds of questions do not address the spectrum of sexual activities that many individuals participate in. They also are not sensitive to gender or sexual orientation and therefore may prompt inaccurate responses or lack of response if the individual completing the measure does not think that the question relates to his or her reality. Other studies use tools that have been developed to measure sexual functioning in people without cancer, and the validity of using these tools in the cancer population is not known.

Quality-of-Life Measures

Although sexual function is a substantive contributor to optimal quality of life (Dahn et al., 2004), many quality-of-life measures have only a limited number of items related to sexual functioning, and these ask about frequency of erections and intercourse and the occurrence of orgasm. In a review of 62 sexual quality-of-life questionnaires, 57 were found to assess sexual functioning from the patient's perspective. The other five assessed sexual functioning from the perspective of the spouse. Of these 57 questionnaires, 57% were designed for specific populations with chronic disease (Arrington, Cofrancesco, & Wu, 2004). In general, these questionnaires were gender-specific and could not be used with both men and women or with both heterosexual and homosexual participants. For example, the Cancer Rehabilitation Evaluation System (CARES) tool was designed to measure quality of life in patients with cancer (breast, prostate, lung, and colorectal) and has three items related to sexual functioning (Schag, Ganz, & Heinrich, 1991).

A number of tools are used specifically in the prostate cancer population that have questions or sections related to sexual functioning. The UCLA Prostate Cancer Index contains seven such questions (Litwin, Fink, Ganz, Leake, & Brook, 1998). The Expanded Prostate Cancer Index Composite (EPIC) scale contains 13 questions related to sexual functioning (Wei, Dunn, Litwin, Sandler, & Sanda, 2000). A prostate cancer–specific module for the European Organization for Research and Treatment of Cancer (EORTC) quality-of-life measure contains six questions on sexual functioning (Borghede & Sullivan, 1996). Clark et al. (1997) included four questions on sexual functioning in a larger questionnaire that also contains measures of masculine image, self-image, and body image. One scale to measure health-related quality of life for men undergoing radiation therapy includes items measuring sexual interest, satisfaction, and impotence (Dale et al., 1999). Another scale for the same population, the QUFW94, contains four questions on this domain (Fransson, Tavelin, & Widmark, 2001). In a study of male Medicare patients, eight questions on sexual functioning were included in the tool that was designed for the study, which is not identified by name (Fowler et al., 1995). The Prostate Cancer Treatment Outcome Questionnaire (PCTO-Q) includes nine questions on sexual functioning (Shrader-Bogen, Kjellberg, McPherson, & Murray, 1997). Sexual consequences for men treated for early prostate cancer are measured via seven questions in a measure developed by Clark and Talcott (2001). Table 23-1 presents a comparison of these tools.

Sexual Function Questionnaires

Several questionnaires exist that are designed to quantify sexual function specifically. Of these, five address patients with cancer: the Potency and Prostatectomy Scale (Hargreave & Stephenson, 1977), the Radical Prostatectomy Questionnaire (Koukouras, Spiliotis, & Scopa, 1991), the Sexual Function–Vaginal Changes Questionnaire (Jensen, Klee, Thranov, & Groenvold, 2003), and the unnamed

Table 23-1. Comparison of Tools Measuring Sexual Function in Prostate Cancer					
Questionnaire	Format	Derived From	Percent of Items Assessing Sexual Function	Internal Consistency	Test-Retest Reliability
Borghede & Sullivan, 1996	Likert scale	Expert opinion, pilot test	24	0.77	Not reported
Clark et al., 1997	Likert scale	Focus groups	23	0.89	Not reported
Dale et al., 1999	Likert scale	Review of literature, clinical experience	34	0.63–0.95	Not reported
Wei et al., 2000 (Expanded Prostate Cancer Index Composite)	Likert scale	UCLA-Prostate Cancer Index and patients	26	0.93	0.91
Fowler et al., 1995	Likert scale, yes/no	Patient interviews for comprehension	33	Not reported	Not reported
Shrader-Bogen et al., 1997 (Prostate Cancer Treatment Outcome Questionnaire)	Likert scale, yes/no, written responses	Not reported	13	0.80–0.93	Not reported
Fransson et al., 2001 (QUFW94)	Likert scale, yes/no, written responses	Questionnaire review, patient and provider interviews	9	0.84	0.94
Clark & Talcott, 2001	Likert scale	Questionnaire review, expert opinion	23	0.92	Not reported
Litwin et al., 1995 (University of California, Los Angeles—Prostate Cancer Index)	Likert scale	Literature review, expert opinion, patient interviews	45	0.65	0.77

measure for women with cervical cancer (Bergmark, Avall-Lundqvist, Dickman, Henningsohn, & Steineck, 1999). Another questionnaire, the Sexual Activity Questionnaire (Thirlaway, Fallowfield, & Cuzick, 1996), was developed to measure the impact of long-term tamoxifen use in women who are at high risk for developing breast cancer but who do not have a breast cancer diagnosis.

One of the most widely used tools for measuring sexual functioning in men is the International Index of Erectile Function (IIEF), which is available in a 15-item or a shortened 5-item format (Rosen et al., 1997). Although not specifically designed for men with prostate cancer, it has been widely used in studies of this population and for many other studies where a measure of erectile function or dysfunction is needed. It also is widely used in clinical practice because it is short and has good reliability and validity.

Measuring Partner/Relationship Status

Some studies measure the status of the primary relationship in the context of the illness and as an adjunct to sexual functioning. The most commonly used tool for this is the Dyadic Adjustment Scale (DAS), which contains 32 items designed to measure adjustment between married or cohabiting couples (Spanier, 1976). The Golombok Rust Inventory of Marital State (GRIMS) is a 28-item scale intended to assess the overall quality of the couple's relationship that also is frequently used (Rust, Bennan, Crowe, & Golombok, 1988).

Qualitative Studies of Sexual Functioning

A number of studies have looked at sexuality and sexual functioning using qualitative methodologies. These studies are rich in their descriptors of sexual changes during cancer treatment and contribute much to nurses' understanding of the patients' and partners' experiences. They use study-specific interview guides for both individual and focus group interviews. One of the major benefits of qualitative interviews is the ability of the skilled interviewer to probe and encourage participants to add detail to their responses. This way, dichotomous or forced responses are avoided, and participants are free to answer in their own words and describe the totality of their experience.

Challenges in Research on Sexual Issues

Although certain cancers (such as prostate) have many measures available to researchers, the same cannot be said for other forms of cancer. It is not wise to merely apply any one of these measures to another kind of cancer, as validity then becomes questionable. In order to be used in research, validity and reliability should be established, and even with measures that have been widely used, this is not necessarily the case (Brucker & Cella, 2003).

Another challenge is the potential for bias in self-report measures, with participants giving responses that may or may not reflect their actual functioning. This same bias is possible when the researcher asks the questions of participants; participants may alter the response to reflect more positively on them because they may be embarrassed to admit to perceived sexual inadequacy in the presence of another person. Problems with language abound, as fairly high literacy levels are needed to complete many of these measures. None of these assessments have a companion measure for the sexual partner to complete, which could increase the validity of the measure. They also tend to focus on desire, erections, arousal, orgasm, and satisfaction and usually do not include questions about nonpenetrative activity or solitary sexual activity such as masturbation. One of the major limitations of measures that are specifically designed to quantify sexual functioning is that typically they are long, and some participants find them difficult and tedious to answer.

Historically, participants often have not answered questions about sexual functioning. This behavior might reflect the fact that people with cancer generally are older and find the questions intrusive or think that they do not apply to them if they are no longer sexually active. In addition, sexual functioning often is not included as a measure of quality of life in studies on individuals with cancer.

Conclusion

The topic of sexuality and cancer is ripe with research opportunities. The little that is known about this topic flows from a limited number of studies, and much still remains unknown. The evidence regarding sexual changes in the context of cancer care and treatment is limited, and failure to find evidence of sexual changes for any one particular disease site is most likely related to a paucity of research in that area, not because sexual changes do not occur.

References

Arrington, R., Cofrancesco, J., & Wu, A.W. (2004). Questionnaires to measure sexual quality of life. *Quality of Life Research, 13,* 1643–1658.

Bergmark, K., Avall-Lundqvist, E., Dickman, P.W., Henningsohn, L., & Steineck, G. (1999). Vaginal changes and sexuality in women with a history of cervical cancer. *New England Journal of Medicine, 340,* 1383–1389.

Borghede, G., & Sullivan, M. (1996). Measurement of quality of life in localized prostatic cancer patients treated with radiotherapy. Development of a prostate cancer-specific module supplementing the EORTC QLQ-C30. *Quality of Life Research, 5,* 212–222.

Brucker, P.S., & Cella, D. (2003). Measuring self-reported sexual function in men with prostate cancer. *Urology, 62,* 596–606.

Clark, J.A., & Talcott, J.A. (2001). Symptom indexes to assess outcomes of treatment for early prostate cancer. *Medical Care, 39,* 1118–1130.

Clark, J.A., Wray, N., Brody, B., Ashton, C., Giesler, B., & Watkins, H. (1997). Dimensions of quality of life expressed by men treated for metastatic prostate cancer. *Social Science and Medicine, 8,* 1299–1309.

Dahn, J.R., Penedo, F.J., Gonzalez, J.S., Esquiabro, M., Antoni, M.H., Roos, B.A., et al. (2004). Sexual functioning and quality of life after prostate cancer treatment: Considering sexual desire. *Urology, 63,* 273–277.

Dale, W., Campbell, T., Ignacio, L., Song, P., Kopnick, M., Mamo, C., et al. (1999). Self-assessed health-related quality of life in men being treated for prostate cancer with radiotherapy: Instrument validation and its relation to patient-assessed bother of symptoms. *Urology, 53,* 359–366.

Fowler, F.J., Jr., Barry, M., Lu-Yao, G., Wasson, J.H., Roman, A., & Wennberg, J. (1995). Effect of radical prostatectomy for prostate cancer on patient quality of life: Results from a Medicare survey. *Urology, 45,* 1007–1015.

Fransson, P., Tavelin, B., & Widmark, A. (2001). Reliability and responsiveness of a prostate cancer questionnaire for radiotherapy-induced side effects. *Supportive Care in Cancer, 9,* 187–198.

Hargreave, T.B., & Stephenson, T. (1977). Potency and prostatectomy. *British Journal of Urology, 49,* 683–688.

Jensen, P., Klee, M., Thranov, I., & Groenvold, M. (2003). Validation of a questionnaire for self-assessment of sexual function and vaginal changes after gynecological cancer. *Psycho-Oncology, 13,* 577–592.

Koukouras, D., Spiliotis, J., & Scopa, C. (1991). Radical consequence in the sexuality of male patients operated for colorectal carcinoma. *European Journal of Surgical Oncology, 17,* 285–288.

Litwin, M.S., Fink, A., Ganz, P.A., Leake, B., & Brook, R. (1998). The UCLA Prostate Cancer Index: Development, reliability, and validity of a health-related quality of life measure. *Medical Care, 36,* 1002–1012.

Litwin, M.S., Hays, R.D., Fink, A., Ganz, P.A., Leake, B., Leach, G.E., et al. (1995). Quality-of-life outcomes in men treated for localized prostate cancer. *JAMA, 273,* 129–135.

Rosen, R., Riley, A., Wagner, G., Osterloh, I., Kirkpatrick, J., & Mishra, A. (1997). The International Index of Erectile Function (IIEF): A multidimensional scale for assessment of erectile dysfunction. *Urology, 49,* 822–830.

Rust, J., Bennan, I., Crowe, M., & Golombok, S. (1988). *The Golombok Rust Inventory of Marital State.* Windsor, Ontario, Canada: City Psychometrics.

Schag, C., Ganz, P.A., & Heinrich, R.L. (1991). CAncer Rehabilitation Evaluation System—short form (CARES-SF): A cancer specific rehabilitation and quality of life instrument. *Cancer, 68,* 1406–1413.

Shrader-Bogen, C.L., Kjellberg, J.L., McPherson, C.P., & Murray, C.L. (1997). Quality of life and treatment outcomes: Prostate carcinoma patients' perspectives after prostatectomy or radiation therapy. *Cancer, 79,* 1977–1986.

Spanier, G. (1976). Measuring dyadic adjustment: New scales for assessing the quality of marriage and similar dyads. *Journal of Marriage and the Family, 38,* 15–28.

Thirlaway, K., Fallowfield, L., & Cuzick, J. (1996). The Sexual Activity Questionnaire: A measure of women's sexual functioning. *Quality of Life Research, 5,* 81–90.

Wei, J.T., Dunn, R., Litwin, M.S., Sandler, H., & Sanda, M.G. (2000). Development and validation of the expanded prostate cancer index composite (EPIC) for comprehensive assessment of health-related quality of life in men with prostate cancer. *Urology, 56,* 899–905.

CHAPTER 24

Resources

Web Sites

- www.cancer.gov/cancertopics/pdq/supportivecare/sexuality/healthprofessional: PDQ® series from the National Cancer Institute that covers sexuality and reproductive issues
- www.cancer.org/docroot/MIT/MIT_7_1x_SexualityforMenandTheirPartners. asp: American Cancer Society Web site; provides information about sexuality for men with cancer and their partners
- www.cancer.org/docroot/MIT/MIT_7_1x_SexualityforWomenandTheirPartners. asp: American Cancer Society Web site; provides information about sexuality for women with cancer and their partners
- www.cancerbackup.org.uk/Resourcessupport/Relationshipscommunication/ Sexuality: Web site from the U.K. organization Cancerbackup; includes information for patients and their partners about sexuality and cancer
- www.mayoclinic.com/health/cancer-treatment/SA00071: Mayo Clinic Web page that contains information about sexuality for women after cancer treatment

Journals

- *Annual Review of Sex Research:* An integrative and interdisciplinary review, this journal is published by the Society for the Scientific Study of Sexuality.

- *Archives of Sexual Behavior:* This is the official publication of the International Academy of Sex Research and is dedicated to the dissemination of information in the field of sexual science. Contributions consist of empirical research (both quantitative and qualitative), theoretical reviews and essays, clinical case reports, letters to the editor, and book reviews.

- *Canadian Journal of Human Sexuality:* This publication is a quarterly, peer-reviewed academic journal focusing on the medical, psychological, social, and educational aspects of human sexuality.

- *Culture, Health and Sexuality:* An international journal for research, intervention, and care, this journal is broad and multidisciplinary in focus, publishing papers that deal with methodologic concerns as well as those that are empirical and conceptual in nature. It offers a forum for debates on policy and practice and adopts a practitioner focus where appropriate. *Culture, Health and Sexuality* takes a genuinely international stance in its consideration of key issues and concerns, as reflected by the composition of the editorial board.

- *Journal of Psychology and Human Sexuality:* This is a scholarly professional journal that publishes original articles about human sexuality. With its psychological focus, this journal encompasses clinical, counseling, educational, social, experimental, psychoendocrinologic, and psychoneuroscience research devoted to the study of human sexuality.

- *Journal of Sex Research:* The *Journal of Sex Research (JSR)* is a scholarly journal devoted to the publication of articles relevant to the variety of disciplines involved in the scientific study of sexuality. *JSR* is published quarterly by the Society for the Scientific Study of Sexuality. It is designed to stimulate research and to promote an interdisciplinary understanding of the diverse topics in contemporary sexual science and publishes empirical reports, theoretical essays, literature reviews, methodologic articles, historical articles, clinical reports, teaching papers, book reviews, and letters to the editor.

- *Journal of Sexual Medicine:* This is the official publication of the International Society for Sexual Medicine. Publishing original research in both basic science and clinical investigations, the *Journal of Sexual Medicine* also features review articles, educational papers, editorials highlighting original research, and meeting information. Special topics include symposia proceedings and the official guidelines from the Second International Consultation on Sexual Dysfunctions in Men and Women.

- *Sexual and Relationship Therapy* (formerly the *Journal of Sex and Marital Therapy*): This journal is an active and contemporary forum reflecting developments emanating from the United States in innovative research and clinical writing. Article topics include therapeutic techniques, outcomes, special clinical and medical problems, the theoretical parameters of sexual functioning, and marital relationships.

- *Sexualities:* This is an international journal that publishes articles, reviews, and scholarly comment on the shifting nature of human sexualities. *Sexualities* adopts a broad, interdisciplinary perspective covering the whole of the social sciences, cultural history, cultural anthropology, and social geography, as well as feminism, gender studies, cultural studies, and lesbian and gay studies.

Books

- Alterowitcz, R., & Alterowitz, B. (2004). *Intimacy with impotence: The couple's guide to better sex after prostate disease.* Cambridge, MA: Da Capo Lifelong Books.
- Britton, P., & Hodgson, H. (2003). *The complete idiot's guide to sensual massage.* Indianapolis, IN: Alpha Books.
- Daniluk, J. (1998). *Women's sexuality across the lifespan.* New York: Guilford Press.
- Ellsworth, P. (2003). *One hundred questions and answers about erectile dysfunction.* Sudbury, MA: Jones and Bartlett.
- Foley, S. (2002). *Sex matters for women: A complete guide to taking care of your sexual self.* New York: Guilford Press.
- Kahane, D.H. (1995). *No less a woman: Femininity, sexuality and breast cancer* (2nd rev. ed.). Alamedam, CA: Hunter House.
- Laken, K. (2002). *Making love again: Hope for couples facing loss of sexual intimacy.* Sandwich, MA: Ant Hill Press.
- Perlman, G., & Drescher, J. (2005). *A gay man's guide to prostate cancer.* Binghamton, MA: Haworth Press.
- Schover, L.R. (1997). *Sexuality and fertility after cancer.* New York: Wiley.

Textbooks

- Hyde, J.S., & DeLamater, J.D. (2002). *Understanding human sexuality* (8th ed.). New York: McGraw-Hill Humanities/Social Sciences/Languages.
- Rathus, S.A., Nevid, J.S., & Fichner-Rathus, L. (2004). *Human sexuality in a world of diversity* (6th ed.). Boston: Allyn & Bacon.
- Westheimer, R.K., & Lopater, S. (2004). *Human sexuality: A psychosocial perspective* (2nd ed.). Philadelphia: Lippincott Williams & Wilkins.

Appendices

APPENDIX A

Exercises to Help Couples

One of the most useful couple-oriented activities for enhancing mutual sexual enjoyment is a series of touching exercises called sensate focus. Masters and Johnson developed this technique, and it has been used as a basic step in treating sexual problems for many years. These exercises can be helpful in reducing anxiety related to performance pressure and in increasing communication and closeness. A modification of this is the sensual massage.

Sensual Massage

Sensual massage omits the genitals and breasts, which are described in the sensate focus section. For sensual massage, begin with facial caressing. Normally, the giver sits and the receiver lies flat on his or her back with the head resting on the giver's thighs. With the hands well lubricated, the giver begins with the chin, and then strokes the cheeks, forehead, and temples. Caress the face as if you were a blind person seeking a mental picture of your partner. Then explore the ear lobes, lips, and the nose before returning to massage the temples for complete relaxation. Rest, talk about the experience, and reverse roles. Massage the remainder of the body tenderly, and be attentive to your feelings. Then reverse roles. The goals of the touching exercise include expressing needs and desires in new ways, finding out how each likes to touch and be touched, and exploring new patterns of pleasuring that do not always have to be sexual.

Sensate Focus Exercises

In the sensate focus touching exercises, partners take turns touching each other while following some essential guidelines. In the following descriptions, we assume that the one doing the touching is a woman and the one being touched is a man. Of course, homosexual as well as heterosexual couples can do these exercises, and in either case, the partners periodically change roles.

Establish ground rules, which might include the following.
- Determine who will be the first giver.
- Establish whether you and your partner will be clothed or unclothed.
- Choose a location where you both will be comfortable, preferably not the bed.
- Dim the lights and play soft music you both enjoy.
- Use plenty of pillows or a comforter.
- If you wish, use baby oils, scented oils, lotions, or powder.
- Tell the giver what feels good and what does not.

The exercises are divided into four progressive stages. Master each stage before moving to the next. Repeat all previous stages each time. The pace depends on your progress and comfort.

Helpful Suggestions

The toucher learns from the one being touched. The one being touched takes the partner's hand and thus controls the degree of pressure as well as the pattern and length of strokes. This is a learning experience for the giver as well as the receiver. The learning hand of the toucher should not be his or her dominant hand. A right-handed person should use the left hand, and a left-handed person should use the right hand.

Do the exercises when you and your partner are rested and are not pressed for time. Do not do the exercises after a heavy meal or when you have had a disagreement. Also, at no time is there to be any attempt to have sexual intercourse, even if the man has his first erection in months. After the session, discuss what you think you have accomplished, and share positive as well as negative feelings with your partner.

Stages of Sensate Focus

The partners take turns being the giver and the receiver. Communication during the exercises is done by guiding the hand of the partner giving the massage. Limit talking until after the exercises are completed.

First stage: Limit touching and stroking to the areas of the body that are not sexually stimulating.

Second stage: Touch, stroke, and explore the sensual responses of the entire body, including the breasts and genitals, without intent to bring about erection or vaginal lubrication. At this stage, some talk may be helpful.

Third stage: Repeat the first two stages. Stroke the penis and clitoris, and probe the vaginal opening with the finger. Note erectile and lubrication responses.

Fourth stage: Repeat the first three stages. Caress and stimulate breasts and genitals. Use a lubricant, especially for the clitoris, the outer lips, and the vaginal opening of the pre- and postmenopausal woman as well as for her partner with less than full erectile response. When the man's erection is firm enough to attempt penetration, the couple will insert the penis and feel it in the vagina.

If the female feels her partner is losing his erection, she can initiate pelvic movements until it returns. The exercise is never over as long as the couple feels comfortable with each other and are enjoying and savoring the good feelings.

The use of baby oil or body lotion is recommended for stages one and two of the sensate focus exercises. A sexual lubricant is helpful during stages three and four when the genitals are touched. Lubricants include Astroglide™ (BioFilm, Inc., Vista, CA) and K-Y Jelly™ (McNeil-PPC, Inc., Fort Washington, PA).

APPENDIX B

Solutions to Case Studies

Chapter 4. Breast Cancer

- What information related to sexuality, if any, should the nurse give to this couple?

  The nurse should tell the couple that along with the usual side effects of radiation, some aspects of sexuality also may be affected. This may be enough to prompt the couple to ask questions, or the nurse may suggest that he or she will provide them with additional information about this in the future when their immediate learning needs have been met.

- What are some of the barriers to listening that women and their partners experience?

  The shock of diagnosis and the overload of information often experienced by women and their partners at this stage of the illness may act as a barrier to listening. Some patients have an overly optimistic perspective and may not want to hear anything negative or may block out the information, as they want to believe that nothing bad will happen to them.

- What anticipatory guidance may be useful for women prior to lumpectomy for breast cancer?

  Patients should be informed that although most of their breast tissue will be conserved, the structure of the breast may be altered significantly. They will have a visible scar and may experience altered sensations in the area of the surgery, including increased sensitivity, burning, or numbness.

- What advice can the nurse give J.R. at this time?

  Her husband's response is not unusual and may be his way of coping with the new circumstances of their life. There is no right or wrong way to cope. He may not actually be withdrawing but rather might be trying to find a new way of coping with the situation. He may benefit from individual counseling as well as some couples counseling.

- What further questions should the nurse ask?

  It would he helpful to ask the patient about her expectations of her husband and how he is meeting or failing these expectations. Assessing her other means of support also is important at this time, along with exploring what kind of touching she is referring to. The patient may mean sexual touching of her breasts or may mean that he avoids any kind of physical contact with her, including hugging or holding her hand when she needs it.

- Who is the best person to refer J.R. to, and when should this be done?

  A referral to a social worker should be made as soon as possible. This professional will be able to identify other resources that may be needed to help this couple with their coping and adaptation. A referral to a support group also may be useful.

Chapter 5. Prostate Cancer

- Why is B.W. apparently reluctant to discuss the topic?

  He may be embarrassed by his wife's openness in talking and asking about this topic. He currently may be experiencing some problems with erectile functioning, and any discussion about it may make him feel uncomfortable. Furthermore, he may come from a conservative background where such topics are not discussed, even with healthcare providers.

- How should the nurse address this?

  The nurse should provide the patient's wife with the information she requests but also should try to engage the patient in a private conversation, noting that he appeared upset when his wife asked questions, and offer him the opportunity to talk about his discomfort or reason for leaving the room. He might want to talk to a male care provider or to someone closer to his own age, and this should be offered to him to ease his discomfort.

- What information can the nurse give his wife that may be helpful?

  The nurse should answer the wife's questions and also give her written information on the topic. She may find these helpful in the future, and her husband may want to read these privately. The nurse also should gently inquire about the patient's response (i.e., leaving the room) and try to assess whether something is happening in the relationship that may need additional counseling.

- Based on these details, would the nurse think that the patient's wife has forgotten what was discussed in the preoperative visit?

  The wife could have either forgotten what was discussed or may have thought at the time that the information did not apply to her husband. Many patients and their partners recall very little about what they were told in the preoperative period.

Chapter 6. Gynecologic Cancer

- When is the most appropriate time to give information to this family?

  The family needs this information immediately. They possibly were given the information at the time they received the diagnosis; however, they may not have been able to listen to and integrate what they were told at that time. It might be necessary to repeat the same information.

- How much should the nurse involve the family in teaching about the surgery and the consequences the patient may be faced with?

  This depends on how involved the patient wants her family to be. A discussion about sexual side effects may be too private; the nurse must ask the patient's permission before including the family in any discussion about sexuality. They may be more interested in issues related to fertility. The healthcare provider always must check with the patient before giving any kind of information to the family.

- What should the nurse tell them?

  This would depend on what they need to know. They might only want to know how long she will be in the hospital and what may happen when she comes home. If they are going to be deeply involved in her physical care, it may be appropriate to give them more detailed information. The nurse also can ask the patient how much she wants her family to know and whether she feels comfortable telling them herself or if she wants the nurse's help with this.

- How should the nurse help G.L. to look at her altered genitalia?

  The nurse should begin by telling her that her genitalia will look different and should offer to support her if she wants to look at herself with a handheld mirror. She may not be comfortable with this, and although the nurse should encourage her, her modesty or fear might make it difficult. The nurse should explain to her that what she sees now will change as healing takes place and the swelling and scars subside.

- What questions should the nurse expect the patient to ask?

  The patient might ask questions about what she will feel like "down there" and whether sex is possible in the future. She also may have questions related to future fertility. She may assume that any chance for a "normal relationship" is now over, and the nurse should explore what she means and provide some anticipatory guidance about dating, disclosure to a partner, etc.

- She asks about the need for birth control. How should the nurse reply?

  None of her reproductive organs have been removed, and it is possible for her to conceive. This question also can lead to a discussion about the physical changes she might expect (e.g., altered sensation, orgasmic capacity), even though she may not be able to ask those questions directly.

Chapter 7. Testicular Cancer

- What can the nurse offer to this man who is obviously greatly distressed at this early stage?

  The nurse can offer general support and validation that he is going through a very traumatic time. He or she could tell him that many men feel this way and that, with time, things will change and his perspective will become more positive.

- How much or how little information is appropriate at this time?

  Addressing his need for information is of paramount importance. He may only want information about the length of his hospital stay because that is all he can cope with. A gentle statement by the nurse about the potential for sexual changes will indicate to the patient and his fiancée that this is a topic that the healthcare provider is willing to talk about and that they can discuss it at a future time. Providing them with written information also would be helpful.

- What strategies may be helpful for this young couple?

A referral to a couples counselor or social worker also may be helpful. He has stated that his fiancée probably will leave him; he is obviously fearful of an uncertain future, and his fears of abandonment may affect his recovery and long-term coping.

Chapter 8. Colorectal Cancer

- How should the nurse integrate this information into the discussion with the patient?

When J.H. is settled comfortably, and after the teaching about chemotherapy has been completed, the nurse may ask her how she is coping with her stoma and external device. Chapter 8 suggests using the "permission" or "bringing up the topic" statements. The nurse can go on to state that many patients in similar situations withdraw physically from their partners; the nurse then can ask her how she is managing. This could either be done with her husband present so that he has the opportunity to share how he is feeling or it can be done in private.

- What should the nurse regard as essential for this couple to know at this stage of the patient's therapy?

The couple should be aware that sexual changes are common in the early stages of recovery and especially during the period when chemotherapy is being given. They need to know that depending on the chemotherapy agents, condoms may need to be used for sexual intercourse. They also need to know where to go for assistance if they experience sexual difficulties.

- What questions would the nurse need to ask to get a deeper understanding of what this couple is facing?

Questions to ask include the following: How is the family coping with illness in the mother? How is the couple coping? How does the couple normally communicate their feelings? What is their past level of sexual functioning, and how has this changed? How important is sex to this couple? What trade-offs are they prepared to make if necessary?

Chapter 9. Hematologic Cancer

- What additional questions should the nurse ask this man?

  The nurse should ask him what he understands about the treatment and what the effect may be on his sexual functioning. The nurse should ask whether he is experiencing any sexual difficulties at the present time and how he and his partner are coping with these. From the phrase he used ("if they are sexually active"), it would appear that this man is not sure whether sexual activity is allowed or possible following the transplant. Depending on his level of knowledge and understanding, information about the potential problems and how to cope with these should be given.

- What anticipatory guidance can be given to him at this time?

  He may experience some erectile and ejaculatory changes, and he may need to consider banking sperm prior to treatment if they want to have children. They need to know that while total body irradiation is given, physical contact will be restricted. While he is receiving chemotherapy, he should use condoms to avoid exposure of his partner to potentially harmful ejaculatory fluid during intercourse. They also should be told that if they have further questions, the nurse will help them to find the answers and will refer them to other members of the team as necessary.

Chapter 10. Cancer of the Head, Neck, and Brain

Case Study 1

- What questions could the nurse ask this patient to gain more information about his fears?

  Questions to ask include the following: What was his level of confidence before his diagnosis and treatment? What is he most afraid of? How might he feel if his greatest fear is realized? How does he cope with life challenges?

- How can the nurse help him to come to terms with the physical changes brought about by his treatment?

  He is wearing a turtleneck sweater and so is probably ashamed or embarrassed by scarring or deformity. The nurse should assess his level of comfort with his changed appearance and suggest he work with the physiotherapist and the social worker to help him to gain a level of acceptance of his physical body.

Case Study 2

- What questions should the nurse ask this young woman?

  The nurse must ensure that the young woman is safe in the house with the patient, because if he threatens her and acts on that threat, she may not be able to keep herself physically safe. She also may need to work with a social worker to help her to cope with the situation. This will be especially vital if she has to leave him, as she will feel guilty for "deserting" a man who is ill and obviously needs help.

- What strategies might the patient's wife use to control the situation, which is very distressing to her?

  She may need to ask a relative or friend to move into the house. She also needs professional support to help her to accept that she may be in some danger and that responding to this danger in the short term is not abandonment but a vital action to prevent her harm. The patient may need to receive medication that will sedate him and help to control his sexual urges that are posing a risk to his wife.

- What referral or other services may be useful for the couple at this time?

  The patient needs an urgent appointment with his oncologist for medication, and his wife needs to see a social worker who can help her to find some degree of safety either in the house or outside the house. She also may need ongoing psychological support, as the situation may not improve.

Chapter 11. Cancer of the Bladder

- How should the nurse respond to the patient's question?

  This man has a need for information, and the nurse should ask him what he specifically wants to know. The nurse can start by telling him that his sex life is going to change, in both the short and long term, and that he or she will be willing to work with him to find answers to his questions and solutions to any problems he may have. He or she should validate his concerns and tell him that most men in his situation have concerns. The nurse then should attempt to answer any questions that he has.

- How should the nurse respond to the wife's obvious discomfort?

  The nurse should state that many women in the wife's situation respond in the same manner, and for them, the survival of the husband is the most important issue. However, she also needs to know that this does not necessarily mean the end of their sex life. The nurse can tell her that these questions do not make her uncomfortable and that she is willing to speak to the woman's husband. The nurse also should let her know that this is a couple's issue, and it is preferable that she participate in the discussion.

- What are some questions the nurse would want to ask regarding sexual functioning?

  Is he having any erectile difficulties? How different is this from his functioning before the surgery? Was this what he expected? Would he like medication to help him attain erections? Has he noticed any changes in his orgasms, and how does he feel about this?

- Should the patient's wife be present for this conversation?

  Ideally, his wife should be there; however, the fact that his wife did not come to this appointment may be an indication that he wants to deal with any changes without her. This is not the ideal situation and may trigger additional questions about the relationship.

Chapter 12. Cancer of the Penis

- What questions should the nurse ask to understand what he means by "harmful"?

  Questions to ask include the following: Is he afraid that sex was a cause of the cancer? Does he think that having sex will cause a recurrence or pain? Is he afraid of transmitting cancer to his wife? These are common fears and myths that people with cancer have, and they need to be addressed by a trusted healthcare professional.

- Why is it important to involve the partner in this discussion?

  She may have the same fears and beliefs and needs to hear exactly what her husband is hearing.

- What would be helpful to know about his previous level of sexual functioning?

  If he had any problems with sexual functioning prior to surgery, they are likely to be worse after the surgery. He should have realistic expectations of any treatment that he is offered.

Chapter 13. The Adolescent With Cancer

• What factors are important in the assessment of this young man?

The nurse needs to assess his understanding of what he is capable of in terms of his sexuality. Has he been told what organs were removed and what effect this will have on his sexual functioning? It is important to ask if he has erections now—during the night, upon awakening, and during the day. He may be able to have only partial erections and may need to use some form of erectile aid to achieve full erections. Because his prostate was removed, he will not have any ejaculate with orgasm; however, depending on the amount of nerve damage and internal scarring, he may be able to have normal erections. The nurse should ask what he means by "perform" to assess whether he is talking about intercourse or some other sexual activity. He should receive all relevant information and not only what the healthcare provider thinks he needs. He also should know that sexual pleasure is possible through activities other than intercourse, so the nurse should ask what he and his girlfriend are doing now to satisfy themselves and each other.

• What anticipatory guidance should he receive?

Because he does not have any ejaculate, he is unlikely to be able to impregnate his partner; however, he remains at risk for sexually transmitted infections and should use condoms. He will need a biopsy to determine if he has any viable sperm in the seminiferous tubules if pregnancy is desired. If he does have sperm, they would be extracted at the appropriate time and used to inseminate his partner.

• Should the nurse's advice be influenced by the fact that he is legally still a minor?

Even though he is under the age of 18 and is legally still a minor, he may be regarded as a mature minor. Nothing is wrong with giving him information when he has asked for it. The healthcare provider is not encouraging sexual behavior; rather, he or she is merely answering his questions.

Chapter 14. The Adult With Cancer

• What specific suggestions or advice can the nurse give to the patient to further encourage his participation in this procedure?

The patient should know that the way he is feeling now may be influenced by the trauma of diagnosis and surgery. It might be very helpful for him to talk to a survivor of testicular cancer who has been through the process and would be able to give him a personal perspective.

- What might be causing the patient's reluctance?

He may be uncomfortable discussing this issue for religious or cultural reasons. Or, he may not be interested in fathering children.

- How should the nurse deal with this?

The nurse should discuss sperm banking in a clear but sensitive manner so that he or she is not making assumptions and thus giving him inappropriate advice. The nurse could ask him if he has beliefs that cause him to think that sperm banking is wrong. The issue may be that he does not want to masturbate because his belief suggests that this is wrong. The healthcare provider also could ask him whether he has thought about fathering children in the future and acknowledge that this is not something that everyone wants. Opening the door to a discussion about his beliefs is as important as identifying the beliefs, and their role in his reluctance to bank sperm is central to his care at this point.

Chapter 15. The Older Adult With Cancer

- The patient does not want to talk about it, but this is an issue for his wife. What should the nurse do in this instance?

It may be helpful for the patient's wife to have a private talk with the nurse or another member of the team (e.g., social worker) to address her concerns. The nurse can explain to the patient that spouses often have their own needs, and she needs support at this time. Most patients would understand this. The healthcare provider also may want to have a private talk with him at another time. The nurse could start the discussion by acknowledging that when he was asked the question about sex, he seemed to get upset. Perhaps he will want to talk about his feelings and concerns without his wife present.

- What are some of the factors that may be contributing to this situation?

Her issues may not be about sex but might be more global. This may be the first time anyone has asked about their coping as a couple. What she may fear is loss of her spouse, and the nurse's question may have brought this to the forefront.

- What are some of the factors that need to be considered when dealing with an older adult couple that may not be applicable to a younger couple?

  It may not be easy for these couples to talk about sex, as they may be conservative or may not know the "correct" words to use. Their sex life may be something that they have never discussed, even with each other. Many older couples think it is not appropriate that they continue to be sexually active and so may be reluctant or embarrassed to discuss the topic.

Chapter 16. The Terminally Ill

- What additional questions should the nurse ask this young woman?

  The nurse should inquire if the patient would like to see this situation remedied and what, if any, solutions she thinks are possible. Has she talked to her husband about this, and how did she interpret his response? She may not be talking about penetrative intercourse but may be regretful of time lost and opportunities not taken for expressing their love for each other.

- What are some strategies that the nurse could suggest to alleviate some of the patient's distress?

  She needs to talk to her husband and needs privacy and time to do this. Family members and friends should be aware of these needs and should provide them with time alone. The patient may find it helpful to make a tape or video recording of herself to leave for her husband where she can talk about her feelings for him and the memories she has of their life together.

- What other healthcare providers may be helpful in dealing with this situation?

  All members of the team may be helpful; what is important is that she has someone within the team that she feels comfortable with. This may not necessarily be someone close in age or the same gender—she may be more comfortable with an older woman who is part of the team or perhaps with one of her friends. Social workers, bereavement counselors, or the family physician also can provide support. The important thing is to identify someone with whom the patient feels most comfortable.

- Could this distress have been prevented? How?

  Some cases occur where this kind of distress can be prevented; however, anticipatory grieving for what is to come is part of the normal process of dying. The perception of time lost or taken away for sexual intimacy may be a sign of overwhelming regret for all the losses she is facing. What could have been prevented is the timing of this discussion so late in the disease process. Many other opportunities to talk about her feelings before she reached the end of her life could have been created, but these were not recognized by her healthcare providers.

Chapter 17. The Effect of the Cancer Experience on Couples

- Should the healthcare provider ask what S.W. is feeling?

  She is obviously in distress, and a gentle probing question may allow the patient to voice her feelings and distress.

- What might the issue be?

  She may be attempting to cope with her diagnosis and might not be able to reach out to her husband for help and support. She is still in the early stage of her recovery and may be feeling overwhelmed. Her adaptation to her illness and the loss of her uterus take place within the context of her relationship with her husband, among others. She may be fearful that he will leave her or there may be a history of conflict or even abuse in the relationship, and these will affect how she copes.

- What are the important questions to ask at this time?

  The patient seems to think that her surgery means that she will not be able to have a sexual life. You need to identify her beliefs and work quickly to dispel any myths or misinformation that she has.

- How should the nurse go about correcting any myths or misconceptions that the patient has?

  The nurse should provide her with factual information about her anatomy and physiology and may need to use diagrams to show her exactly what organs were removed and how these are or are not involved in sexual functioning. The patient's beliefs may be erroneous; however, beliefs are strong and long lasting, and it may take time and education to change them.

- Would a referral for sex therapy be helpful at this point?

  Sex therapy may be very helpful because some deep-seated problems with this couple may exist, which the sex therapist can address with the woman alone and with the couple at some future time.

Chapter 18. Gay and Lesbian Patients

- What assumptions has the nurse made in this case?

  The nurse has assumed that the patient is heterosexual and married and that he has a son.

- What clues or cues did the nurse ignore or misinterpret?

  The nurse assumed that because the patient was wearing a ring on his left hand, this meant he was married to a woman. The nurse also assumed that his young male visitor must be his son. Although the healthcare provider noticed that the patient seemed abnormally tense, she did not ask him why this was so and also ignored his rather terse response to the query about side effects.

- If she could go back to the beginning of this interaction, what, if anything, should the nurse do differently?

  A gentle question such as, "You seem really tense. Is there something that I should know to better be able to provide you with care?" may have helped earlier in the conversation. She also could have asked him about who will be providing him with support during and after his surgery and during recovery.

- How should nurses deal with a patient who appears reluctant to discuss a sensitive topic such as sexuality with them?

  It often is enough for nurses to raise the topic, indicate that they are willing to talk about it, and leave it up to the patient to initiate another conversation when ready. This is what the "permission" and "bringing up the topic" stages of the PLISSIT and BETTER models describe.

Index

The letter f after a page number indicates that relevant content appears in a figure; the letter t, in a table.